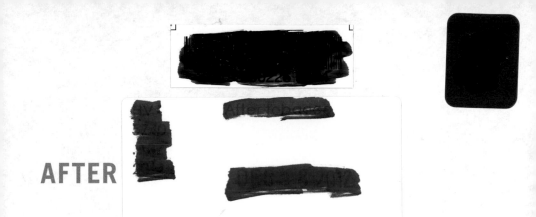

AFTER

D0427828

AFTER TOBACCO

WHAT WOULD HAPPEN IF AMERICANS STOPPED SMOKING?

EDITED BY

Peter Bearman,
Kathryn M. Neckerman,
and Leslie Wright

COLUMBIA UNIVERSITY PRESS ■ NEW YORK

COLUMBIA UNIVERSITY PRESS
Publishers Since 1893
New York   Chichester, West Sussex

Library of Congress Cataloging-in-Publication Data

After tobacco : what would happen if Americans stopped smoking? / edited by Peter
   Bearman, Kathryn M. Neckerman, and Leslie Wright.
       p.   cm.
    Includes bibliographical references and index.
    ISBN 978-0-231-15776-6 (cloth : alk. paper)—ISBN 978-0-231-15777-3 (pbk. : alk. paper)
    1. Smoking cessation—Economic aspects—United States.   2. Smoking cessation—
Social aspects—United States.   3. Smoking—Health aspects—United States.   4. Tobacco—
United States.   I. Bearman, Peter S., 1956–   II. Neckerman, Kathryn M.   III. Wright,
Leslie, 1968–
    HV5740.A37   2011
    362.29'60973—dc22   2011008584

Columbia University Press books are printed on permanent
and durable acid-free paper.

This book is printed on paper with recycled content.

Printed in the United States of America
c 10   9   8   7   6   5   4   3   2   1
p 10   9   8   7   6   5   4   3   2   1

References to Internet Web sites (URLs) were accurate at the time of writing. Neither the author
nor Columbia University Press is responsible for URLs that may have expired or changed since
the manuscript was prepared.

CONTENTS

PART 2 HEALTH AND LONGEVITY

PART 3 LAW AND SOCIETY

PART 4 EPILOGUE

AFTER TOBACCO

1

INTRODUCTION

PETER BEARMAN, KATHRYN M. NECKERMAN, AND LESLIE WRIGHT

In 2007, the Institute of Medicine's (IOM) Committee on Reducing Tobacco Use called for dramatic steps to reduce smoking to levels so low that tobacco use would no longer have a significant impact on the public health. In its report, "Ending the Tobacco Problem: A Blueprint for the Nation," the IOM Committee advocated more vigorous use of conventional policies, such as cigarette taxes and bans on smoking in public places. In addition, the report proposed more innovative steps, such as prohibiting the sale of cigarettes except by licensed nonprofit vendors.

The IOM's report was released at a time of significant change in tobacco control policy. In 1998, the four largest tobacco companies signed a Master Settlement Agreement with 46 states, agreeing to restrict advertising and to pay the states a total of $206 billion over the next 25 years. This agreement was followed in short order by an end to the 70-year-old program of price supports for tobacco farmers, the activation of the Framework Convention on Tobacco Control, the release of the U.S. Surgeon General's report on secondhand smoke, and a decision against the tobacco industry in a racketeering case brought by the Department of Justice. Most recently, Congress enacted a large increase in the federal cigarette tax, passed a new law intended to curb cigarette sales over the Internet, and granted the Food and Drug Administration regulatory authority over cigarettes.

State and local governments have been active as well. Between 2002 and 2008, four out of five states raised tobacco tax rates, and the average tax rate nearly doubled. States also extended "clean air" laws, with 17 states banning smoking in the workplace, 14 states banning smoking in restaurants, and 8 states banning smoking in bars between 2004 and 2007. City governments also took more vigorous steps to reduce smoking. New York City, for instance, raised cigarette taxes to $1.50 and mounted an extensive anti-smoking campaign that lowered smoking rates by 11 percent in just one year.

Despite these efforts, smoking rates remain high nationwide, with one out of five adults smoking, a far higher rate than the federal government's "Healthy People 2010" goal of 12 percent. Achieving a significant reduction in smoking will require bolder measures, and this means we must address the reasons that some people oppose tobacco control. Although few people doubt that smoking is damaging to health, initiatives to reduce smoking raise controversy because of concern about the economic and social consequences of these measures. Retail and hospitality trade associations and state or local business associations often oppose smoking bans in public places or increases in tobacco excise taxes because they fear a loss of sales. Because tobacco farming and cigarette manufacturing are concentrated in southeastern states such as Kentucky, North Carolina, and Virginia, policymakers in those states worry about the impact of reducing smoking on the regional economy.

Although these stakeholders come most readily to mind, there are other ways as well in which tobacco control could be costly or disruptive. For instance, high excise taxes allow vast profits to be made from smuggling, suggesting that raising excise tax rates could lead to an increase in crime. If smoking rates fell, more Americans would survive to retirement age, perhaps worsening the financial woes of Social Security. The large tobacco companies have sought to improve public relations through philanthropy, often targeting charitable giving to minority or disadvantaged communities, raising questions about how a decline in the industry might affect nonprofits that depend on this largesse. By some estimates, persons with a mental illness smoke nearly half of all cigarettes sold in the United States today; it is unclear what would happen if taxes and regulations put cigarettes out of reach for this vulnerable population. Tobacco control policies could stigmatize those who continue to smoke, leading smokers to conceal their smoking from family, friends, and doctors. As these examples suggest, tobacco control policy touches many aspects of American life. Unfortunately, these potential consequences of tobacco control are poorly understood.

It was because of these gaps in knowledge that the American Legacy Foundation invited Columbia University's Institute for Social and Economic Research and Policy (ISERP) to commission a series of studies of the economic and social impacts of tobacco control policy. To ensure the objectivity and scientific soundness of the commissioned studies, the chapter proposals and completed chapters underwent peer review, with reviewers asked to evaluate the scientific validity of the research and to identify any bias in research methods or presentation of findings. ISERP hosted two meetings of the authors, the first to discuss proposed analyses and the second to report preliminary results.

This book is the result. *After Tobacco* offers the most comprehensive analysis to date of what tobacco control policy could mean for a wide range of stakeholders. The first and longest section of the book considers the economic impacts of reducing smoking rates. This section includes chapters on tobacco farmers, cigarette factory workers, the southeastern regional economy, tobacco retailers, the hospitality industry, nonprofit organizations, and state governments. The second section considers how a reduction in smoking would affect mortality, medical care costs, and Social Security. The final section of the book considers the implications of a more vigorous tobacco control policy for law enforcement and for social stigma, mentally ill populations, and health disparities.

Most chapters are organized around a set of alternative scenarios about the course of tobacco policy between 2005 and 2025. As a baseline, we assumed that tobacco control policy would remain unchanged over this period, with tobacco excise tax rates adjusted for inflation. We compared this baseline or "status quo" scenario with two alternative scenarios, both set to start in 2006. The first is the "IOM scenario," which parallels a set of policies recommended in the IOM's report, "Ending the Tobacco Problem" (2007). These policies include a $2 per pack increase in excise tax rates; nationwide restrictions on smoking in restaurants, bars, and workplaces; stronger enforcement of measures restricting underage purchase of cigarettes; and expanded support for smoking cessation, media campaigns, and school-based prevention programs. Our IOM scenario employs conventional policy tools, scaling up existing programs and enforcing existing laws more widely and consistently. Because these policy tools are well established, we can draw on a strong base of knowledge about their impacts on smoking.

The second scenario, the "high-impact scenario," addresses less conventional policy or medical developments that could reduce smoking rates more rapidly. Such developments might include a mandated reduction in the nicotine content of cigarettes or new kinds of pharmacotherapy that help smokers quit. Because most smokers say they want to stop, smoking rates could fall quickly if nicotine levels in cigarettes were reduced or new medications to treat addiction became available. Other policy options might include more compelling health warnings on cigarettes, a ban on visual advertising and promotion of cigarettes in retail settings, and restrictions on the number of stores licensed to sell tobacco products. Because the likely effects of these more innovative developments are unknown, we could not draw on existing studies to project their implications for smoking rates. Instead, we selected some simple parameters to represent a rapid reduction in smoking rates. The high-impact scenario assumes that some combination of policy changes and/or medical developments lead to no new smoking initiation under the age of 18, a doubling of the quit rate among adults under age 40, and a reduction by half in smoking prevalence rates between 2005 and 2010.

In addition to the baseline, IOM, and high-impact policy scenarios, the three chapters on health and longevity consider a fourth, "100 percent cessation," scenario in which all smokers stopped smoking in 2006. This scenario is particularly relevant in studies of health and related outcomes because tobacco-related illness has a long latency period: most people begin smoking as teenagers or young adults, whereas tobacco-related illness typically does not appear until middle age. Likewise, although health begins to improve immediately after people stop smoking, former smokers still have an elevated risk of illness and mortality for years after they quit. Because of this time lag between changes in smoking and effects on health, the impact of tobacco control policies on health and related outcomes can take years to appear. For these outcomes, it is useful to set an outer bound on the near-term consequences of tobacco control policy.

All of these scenarios take us outside the normal parameters of tobacco control policy. Even the IOM scenario—the most moderate—assumes a sharp increase in excise tax rates and a nationwide adoption of smoking bans in workplaces, restaurants, bars, and other public places. The projected declines in smoking rates are also unprecedented. The IOM scenario is projected to reduce smoking rates by 23 percent within five years, the high-impact scenario by 62 percent within the same period. Such dramatic reductions in smoking would have significant benefits for health. However, the policies needed to bring about such a reduction are unlikely to be adopted until we understand their potential costs. Thus it is critical that we examine the consequences of tobacco control policy measures that seem unlikely or even unthinkable.

OUTLINE

An essential first step is to define the policy scenarios and describe how they are likely to affect smoking between 2005 and 2025. In chapter 2, David Levy and Elizabeth Mumford describe SimSmoke, the simulation model they use to project smoking patterns under the three scenarios. SimSmoke models the effects of six types of policies: tobacco excise tax rates, bans on smoking in public venues, youth access restrictions, school-based anti-smoking initiatives, quitlines and other cessation programs, and media campaigns. The SimSmoke model is based on research about how these policies affect smoking rates. Using SimSmoke, the authors project smoking patterns between 2005 and 2025 under the three main policy scenarios. For most chapters in the book, these projections of smoking prevalence (the percentage of the adult population who smoke) and cigarette consumption are the point of departure.

Next, we examine the economic consequences of tobacco control measures. The first three chapters in part 1 focus on tobacco farming and cigarette production and on the southeastern region where these activities are concentrated. In chapter 3, Daniel Sumner and Julian Alston review trends in tobacco agriculture and policy, including the recent dismantling of the tobacco price support program, and model the implications of the three policy scenarios for farm yield and revenue. In chapter 4, Javier Espinosa and William Evans examine the impact of tobacco control policy on cigarette factory workers. As the authors point out, employment in cigarette manufacturing has fallen much more steeply than cigarette consumption has, in part because labor-saving technology has made cigarette manufacturing more efficient. Their chapter projects the implications of falling smoking rates for the highly paid blue-collar employees of cigarette manufacturing plants. A third chapter focusing on the southeastern region (chapter 5), by Kathryn Neckerman and Christopher Weiss, considers the prospects for "tobacco-dependent communities"—counties in which a large share of income has historically been generated by tobacco farming or cigarette production.

The four chapters that follow consider economic impacts of tobacco control for other stakeholders. In chapter 6, Kurt Ribisl, William Evans, and Ellen Feighery examine the implications of tobacco control policy for retailers who sell tobacco. For the three policy scenarios, they project employment in the retail sector overall and also for tobacco stores; convenience stores; beer, wine, and liquor stores; and general merchandise stores and supermarkets. Chapter 7, by Andrew Hyland, Mark Travers, and Brian Fix, considers the hospitality industry; the authors conduct a systematic review of previous studies and carry out their own state-level analysis of the implications of clean air laws for restaurants, bars, and other hospitality businesses. In chapter 8, Patrick Rooney and Heidi Frederick consider patterns of charitable giving by the large tobacco companies, placing these donations in the context of corporate philanthropy and more generally in the context of revenue streams to nonprofit organizations. In the last chapter in this section, Howard Chernick examines the likely impact of tobacco control policies on state tax revenues, taking into account both the increase in tax rates and the likely decline in smoking as new tobacco control policies are implemented.

In part 2, three chapters examine how reducing smoking would influence health and longevity and, thereby, medical care expenditures and Social Security costs. The first of these chapters, by Benjamin Apelberg and Jonathan Samet, considers the impact of tobacco control measures on mortality from the major smoking-related illnesses. The authors project trends in mortality between 2005 and 2025 under the status quo, IOM, and high-impact scenarios considered earlier; they also model the effects of the 100 percent cessation scenario, in which all Americans are assumed to have quit smoking in 2006. Chapter 11 presents work by Douglas Levy and Joseph Newhouse on the implications of reductions in smoking for medical care expenditures. They examine how a decline in smoking would affect health care costs overall and separately by payer, including private insurance, Medicare, and Medicaid. They also examine the costs of neonatal care for infants with prenatal exposure to smoke and the costs of smoking-related disease among residents of nursing homes. In chapter 12, Michael Hurd, Yuhui Zheng, Federico Girosi, and Dana Goldman examine the implications of tobacco policy for Social Security. To address current concerns about the solvency of the Social Security trust fund, they project the impact of declining smoking rates on Social Security taxes and benefits all the way to 2050.

The four chapters in part 3 explore some social implications of tobacco control policy. The first of these chapters, by Frank Chaloupka, Philip Cook, Richard Peck, and John Tauras, addresses the concern that stricter enforcement of excise taxes or anti-smoking regulations would lead either to prohibitive enforcement costs or to a surge in criminal activity. The next chapter, by Jennifer Stuber, Sandro Galea, and Bruce Link, considers the role of stigma in tobacco control policy. They point out that some tobacco control policies may stigmatize smokers through exclusion (e.g., smoking bans in restaurants or workplaces) or negative stereotyping and discuss new evidence about the relation of stigma to smoking cessation. Chapter 15, by Jill Williams, Cristine Delnevo, and Douglas Ziedonis, examines the population of smokers with serious mental illness or multiple addictions. The authors challenge health care providers to develop smoking cessation programs tailored to the needs of this vulnerable population. Chapter 16, by Edith Balbach, Cathy Hartman, and Elizabeth Barbeau, considers how vigorous new anti-smoking policies might affect disparities in smoking. Smoking rates are higher among those with less education and lower income; Balbach and colleagues consider whether more vigorous tobacco control policies might narrow or widen these disparities.

In the final chapter, the editors summarize the results of these studies and consider their implications for research and public policy.

LIMITATIONS

There are some questions this book does not consider. For instance, estimates of the health benefits from reducing smoking do not include the impact on illness and quality of life or the gains from reducing exposure to secondhand smoke. For both these reasons, a reduction in smoking will have greater benefits for health than we estimate here. Nor do we consider directly how former smokers might spend the money they previously spent on cigarettes. When people stop smoking, sales of tobacco products fall, but industries such as food, apparel, and entertainment are likely to benefit. Reducing smoking could have economic benefits that, for the most part, we do not consider.

A second limitation is inherent in any attempt to project future events: it is impossible to consider all the contingencies that might affect those events. For example, the income of tobacco farmers and cigarette manufacturers depends not only on demand from the U.S. market but also on cigarette exports to other countries. Authors in this volume make assumptions about future trends in cigarette exports, but these trends could be affected by unexpected developments in trade policy, global anti-smoking efforts, international cigarette production, or economic growth in developing nations. Likewise, the effect of tobacco control on mortality trends could be affected by scientific advances in the treatment of cancer or heart disease.

Such limitations notwithstanding, this book makes a significant contribution to policy debates by estimating the magnitude and direction of the impacts of tobacco control for a wide range of stakeholders and provides a valuable resource for policymakers at all levels of government. Achieving a significant reduction in smoking rates will require sustained political commitment at the federal level and also at the state and local levels of government, where key decisions are made about cigarette taxes, clean air regulations, and public health services. Over the last 10 to 15 years all levels of government have taken important steps to curb smoking, but more vigorous action will be needed to address the health harms of tobacco, and the steps ahead may be more difficult. In its 2007 report the IOM Committee speculated that the recent drive to curb smoking might have lost its momentum, a victim of shifting public priorities. At this writing, such political obstacles were compounded by an economic downturn in which states faced budgetary pressure to curb spending on smoking prevention and cessation. This book will help policymakers at all levels of government understand how reducing smoking rates will affect their constituencies.

2

TRENDS IN SMOKING RATES UNDER DIFFERENT TOBACCO CONTROL POLICIES: RESULTS FROM THE SIMSMOKE TOBACCO POLICY SIMULATION MODEL

DAVID T. LEVY AND ELIZABETH MUMFORD

Although smoking rates have declined over the last several decades, this decline has only been a gradual one. As the recent report from the Institute of Medicine (IOM) describes, a more vigorous package of policies could reduce smoking rates more dramatically, with correspondingly large benefits for public health (Hopkins et al. 2001; Institute of Medicine 2007; Levy, Chaloupka, and Gitchell 2004; U.S. Department of Health and Human Services 2000). The purpose of this volume is to project the economic and social consequences of more vigorous tobacco control policies. A necessary first step in this endeavor is to understand exactly how these more vigorous policies are likely to affect smoking behavior. That is the topic of this chapter.

To project the impact of tobacco control policy changes over time, we use a tobacco control policy simulation model known as SimSmoke. Simulation models are being used more and more in public health to estimate how the effects of public policies will unfold over time in complex social systems (Homer and Hirsch 2006). Simulation models of smoking behaviors date back at least to the 1980s (Roberts et al. 1982) and have become more sophisticated with methodological advances in simulation (see, for instance, Ahmad 2005; Ahmad and Franz 2008; Mendez and Warner 2004; Mendez, Warner, and Courant 1998; Orme et al. 2001; Tengs, Osgood, and Lin 2001; Tengs et al. 2004). The SimSmoke model is well suited to our purpose here because it identifies the effects of specific tobacco control policies and considers a broader ar-

THE SIMSMOKE MODEL

The SimSmoke model was originally developed to examine the effect of tobacco control policies for the United States (Levy, Cummings, and Hyland 2000a; Levy et al. 2002) and has subsequently been applied to individual states (Levy, Nikolayev, and Mumford 2004; Levy et al. 2007) and nations (Ferrante et al. 2007; Levy, Bales, and Nikolayev 2006; Levy et al. 2005). SimSmoke projects smoking prevalence over time and estimates the effect of tobacco control policies on those rates. The development of SimSmoke, in terms of the tobacco control policies selected as inputs and the projected smoking and health outcomes, has been documented (Levy, Cummings, and Hyland 2000a, 2000b; Levy and Friend 2001, 2002a, 2002b; Levy, Friend, and Polishchuk 2001; Levy et al. 2001). Validation has been conducted at the national level and for selected states. The U.S. model predicted smoking prevalence rates well over the 1993–2003 time period, with most of the changes in trend over that time period related to price changes (Levy, Nikolayev, and Mumford 2005a). Models for the states of California and Arizona predict smoking prevalence well and indicate that an important part of the impact is explained by the media campaigns/comprehensive programs implemented in the states (Levy, Nikolayev, and Mumford 2004; Levy et al. 2007). With this foundation, other reports have considered the future impact of selected policies in projecting smoking and mortality outcomes (Levy, Mumford, and Pesin 2003; Levy, Nikolayev, and Mumford 2005b).

Previous analyses using SimSmoke have focused on smoking prevalence, as influenced over time by initiation and cessation rates and the effect of policies on these rates. We have recently extended the model (Levy and Mumford 2007) to consider trends in the average quantity smoked per smoker ("quantity") and per-capita consumption (PCC). These other smoking measures reflect the intensity of smoking and overall consumption relative to the population and have important implications for communities, the economy, and health, as described in future chapters. SimSmoke predicts well the quantity and PCC measures over the years 1993 through 2004 (Levy and Mumford 2007).

ray of policies than do the other models (Levy, Cummings, and Hyland 2000a; Levy et al. 2002).

This chapter considers the effect of individual policies and a combination of different policies on smoking prevalence (the proportion of adults who are smokers), quantity smoked, and total and per-capita consumption (PCC). We examine three policy scenarios, introduced in the previous chapter:

- *Status quo*—Tobacco control policies are frozen in place as of the beginning of 2006, with excise tax rates assumed to be adjusted for inflation;
- *IOM scenario*—The IOM report includes a range of policy recommendations, and our IOM scenario represents a package of the strongest policies; and

- *High-impact scenario*—This scenario is included in order to cover possible (although not necessarily likely) developments that could drive smoking rates even lower than the IOM scenario.

Using the SimSmoke model, this chapter examines how these three scenarios would be likely to influence smoking patterns between 2005 and 2025. Our estimates of smoking rates and tobacco consumption provide the basis for projections of the social and economic impact of tobacco control policy in the chapters to follow.

HOW THE SIMSMOKE MODEL WORKS

The SimSmoke simulation model begins with the number of current smokers, never smokers, and ex-smokers by age and gender for the United States in the baseline year (figure 2.1). These numbers are projected to change over time through the operation of three types of modules. In the population module, the entire U.S. population evolves from 2002 to 2025 through fertility and mortality. The smoking module divides this population into current smokers, never smokers, and ex-smokers, and these numbers evolve between 2002 and 2025 through smoking initiation, cessation, and relapse. Lastly, SimSmoke includes six policy modules, which it uses to project changes over time in the populations of current smokers, never smokers, and ex-smokers under alternative policy scenarios. Each of the six policy modules is based on estimates of how the given policy changes smoking initiation and cessation. The policy parameters in the model were initially derived from thorough reviews of the literature and the advice of an expert panel and more recently underwent review by the IOM Committee. Although the model was designed to estimate smoking prevalence, we have adapted it to predict the effects of policy changes on quantity smoked and PCC. (Readers can consult appendix 2.1 as well as the referenced papers for more information.)

In developing the model, we chose 2002 as our baseline year. This allowed us to establish baseline smoking measures following several years without large, destabilizing changes in market or policy conditions. (Prices changed significantly in 1998–1999 but were relatively stable for several years after that.) For the analyses reported here, we track the effect of policies implemented between 2002 and 2005, up to the point where our alternative policy scenarios begin in 2006. Smoking prevalence is estimated as 21.1 percent in 2002, falling to 20.4 percent in 2005. This small decline reflects long-run trends, including policies implemented before 2002 as well as those implemented between 2002 and 2005. Over that three-year period, average cigarette prices increased by about 14 percent, and several states implemented clean air laws. All three policy sce-

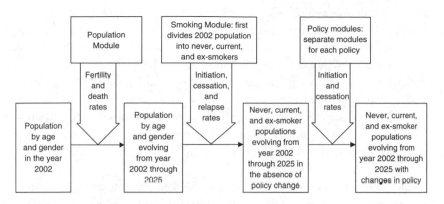

FIGURE 2.1 Structure of the SimSmoke Model

narios begin with these same smoking rates in 2006. For the status quo scenario, we projected smoking rates between 2006 and 2025 assuming no further changes in tobacco control policy.

SimSmoke defines smokers as individuals who have smoked more than 100 cigarettes in their lifetime and are currently smoking. The model does not consider experimenters or the transition from initial use to becoming an established smoker. Never smokers are individuals who have smoked fewer than 100 cigarettes in their lifetime. Once a smoker, an individual can remain a smoker or become an ex-smoker. Ex-smokers are defined as those who have smoked more than 100 cigarettes in their lifetime but have not smoked in the past 30 days. The model distinguishes 16 categories of ex-smokers, corresponding to years since last smoking, because relative health risks from smoking decline with years since quitting. Figure 2.2 displays the transitions related to smoking status.

Because SimSmoke measures initiation, cessation, and policy effects in percentage terms relative to initial levels of smoking prevalence, changes in prevalence depend on initial levels and are best analyzed in terms of percentage changes. The percentage change in prevalence includes two components: status quo changes—those that would have occurred even without any policy changes—and policy-induced changes (Levy, Nikolayev, and Mumford 2005a).

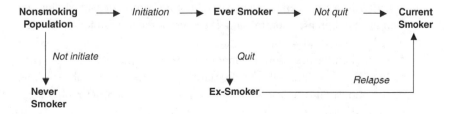

FIGURE 2.2 Evolution of Smokers

Status quo changes in prevalence tend to be relatively gradual and are calculated by holding constant all policies from the baseline year. Changes in smoking patterns occur under the status quo model, reflecting, for instance, changes in the age distribution of the population or policy change from earlier periods. Policy-induced changes are the deviation from the status quo trend as a result of the changes in policies implemented over the same period, in our case 2006–2025. Changes in policy generally lead to more abrupt changes in smoking trends in the year in which they are implemented, with continuing effects in future periods. To simplify, we assume all policies were implemented on January 1.

SimSmoke tracks the average quantity smoked per smoker in addition to prevalence. As with prevalence, trends in quantity have two components: status quo and policy-induced changes. Based on studies that consider the effect of policies on quantity smoked, quantity changes were found to be similar in percentage terms to the effects on prevalence for taxes, clean air laws, and media/comprehensive campaigns and are, therefore, estimated as having the same effects as those for prevalence as described below.

Per-capita consumption is also tracked. From the initial level of PCC, percentage changes are tracked as the sum of percentage changes in prevalence and percentage changes in quantity.

MODELING THE IOM POLICY SCENARIO

Our analysis examines the effect on smoking of adopting a set of policies recommended by the IOM Committee. Policy changes are made in the year 2006 and maintained in all future years. We consider changes in the following policies, individually and in combination:

- Across-the-board tax increases of $2.00. We assume these taxes are indexed to inflation so that their value is maintained over time.
- A clean air policy that bans smoking at all worksites, which includes bars, restaurants, and retail stores, plus increased compliance through enforcement and publicity from other policies (especially media policies regarding secondhand smoke).
- An intensive media campaign as part of a more comprehensive strategy (at Centers for Disease Control and Prevention–recommended levels), directed at adults and youth in all states.
- A comprehensive cessation treatment policy with full coverage of pharmacotherapy and behavioral therapy, training and mandated tobacco brief interventions, and multisession quitlines with free nicotine replacement therapy. We assume that the policies are well publicized.

- School-based prevention education consisting of well-tested programs applied through middle and high school and combined with a youth-oriented media campaign.
- A well-publicized youth access policy conducted at a high enforcement level and with high penalties.

The IOM scenario includes the simultaneous implementation of all these policies in 2006.

We used the six policy modules to project smoking rates under the IOM policy scenario from 2006 forward. Some policies were already in place in individual states; the effects of these future policies will be reduced to the extent that states have already implemented them. To indicate the degree of uncertainty, we provide lower and upper bounds on the effect size parameters of the different policies. We rely on meta-analyses and reviews where available, exercising caution in their use because the results may not be directly relevant to the parameters in the model. For example, the observed effects may depend on how the policy is implemented or how outcomes or policy indicators are measured. A description of policies and their effect sizes and bounds can be found in table 2.1. The remainder of this section discusses each policy in more detail.

EXCISE TAXES Price and tax changes are relatively well defined and easy to measure, and there is strong evidence that price policy is effective at reducing smoking rates, especially among the young (Hopkins et al. 2001; Levy, Chaloupka, and Gitchell 2004). Reviews find that price elasticities (i.e., the percentage change in consumption from a 1 percent increase in price) fall in the range of −0.2 to −0.5 (Chaloupka and Warner 1999; Hopkins et al. 2001; U.S. Department of Health and Human Services 1994). About half of the effect of price increases is on smoking prevalence and half on quantity smoked for continuing smokers. A meta-analysis (Gallet and List 2003) found that total price elasticities, including both quantity and prevalence effects, center around −0.48. As SimSmoke estimates, elasticities were higher over the long run and for younger individuals. More recently published studies, however, find lower elasticities, suggesting that the relation between price and smoking behaviors may have shifted.

Future price or tax effects depend on a number of contingencies. Effects are likely to be stronger in states where taxes were low at the outset. As of early 2010, state excise taxes on cigarettes ranged from a low of 7 cents per pack in South Carolina to a high of $3.46 per pack in Rhode Island. The same size tax increase will yield a larger percentage increase in cigarette taxes in low-tax states and thus a larger decrease in smoking prevalence. On the other hand, price elasticity could fall as more consumers shop online for cigarettes, assuming they can continue to evade tobacco taxes by doing so. The effect of tax increases may also be lower if

TABLE 2.1 Policy Descriptions and Parameters for SimSmoke Projections

POLICY	DESCRIPTION	PERCENTAGE EFFECT (WITH BOUNDS IN PARENTHESES)[a]
Tax Policy		
Most Recent Price	The state level average price for a pack of cigarettes is computed as the weighted average of single pack, carton, and vending machine cigarette prices, including state excise taxes. Prices of both branded and generic cigarettes are used in the average. Future price changes depend on the tax rate, measured as actual average taxes per pack, and the inflation rate, based on the consumer price index.	Elasticity −0.6 (−0.4, −0.8) ages 10–17 −0.3 (−0.2, −0.4) ages 18–24 −0.2 (−0.13, −0.27) ages 25–34 −0.1 (−0.07, −0.13) ages 35 and above
Clean Air Laws		
Worksite Total Ban, well enforced and publicized	Ban in all indoor worksites in all areas, with strong public acceptance and enforcement.	−7% (−5.25%, −8.75%)
Restaurant Total Ban	Ban in all restaurants in all areas, with strong public acceptance and enforcement.	−2% (−1%, −3%)
Other Places Bans	Ban in three of four (government buildings, retail stores, public transportation, and elevators).	−1% (−0.5%, −1.5%)
Mass Media/Comprehensive Campaigns		
Highly publicized media campaign	Campaign publicized heavily on TV (at least two months of the year) and at least some other media, with a social marketing approach.	−6% (−3%, −15%)

TABLE 2.1 *(Continued)*

POLICY	DESCRIPTION	PERCENTAGE EFFECT (WITH BOUNDS IN PARENTHESES)[a]
Cessation Treatment Policy		
Comprehensive program	A proactive quitline with publicity through the media campaign and free nicotine replacement therapy, mandated treatment access, and brief interventions.	−3.1% (−0.7%, −6.1%) in first year, increasing to −9.7% (−2.4%, −17.9%) after 20 years[b]
School Education/ Youth Media Campaign		
Comprehensive curriculum/media	Comprehensive, well-designed school curriculum with community media program targeted to youth.	−10% (0, −20%) for educational campaign through age 17[c] −10% (0, −20%) for media campaign through age 17[c]
Youth Access Restrictions		
Strongly enforced and publicized	Compliance checks are conducted four times per year per outlet, penalties are potent and enforced, and with heavy publicity and community involvement.	−20% (−0%, −40%) for ages 16–17 −30% (0%, −40%) for ages < 16[c]

[a] Unless otherwise indicated, the effects are on prevalence in the first year and on initiation and first-year quit rates during the years that the policy is in effect. Note that the predicted effects will also depend on the policies previously in effect.
[b] Affects prevalence in the first year and first-year quit rates in future years.
[c] Affects prevalence in the first year and initiation rates in future years.

cigarette manufacturers do not pass the tax increase on to consumers (as they have generally done in previous years) or if they offset the price increase with discounting or use other marketing practices to increase demand.

In the price/tax module (Levy, Cummings, and Hyland 2000b), policy effects operate through price. Price effects are modeled as age-specific constant proportional effects on prevalence, initiation, and cessation rates (Levy, Cummings, and Hyland 2000b). Based on economic theory, cigarette use is influenced by changes in the retail price relative to the prices of other goods. Because younger individuals are more heavily influenced by prices, SimSmoke assigns larger price elasticities for teenagers and younger adults (see table 2.1). Based on the recent evidence about changes in price elasticities, these estimates have been lowered since our earlier work (Levy, Cummings, and Hyland 2000b). We consider bounds that range between 33 percent above and 33 percent below the age-specific elasticities, similar to the consensus range observed in previous reviews (Chaloupka and Warner 1999; Hopkins et al. 2001).

CLEAN AIR LAWS Clean air laws include bans on smoking at worksites as well as restaurants, bars, and other public venues. There is strong evidence that worksite restrictions reduce the quantity smoked, but evidence about the effect on smoking prevalence is not as consistent (Hopkins et al. 2001; Levy, Chaloupka, and Gitchell 2004). A 2002 review concluded that worksite laws reduced smoking prevalence by 3.8 percentage points (Fichtenberg and Glantz 2002a); this figure is consistent with the results of more recent reviews, although the variation in study design and outcome measures remains a challenge (Hopkins et al. 2010).

SimSmoke models the effect of clean air laws at worksites, restaurants, and other public places (Levy, Friend, and Polishchuk 2001). Because of gender and age differences in labor force participation, women experience 80 percent of the workplace effect that men do; effects are stronger as age increases from 25 to 40 and then diminish for older individuals. The module projects a 10 percent reduction in prevalence rates with all policies fully implemented and with strong enforcement and media publicity. Among the three venues, clean air laws at worksites are expected to have the largest effect, accounting for a 7 percent decline, with a 2 percent decline for restaurant and bar laws, and 1 percent for laws covering other places. We use bounds of 25 percent below and 25 percent above the effect size for worksite laws based on the review by Fichtenberg and Glantz (2002a). The range is higher (50 percent of the effect size) for restaurants and other public places, for which the evidence base is weaker.

The model accounts for the fact that many states have already adopted clean air laws (see chapter 7). The model also takes into account the many private worksites that already had smoking bans. By 2005, we estimate, 72 percent of worksites had strict bans (up from 67 percent in 2002), and 36 percent of restaurants and 31 percent of other public places were covered. We assume that enforcement and publicity were at half the maximum level between 2002 and 2005.

MASS MEDIA/COMPREHENSIVE CAMPAIGNS Although states using media campaigns as part of their tobacco control programs have shown a decline in smoking rates, the specific role of media campaigns is less clear (Friend and Levy 2002; Hopkins et al. 2001; Secker-Walker et al. 2002). A review by Hopkins et al. (2001) found a drop in smoking prevalence of 3.4 percentage points (about 13 percent in relative terms) but with a broad range of effects. A meta-analysis of the effect of media campaigns (Snyder et al. 2004) considered smoking campaigns and found a reduction of 16 percent among adults. A study that considered variation across states and over time (Farrelly, Pechacek, and Chaloupka 2003) estimated that tobacco control expenditures at high levels, including media campaigns, would reduce per-capita tobacco consumption among adults by 8 percent.

The SimSmoke mass media policy module is based largely on the experience in Massachusetts and California. Our model assumes that media expenditures have a nonlinear effect: these policies begin to have an effect when they reach a certain threshold but show diminishing returns as expenditures increase further (Levy and Friend 2001). We also assume that the effects of media campaigns depend on other policies. Comprehensive strategies including cessation treatment and excise tax increases generate publicity, which reinforces the media campaign, thus increasing its potential to change attitudes toward smoking. SimSmoke projects that a well-publicized mass media campaign using a social marketing approach and directed at all smokers would yield a 6 percent reduction in smoking prevalence. Our bounds for media campaign effect sizes range from 3 percent to 15 percent based on the Hopkins et al. (2001) and Snyder et al. (2004) reviews.

To incorporate the effect of past media campaigns, state per-capita media expenditures in 2002 were used to estimate annual reductions in smoking rates by state between 2002 and 2005. (Because information on media expenditures was not consistently available for more recent years, we began with 2002 data and assumed a 1.5 percent reduction in expenditures between 2002 and 2005.) These annual reductions were then weighted by the number of smokers in a state, with separate estimates for campaigns directed at youth and all ages.

CESSATION TREATMENT POLICIES There is strong evidence that individual cessation treatments can help reduce smoking rates, but evidence about effect sizes is based on just a few studies of very different programs (Hopkins et al. 2001; Levy, Chaloupka, and Gitchell 2004). Not surprisingly, estimates of program effectiveness vary widely as well (Hopkins et al. 2001; Kaper et al. 2005a). There are more studies of quitlines (Hopkins et al. 2001; Levy, Chaloupka, and Gitchell 2004; Stead, Perera, and Lancaster 2006), but here as well, policies and outcomes vary considerably from study to study.

An earlier version of SimSmoke modeled the effects of mandated brief interventions by health care providers as well as complete financial coverage of an array of cessation treatments (Levy and Friend 2002a, 2002b). The cessation treatment module was revised based on the IOM report to consider a more inclusive policy and now considers the effect of well-publicized quitlines (e.g., through a media campaign) that encourage follow-up with multiple sessions. We assume that quitline callers can obtain free nicotine replacement therapy (NRT) for a limited period of time. We estimate that well-publicized quitlines and "free NRT" will attract 6 percent of smokers, with a range of 3 to 9 percent (An et al. 2006; Cummings et al. 2006a, 2006b; Metzger, Mostashari, and Kerker 2005; Miller et al. 2005; Swartz et al. 2005; West et al. 2005). Of these, 30 percent are assumed to be new quit attempts (Kaper et al. 2005b) with a range of 15 to 45 percent. Because cessation treatments would be covered by insurance, we assume that an additional 4 percent of smokers would use pharmacological treatment alone (range of 2 to 6 percent), an additional 2 percent would use behavioral treatment alone (range of 1 to 3 percent), and an additional 3 percent would use combined pharmacotherapy and behavioral treatment (range of 1 to 5 percent). Half (range of 25 to 75 percent) of those who use treatments as a result of the policy would not otherwise have made a quit attempt. In addition, brief interventions by health care providers increase the use of new treatments by 10 percent (range of 0 to 20 percent).

The module assumes a direct effect of cessation treatment on prevalence as well as a sustained effect on future one-year quit rates. Because of uncertainty about overall effects and the disparate nature of the policies examined in past studies, we consider ranges over parameters within the cessation treatment model. The model assumes that use of behavioral or pharmacotherapies alone doubles quit rates and that their combined use quadruples quit rates (Fiore et al. 2000). The combined policies are projected to increase quit attempts in the first year from 45 percent to 63 percent of smokers and to raise the likelihood of success for each attempt from 8.9 percent to 11.4 percent. Under these conditions, smoking prevalence would drop by 3.1 percent in the first year, and the effects would grow substantially over time. (For a more detailed discussion of the basis of these parameters, see appendix 2.1.)

Like the other modules, the cessation treatment module takes into account the baseline level of treatment coverage and health care involvement in 2002. The SimSmoke model assumes that about half of all smokers were receiving brief interventions from their health care providers at baseline. In 2002, 14.6 percent of adults did not have health insurance coverage in the previous year, 71 percent were covered by private insurance, 11 percent by Medicaid, and 13.5 percent by Medicare (ferrer.bls.census.gov/macro/032002/health/h02_001.htm). By 2003 (Centers for Disease Control and Prevention 2004b), 36 Medicaid programs covered some counseling or medication for all Medicaid recipients, but only New Jersey and Oregon offered comprehensive coverage, and Medicare did not provide coverage. Measures of insurance coverage by private payers were more limited (Levy and Friend 2002a). A study of managed care organizations (McPhillips-Tangum et al. 2002) found that 59 percent of plans covered pharmacotherapy and 86 percent covered behavioral therapy. Overall, less than 20 percent of the population was covered for both pharmacotherapy and behavioral therapy, and these benefits were not well publicized. At that time, about 40 states had quitlines, but they were not widely publicized and did not provide free pharmacotherapy (www.cdc.gov/tobacco/quit/Quitlines/Appendix .pdf).

SCHOOL-BASED PREVENTION PROGRAMS AND YOUTH MEDIA CAMPAIGNS

School-based prevention programs include well-tested programs applied in middle and high school. Evidence about the efficacy of school-based prevention programs has been mixed (Levy, Chaloupka, and Gitchell 2004; Skara and Sussman 2003; Thomas and Perera 2006). For education programs alone, many studies find no effects, especially over longer periods of time, whereas others have reported large effects (Levy, Chaloupka, and Gitchell 2004). School-based programs tend to be more effective in combination with sustained media campaigns directed at youth (Friend and Levy 2002; Levy, Chaloupka, and Gitchell 2004; Sowden and Arblaster 1999). For media campaigns, Hopkins et al. (2001) found a broad range of results with a median reduction of 2.4 percentage points for media campaigns when combined with other programs—roughly a 10 percent decline. The American Legacy Foundation media campaign (Farrelly et al. 2005a) yielded a 7 percent relative reduction in youth smoking prevalence; a meta analysis by Snyder et al. (2004) found similar results.

Although most studies of youth policies use the 30-day prevalence measure of smoking, SimSmoke models the number of established smokers; therefore we developed estimates of initiation rates into established smoking. Based on the IOM review on school programs, it is estimated that sustained school programs alone reduce smoking rates by 10 percent, or by 20 percent if accompanied by a sustained media campaign aimed at youth. Given the broad range of results for education programs, we selected a lower bound of zero (no effect) and an upper bound of 20 percent; the latter assumes that the more successful programs can be replicated and that their effects are long-term. The 10 percent incremental effect of media campaigns reflects the synergies from implementing the campaign in conjunction with the educational programs and is thus higher than the effect of a youth media campaign alone. For media campaigns we consider the same bounds of 0 percent to 20 percent, based on the lack of clear evidence from some of the reviews and the upper bound implied by the Snyder review.

The effects of school programs and media campaigns are modeled as across-the-board reductions in initiation rates at all ages through age 24, with no differences by gender. To incorporate the lag between the programs and their ultimate effect on initiation, the program affects initiation rates of youth through age 15 in the first year that the program is in effect, through age 16 the second year that the program is in effect, and so on through age 24, the last age of initiation.

Because current school-based programs are generally not implemented in a consistent manner, do not use well-tested formats, and are not continuously applied throughout middle and high school, we assume they have no measurable effect. Therefore, the IOM education policy is expected to produce the entire effect described above. Based on the American Legacy Foundation's youth media campaign, we estimate that youth campaigns reduced smoking prevalence by 5 percent for the years 2002 through 2005. The effect of the IOM scenario youth media component is the difference between the effect of existing campaigns and the additional effect caused by synergy with school-based programming.

YOUTH ACCESS Evidence on the effectiveness of youth access policies is weak, with mixed effects across studies (Hopkins et al. 2001; Levy, Chaloupka, and Gitchell 2004). For youth access interventions supported by community mobilization, Hopkins et al. (2001) found a median decrease of 5.8 percentage points. However, some meta-analyses fail to find significant effects of youth access policies on smoking prevalence (Fichtenberg and Glantz 2002b; Stead and Lancaster 2000).

The SimSmoke youth access module considers the effect of bans on self-service and vending machines as well as three components of retail compliance (compliance checks, penalties, and community mobilization). The module also takes into account that, as retail sales to youth are reduced, youth can obtain cigarettes through social sources (family members or friends) or theft. Policy effectiveness is likely to depend on strong adult programs (especially directed at those ages 18 to 20) because adults are important sources of cigarettes for youth; thus community mobilization plays an important role. With a strongly enforced and publicized campaign (compliance checks are conducted four times per year per outlet, penalties are potent and enforced, and there are heavy publicity and community involvement), the model yields a 20 percent reduction in both smoking prevalence and future initiation among 16- to 17-year-olds and a 30 percent reduction among those 10–15 years of age (Levy and Friend 2000; Levy et al. 2001). These policies work through the prevalence and initiation rate but do not affect cessation, since cessation does not enter the model until after age 24. Based on the lack of consistent evidence in meta-analyses, the lower bound is set at zero, or no effects. The upper-bound effect is set at 40 percent, consistent with the results of some intensive campaigns with strong community involvement (Levy et al. 2001).

Data from the Substance Abuse and Mental Health Administration (prevention .samhsa.gov/tobacco/01synartable.asp) indicate a 15 percent noncompliance rate among retailers, but these figures may be understated because compliance rates are used to determine federal funding for substance abuse programs. Based on compliance rates and programs in effect, we estimate that states on average have a low enforcement policy.

HIGH-IMPACT SCENARIO

In addition to the status quo and IOM scenarios, we include a high-impact scenario to cover possible if unlikely developments that could drive prevalence even lower than the IOM's recommended policies would. This scenario incorporates the IOM policy recommendations discussed previously, but it also assumes new policy/medical developments such as major advances in pharmacotherapy, stringent FDA regulation of the nicotine content of cigarettes, or a more significant restriction in youth access. We do not identify these new policy/medical developments because we lack the empirical evidence to model their effects in the way that more conventional policies are modeled for the IOM scenario. Instead, the high-impact scenario is defined by its outcomes: we assume a package of policies that results in (1) no new initiation under the age of 18, (2) a doubling of the quit rate for adults under age 40, and (3) a reduction by half in prevalence by 2010 (a 13 percent annual reduction). The policies underlying the high-impact scenario are assumed to have their primary effect on initiation. We assume there is no effect on the average quantity smoked over and above the reductions stemming from the IOM scenario. Although the policy and medical developments reflected in the high-impact scenario could mean downward pressure on quantity smoked, it is also plausible that those who continue to smoke in the face of those developments might be "hard-core" smokers who smoke as much or more than those who have quit.

RESULTS

This section reports projections of the proportions of smokers and ex-smokers, quantity smoked, and total and PCC between 2006 and 2025 under the three policy scenarios. We examine smoking rates for the adult population (ages 18 and older) as well as some breakdowns by age and gender. To facilitate comparison with existing data series, we scaled the 2004 SimSmoke estimates to equal the estimates most commonly used for policy purposes. We set the adult smoking prevalence and PCC measures equal, respectively, to the National Health Interview Survey and USDA estimates for 2004, the most recent year for which data were available at the time we carried out this analysis. Results for smoking prevalence are presented in detail to illustrate the approach. We first compare results across the three scenarios, then examine the six policies in the IOM scenario to compare their individual impact on smoking. The effects of these policies are presented relative to the status quo level in the same year (i.e., [Policy rate$_t$ − status quo rate$_t$]/status quo rate$_t$).

SMOKING PREVALENCE

Table 2.2 and figure 2.3 display estimates of smoking prevalence under the status quo and the other two policy scenarios for the adult (ages 18 and older) population. Under the status quo scenario, adult smoking prevalence is projected to

TABLE 2.2 SimSmoke Projections of Smoking Prevalence Under Three Policy Scenarios, by Gender and Age, 2005–2025

POLICY/YEAR	2005	2006[a]	2010	CHANGE VS. STATUS QUO (%) (2010)[b]	2015	2020	2025	CHANGE VS. STATUS QUO (%) (2025)[b]
Ages 18 and above								
Status quo	20.4%	20.2%	19.3%	—	18.2%	17.2%	16.2%	—
IOM recommendations	20.4%	16.6%	14.9%	−22.6%	13.1%	11.6%	10.4%	−36.1%
High-impact scenario	20.4%	14.5%	7.4%	−61.8%	6.9%	6.3%	5.7%	−64.8%
Males aged 18 and above								
Status quo	22.8%	22.5%	21.5%	—	20.2%	19.0%	17.9%	—
IOM recommendations	22.8%	18.6%	16.7%	−22.4%	14.6%	12.9%	11.5%	−35.7%
High-impact scenario	22.8%	16.1%	8.3%	−61.6%	7.8%	7.0%	6.4%	−64.1%
Females aged 18 and above								
Status quo	18.1%	17.9%	17.1%	—	16.1%	15.2%	14.3%	—
IOM recommendations	18.1%	14.7%	13.2%	−22.6%	11.6%	10.2%	9.2%	−36.0%
High-impact scenario	18.1%	12.8%	6.5%	−61.7%	6.1%	5.5%	5.1%	−64.8%

Ages 15–17								
Status quo	3.8%	3.6%	3.4%	—	3.4%	3.4%	3.4%	—
IOM recommendations	3.8%	1.9%	1.4%	−58.5%	1.4%	1.4%	1.4%	−59.1%
High-impact scenario	3.8%	1.7%	0.1%	−97.6%	0.0%	0.0%	0.0%	−100.0%
Ages 18–24								
Status quo	26.5%	26.4%	23.0%	—	22.6%	22.3%	22.5%	—
IOM recommendations	26.5%	20.6%	16.5%	−28.0%	13.3%	13.1%	13.2%	−41.1%
High-impact scenario	26.5%	18.0%	8.9%	−61.2%	9.0%	8.8%	8.9%	−60.2%
Ages 25–44								
Status quo	22.6%	22.2%	21.7%	—	20.6%	20.0%	19.5%	—
IOM recommendations	22.6%	18.3%	16.6%	−23.6%	14.7%	12.8%	11.5%	−41.1%
High-impact scenario	22.6%	15.9%	7.3%	−66.5%	6.3%	5.6%	5.2%	−73.5%
Ages 45–64								
Status quo	20.9%	20.7%	19.9%	—	18.4%	16.6%	15.0%	—
IOM recommendations	20.9%	17.4%	16.0%	−19.9%	14.2%	12.2%	10.6%	−29.7%
High-impact scenario	20.9%	15.1%	8.3%	−58.3%	7.8%	6.9%	5.9%	−61.0%

TABLE 2.2 (*Continued*)

POLICY/YEAR	2005	2006[a]	2010	CHANGE VS. STATUS QUO (%)[b] (2010)[b]	2015	2020	2025	CHANGE VS. STATUS QUO (%)[b] (2025)[b]
Ages 65+								
Status quo	9.7%	9.9%	10.4%	—	10.9%	10.9%	10.5%	—
IOM recommendations	9.7%	8.3%	8.3%	−19.9%	8.3%	7.9%	7.3%	−30.1%
High-impact scenario	9.7%	7.2%	4.6%	−55.9%	5.1%	5.1%	4.8%	−53.9%

[a] Policies are implemented and maintained from year 2006 forward.
[b] Percentage changes calculated relative to the status quo rate as (Policy rate − status quo rate)/status quo rate.
Source: SimSmoke model "U.S. 2002."

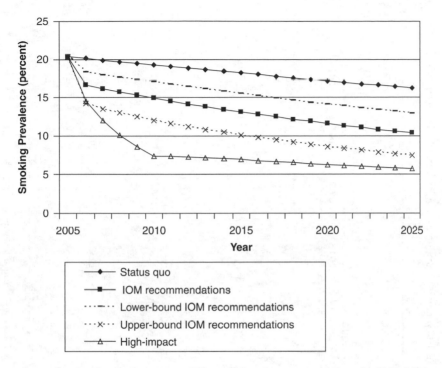

FIGURE 2.3 SimSmoke Projection of Three Policy Scenarios and Bounds, 2005–2025

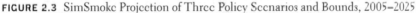

Source: SimSmoke model (see appendix 2.1 for more detail).

decline from 20.4 percent in 2005 to 19.3 percent in 2010 and 16.2 percent in 2025. The reduction in smoking prevalence under the status quo scenario is explained by stricter public policies implemented prior to 2005 as well as long-term demographic trends. In the earlier years, as table 2.2 shows, the largest reductions in smoking prevalence are among those under age 24, due to reduced initiation, and among the 45- to 64-year-old age groups, due to higher cessation rates within those groups. Over time, the reductions in smoking among the young are shifted to older age groups.

Under the IOM scenario, the smoking rate is projected to fall to 14.9 percent by 2010 and to 10.4 percent by 2025, representing (respectively) a 22.6 percent and a 36.1 percent reduction below the status quo projections for the corresponding years. (Our uncertainty bounds, shown in figure 2.3, are between 12.4 percent and 36.9 percent and respectively reflect the lower and upper bounds for each of the individual policies.) Projected declines in smoking do not differ by gender. The impact of individual policies differs by age, however, with the biggest impact seen among 15- to 17-year-olds, who are most sensitive to the tax

TABLE 2.3 SimSmoke Projections of Prevalence of Ex-Smoking by Duration of Abstinence Under Three Policy Scenarios, Population Aged 18 and Above, 2005–2025

POLICY/YEAR	2005	2006[a]	2010	CHANGE VS. STATUS QUO (%)[b] (2010)[b]	2015	2020	2025	CHANGE VS. STATUS QUO (%)[b] (2025)[b]
Ex-smoker <2 years prevalence								
Status quo	2.4%	2.3%	2.1%	–	2.0%	1.9%	1.8%	–
IOM recommendations	2.4%	5.1%	2.4%	16.2%	2.2%	2.0%	1.7%	–5.0%
High-impact scenario	2.4%	6.9%	5.3%	154.6%	1.5%	1.4%	1.3%	–31.6%
Ex-smoker 3–15 years prevalence								
Status quo	8.2%	8.1%	7.4%	–	6.4%	5.8%	5.6%	–
IOM recommendations	8.2%	8.1%	10.1%	37.0%	9.2%	8.6%	5.9%	5.6%
High-impact scenario	8.2%	8.1%	13.3%	80.8%	14.5%	12.5%	4.8%	–15.5%
Ex-smoker 16+ years prevalence								
Status quo	9.5%	9.5%	9.9%	–	10.3%	10.4%	10.1%	–
IOM recommendations	9.5%	9.6%	9.9%	0.1%	10.3%	10.4%	12.3%	21.7%
High-impact scenario	9.5%	9.6%	9.9%	0.0%	10.3%	10.4%	16.4%	62.5%

[a] Policies are implemented and maintained from year 2006 forward.
[b] Percentage changes calculated relative to the status quo rate in the same year as (Policy rate – status quo rate)/status quo rate.
Source: SimSmoke model "U.S. 2002."

increases and are the only age group affected by school education and youth access policies.

The high-impact scenario leads to a steeper decline in smoking prevalence. We project that smoking rates would decline to 7.4 percent by 2010 and to 5.7 percent by 2025; both of these rates are more than 60 percent lower than the status quo projection for the corresponding years. The sharp reduction after 2006 reflects an immediate impact on cessation by factors such as advances in cessation treatment and reduced addictiveness of tobacco products. Further reductions follow through the impact on future initiation and cessation rates. By construction, the impact is greatest among youth, with prevalence dropping to zero.

Table 2.3 shows the population of ex-smokers. Under the status quo scenario, the proportion of ex-smokers is projected to decline from 20.0 percent of the population in 2005 to 17.6 percent in 2025. Although past policies will continue to induce more people to quit, this increase in numbers of ex-smokers is offset by the aging of older cohorts, which have a higher prevalence of ex-smokers. Initially, under both the IOM and high-impact scenarios, we observe large increases in the proportion of recent ex-smokers. By 2025, time since cessation has increased for these ex-smokers, leading to an increase in the size of the population that has quit more than 15 years ago. Thus a sizable group of individuals would have health risks substantially lower than those of smokers but higher than those of never smokers.

EFFECTS OF SPECIFIC IOM POLICIES

Table 2.4 shows the estimated effects of individual IOM policies on smoking prevalence, and figure 2.4 displays the effect of each individual policy as a percentage of the total effect of the IOM scenario in 2010 and in 2025.

TAXES Of the six tobacco control policies modeled, tobacco excise taxes are typically estimated to have the most pronounced effect on smoking prevalence in recent years (Levy, Chaloupka, and Gitchell 2004). However, the same absolute increase in taxes has a smaller percentage effect in 2005 than in earlier years because prices are now higher, and the tax increase represents a smaller relative increase (Levy, Nikolayev, and Mumford 2005b). As table 2.4 indicates, an increase in the average tax rate of $2.00 is projected to result in a 7.1 percent relative reduction in adult smoking prevalence compared to the status quo by 2010 and a relative reduction of 10.8 percent by 2025. The apparent growth in the effect of price on adult smoking prevalence over time is primarily because youth are more responsive to price increases than adults; the effects on adult prevalence increase as those youth initiating under the higher price age into adulthood.

TABLE 2.4 SimSmoke Projections of Selected Policy Effects on Smoking Prevalence Under IOM Policy Measures, Total Population Aged 18+, 2005–2025

POLICY/YEAR	2005	2006[a]	2010	CHANGE VS. STATUS QUO (%) (2010)[b]	2015	2025	CHANGE VS. STATUS QUO (%) (2025)[b]
Status quo scenario	20.4%	20.2%	19.3%	—	18.2%	16.2%	—
IOM policy measures							
$2.00 tax increase	20.4%	19.0%	17.9%	−7.1%	16.7%	14.5%	−10.8%
Clean air laws	20.4%	19.3%	18.4%	−4.9%	17.3%	15.3%	−5.8%
Media/comprehensive campaign	20.4%	19.1%	18.2%	−5.7%	17.1%	15.1%	−6.7%
Cessation treatment	20.4%	19.6%	18.2%	−5.6%	16.9%	14.6%	−9.7%
School ed/media	20.4%	20.2%	19.2%	−0.4%	17.8%	15.3%	−5.4%
Youth access policy	20.4%	20.2%	19.2%	−0.7%	17.9%	15.7%	−3.2%

[a] Policies are implemented and maintained from year 2006 forward.
[b] Percentage changes calculated relative to the status quo rate as (Policy rate − status quo rate)/status quo rate.
Source: SimSmoke model "U.S. 2002."

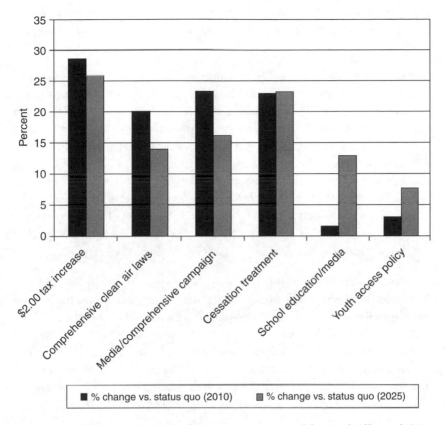

FIGURE 2.4 Effect of Individual Policies as a Percentage of the Total Effects of IOM-Recommended Policies, 2010 and 2025

Source: SimSmoke model (see appendix 2.1 for more detail).

CLEAN AIR POLICIES Clean air policies have a similar but smaller effect on smoking prevalence, leading to a 4.9 percent lower smoking rate in 2010 (relative to the status quo), and a 5.8 percent drop by 2025, largely as a result of higher cessation rates. These estimates take into account the fact that many states and firms have already implemented smoking restrictions. We assume clean air laws will have the strongest effect on 25- to 64-year-olds, and particularly 35- to 44-year-olds, because employment rates are so high for this group.

MASS MEDIA We project that a vigorous media campaign, implemented at a high intensity along with other programs and maintained over time, will lead to a 5.7 percent decline in adult smoking rates by 2010 and a 6.7 percent decline by

2025, both relative to the status quo. Media campaigns are projected to have similar effects as clean air laws and the tax increase, with all age groups affected similarly.

CESSATION POLICIES A policy of mandated brief interventions delivered by health care providers along with full financial coverage of cessation treatments and well-publicized quitlines with free NRT have relatively small effects in the early years of the projection. Their impact grows over time, however, through increased cessation rates, which affect those older than age 24 and are more influential for those over age 35 (Levy and Friend 2002a). These policies might also be an important influence on more addicted smokers, who smoke larger quantities and may be less amenable to quitting as a result of other policies (Levy, Chaloupka, and Gitchell 2004). The combined cessation policies are projected to reduce adult smoking prevalence by a relative value of 5.6 percent by 2010 over the status quo scenario and by 9.7 percent relative to status quo by 2025.

SCHOOL-BASED PREVENTION EDUCATION AND YOUTH MEDIA CAMPAIGN
We model the effects of a sustained school program combined with a media campaign directed at youth. School-based programs are projected to lead to a 15 percent reduction in smoking prevalence, relative to the status quo, among those aged 10 to 17. These programs only directly affect youth, but they have an indirect effect on adult prevalence rates as those affected as teenagers age into the adult population. We project that this policy will lead to a decline in adult smoking prevalence, relative to the status quo, of 0.4 percent by 2010 and 5.4 percent by 2025.

YOUTH ACCESS POLICIES We model a policy of strict control of youth access (bans on access to self-service and vending machines in addition to strict retail compliance checks, penalties for noncompliance, and a high level of publicity). Initially, youth smoking rates drop by about 22 percent, and this effect stays roughly constant over time. These policies have an indirect effect on adult smoking rates, which are 0.7 percent lower than in the status quo by 2010 and 3.2 percent lower by 2025 as more youth age into the adult population.

As figure 2.4 shows, the excise tax increase, clean air laws, the high-intensity media campaign, and cessation treatment policies are projected to have roughly similar effects in 2010. In 2025, excise taxes and cessation treatments have about the same relative effect, while clean air laws and media campaigns decline in importance, and youth-oriented policies are expected to account for a larger share of the total IOM effect.

OTHER SMOKING MEASURES

As table 2.5 shows, the average quantity smoked per smoker (AQSS) is projected to drop under the status quo scenario by 0.5 percent per year. Compared with

TABLE 2.5 SimSmoke Projections of Total Average Quantity Smoked per Smoker in Cigarettes per Day Under Three Policy Scenarios, 2005–2025

AGE/YEAR	2005	2006[a]	2010	CHANGE VS. STATUS QUO (%)[b] (2010)	2015	2020	2025	CHANGE VS. STATUS QUO (%)[b] (2025)
Total Ages 18+								
Status quo	14.7	14.6	14.4	–	14.0	13.6	13.2	–
IOM recommendations	14.7	12.1	12.0	–16.9%	11.7	11.4	11.1	–16.4%
High-impact scenario	14.7	12.1	12.0	–16.9%	11.7	11.4	11.1	–16.4%
Ages 15–17								
Status quo	8.4	8.3	8.2	–	8.0	7.8	7.6	–
IOM recommendations	8.4	4.5	4.4	–45.8%	4.3	4.2	4.1	–45.9%
High-impact scenario	8.4	4.5	4.4	–45.8%	4.3	4.2	4.1	–45.9%
Ages 18–24								
Status quo	11.4	11.3	11.1	–	10.8	10.6	10.3	–
IOM recommendations	11.4	8.7	8.6	–22.6%	8.4	8.2	8.0	–22.6%
High-impact scenario	11.4	8.7	8.6	–22.6%	8.4	8.2	8.0	–22.6%

TABLE 2.5 *(Continued)*

AGE/YEAR	2005	2006[a]	2010	CHANGE VS. STATUS QUO (%)[b] (2010)	2015	2020	2025	CHANGE VS. STATUS QUO (%)[b] (2025)
Ages 25–44								
Status quo	14.2	14.0	13.7	—	13.2	13.0	12.7	—
IOM recommendations	14.2	11.6	11.3	-17.5%	10.9	10.7	10.5	-17.1%
High-impact scenario	14.2	11.6	11.3	-17.5%	10.9	10.7	10.5	-17.1%
Ages 45–64								
Status quo	17.0	16.9	16.6	—	16.2	15.8	15.4	—
IOM recommendations	17.0	14.1	13.9	-16.1%	13.6	13.3	12.9	-16.1%
High-impact scenario	17.0	14.1	13.9	-16.1%	13.6	13.3	12.9	-16.1%
Ages 65+								
Status quo	14.6	14.4	14.3	—	14.0	13.6	13.2	—
IOM recommendations	14.6	12.1	12.0	-16.2%	11.7	11.4	11.1	-16.2%
High-impact scenario	14.6	12.1	12.0	-16.2%	11.7	11.4	11.1	-16.2%

[a] Policies are implemented and maintained from year 2006 forward.
[b] Percentage changes calculated relative to the status quo rate as (Policy rate − status quo rate)/ status quo rate.
Source: SimSmoke model "U.S. 2002."

2005, the status quo reduction yields a 2.1 percent reduction by 2010 and a 10 percent reduction by 2025. This predicted change does not differ by age or gender. The predicted effects of the IOM and high-impact scenarios on quantity smoked are identical. Relative to the status quo scenario, quantity smoked is expected to drop by 16.9 percent within five years. (The reduction in quantity is slightly less in 2025 [16.4 percent] than in 2010 [16.9 percent] because of the timing of policy effects; reductions due to the policy scenarios take place in the immediate years following the policy change, but the reduction in quantity predicted by the status quo scenario takes place more gradually over time.) Greater reductions are projected for younger smokers, with a relative reduction in AQSS of 45.8 percent among 15- to 17-year-olds and 22.6 percent among 18- to 24-year-olds.

Table 2.6 shows projections of total and PCC; PCC is equivalent to total consumption divided by the total U.S. population aged 18 and above. Because total population increases over time, PCC falls faster than total consumption under the status quo case. Because we based our projections on USDA data, which do not distinguish consumption by demographic category, these projections do not include breakdowns by age and gender. Under the IOM scenario, the estimated PCC is 39.6 percent lower than in the status quo scenario in 2010 and 50.2 percent lower in 2025. The high-impact scenario yields a 75.3 percent reduction relative to the status quo by 2010; there is little further decline between 2010 and 2025.

SUMMARY AND DISCUSSION

If tobacco control policies had been maintained at their 2005 levels, the Sim-Smoke model projects a reduction in adult smoking prevalence from 21 percent in 2004 to about 19 percent by 2010. The decline occurs as a result of the aging of older cohorts and the effects of policies implemented between 2002 and 2005. By 2025, under the status quo scenario, the smoking rate would be projected to fall to 16 percent. This reduction assumes that the initiation, cessation, and relapse rates estimated for 2005 remain constant over time.

In addition to this status quo scenario, we developed projections for two policy scenarios. First, we considered a best-case scenario of policies recommended by the IOM Committee. Under this IOM scenario we project that smoking prevalence would fall to about 15 percent by 2010 and to about 10 percent by 2025, in other words, 23 percent and 36 percent (respectively) below the status quo level of the corresponding years. The impact of the comprehensive set of IOM policies over a 20-year period provides strong encouragement for their implementation. Second, we considered a high-impact scenario in

TABLE 2.6 SimSmoke Projections of Total and Per-Capita Consumption Under Three Policy Scenarios, Ages 18+, 2005–2025

POLICY/YEAR	2005	2006[a]	2010	CHANGE VS. STATUS QUO (%)[b] (2025)	2015	2020	2025	CHANGE VS. STATUS QUO (%)[b] (2025)
Total Consumption (million packs per year)								
Status quo	19,377	19,303	18,910	–	18,271	17,459	16,770	–
IOM recommendations	19,377	12,399	11,418	−39.6%	10,249	9,184	8,356	−50.2%
High-impact scenario	19,377	11,575	4,669	−75.3%	4,481	4,122	3,815	−77.2%
PCC (packs per year per capita)								
Status quo	88.8	87.5	81.9	–	75.4	69.2	63.7	–
IOM recommendations	88.8	56.2	49.5	−39.6%	42.3	36.4	31.8	−50.2%
High-impact scenario	88.8	52.5	20.2	−75.3%	18.5	16.3	14.5	−77.2%

[a] Policies are implemented and maintained from year 2006 forward.
[b] Percentage changes calculated relative to the status quo rate as (Policy rate − status quo rate)/status quo rate.
Source: SimSmoke model "U.S. 2002."

which smoking rates would fall much more rapidly. Although the policy assumptions that underlie the high-impact scenario are unlikely to occur in the near future, exploring the potential for rapid progress in tobacco control is instructive in terms of the best or worse that various stakeholders might anticipate. SimSmoke projects that the smoking rate would fall to about 7.5 percent by 2010 and less than 6 percent by 2025 if the high-impact scenario has been implemented in 2006.

The average quantity smoked by the remaining smokers is projected to fall by more modest amounts under the IOM and high-impact scenarios. Reductions in quantity are projected to occur relatively soon after a policy change, whereas changes in prevalence tend to build over time, especially for policies that have a greater effect on the young. Over time, trends in PCC will reflect changes in prevalence as well as changes in quantity smoked by remaining smokers, so that larger changes are projected in this measure than in prevalence. Relative to the status quo, we project that by 2025 PCC would fall by 50 percent under the IOM scenario and by 77 percent under the high-impact scenario.

These projections are based on the SimSmoke model, which has been developed and vetted over a number of years. It is important to point out, however, that the model is only as good as our knowledge of the effects of tobacco control policies. The strength of evidence for each of these policies varies greatly (Hopkins et al. 2001; Levy, Nikolayev, and Mumford 2004). The evidence for the effects of taxes and clean air policies is stronger than that for media policies; the evidence for youth access policies is even weaker and less consistent. Our uncertainty bounds for the six IOM policies suggest that IOM policy effects in relative terms may be about 40 percent less or 50 percent greater than the effect projected for 2025. As new empirical studies are conducted, information from those studies can be incorporated into simulation models and the model further validated.

Previous applications of SimSmoke to Arizona, California, and the entire United States provide some assurance that the parameters and assumptions underlying the current model are valid (Levy, Nikolayev, and Mumford 2004, 2005a; Levy et al. 2007). However, it should be noted that the model overpredicts the effect of policies on 18- to 24-year-old smokers and underpredicts the effect of policies on those over age 65, suggesting the need for further study. Unless policies are directed at younger adults, smoking initiation may be delayed to older ages.

Knowledge about the synergistic effect of policies is also weak. A few empirical studies consider simultaneously the effect of two tobacco control policies (Farrelly, Pechachek, and Chaloupka 2003; Hu et al. 1995; Miller et al. 2005), but most examine the effect of only one policy, thus making it difficult to learn how multiple policies interact with one another. In the absence of empirical studies that consider the effect of multiple policies simultaneously, simulation models provide an alternative approach that combines information from different studies and draws on theories from social science to model policy effects. As simulations are conducted for different states in the United States and for nations other than the United States, we may be better able to identify the effect of different policies individually and in combination.

The impact that an array of tobacco control policies has on different sectors of the population can be exceedingly complex. SimSmoke makes some important simplifications that make the model more tractable but also add potential limitations.

First, the model assumes that most policies have a direct effect on cessation through a decrease in prevalence that occurs largely in the first year. In future years the effects of policy are maintained or increased through effects on the initiation and cessation rates. This assumption of rapid implementation is obviously unrealistic but is acceptable in this context because our focus is on effects over the 20-year time horizon: our intent is not to predict smoking patterns but to describe a series of what-if scenarios for later chapters to build on, setting best- and worst-case scenarios for stakeholders. Nevertheless, knowledge about the time patterns of policy implementation and individual response will help to improve the predictive utility of the model. The model also might be extended to consider the steps in the progression to smoking initiation and to smoking cessation, rather than just simple initiation and cessation. The increasing smoking rate of young adults relative to youth suggests that the progression to established smoking may have changed during the 1990s (Centers for Disease Control and Prevention 2002).

In addition, in this chapter we do not consider the implications of immigration patterns for smoking or estimate smoking prevalence by socioeconomic or racial/ethnic category. As Balbach and colleagues discuss in chapter 16, the evidence about how policy effects might differ by social class or race/ethnicity is weak. Currently, a higher percentage of those with lower income/education status are smokers. These smokers may be less responsive to some policies, for example, media campaigns, but evidence indicates that they are more responsive to others, such as tax increases (Farrelly and Bray 1998). With proper targeting, cessation treatments and media campaigns might be more effectively directed to these groups.

SimSmoke is also limited in that it does not provide state-specific estimates of the effects of smoking rates or the effects of policies. It is likely that more vigorous policies would have larger effects in states where tobacco control policies are currently weak: for instance, a $2 increase in the excise tax is a much larger percentage change for states in which taxes are currently low.

A further simplification is that policies are modeled as having a unidirectional effect on smoking rates. As such, SimSmoke does not explicitly model potential feedbacks through industry practices, social norms and attitudes, and peer and family behaviors. As policies are implemented, the tobacco industry might strategically adjust its pricing, marketing practices, or product lines. In particular, the projections of the high-impact scenario presume that strong regulations and treatment progress are not negated by actions of tobacco manufacturers. In addition, although it allows for some of the synergies that might be caused by changing social norms, SimSmoke does not explicitly model attitudes or norms. An increase in social norms against smoking may enhance the effects of tobacco control policies and promote further policy change, which could in turn accelerate the decline in smoking. In particular, reductions in peer and adult smoking may "spill over" and reduce subsequent initiation.

The PCC and quantity models are subject to some additional limitations. In particular, the evidence on the effects of policy on the average quantity of cigarettes smoked is much sparser than the effects on prevalence, and the quantity effects depend on the prevalence effects in the model, thus compounding any potential errors. The PCC data are subject to seasonal and inventory changes (Chandra and Chaloupka 2003; Gilpin et al. 2001), omit untaxed sales, and include cigarettes purchased but not smoked. However, because the PCC measure includes all taxable sales, it remains a relatively accurate measurement of consumption.

With these caveats in mind, the SimSmoke model suggests that policies can have a large impact on smoking rates. If the IOM policies had been implemented in 2006, we project that smoking rates would have dropped to about 15 percent by 2010. Evidence from California, which has had strong tobacco control policies, suggests that this projection is attainable (Gilpin et al. 2003). Maintaining policies at high levels could reduce smoking prevalence in the United States to about 10 percent by 2025—a target in line with *Healthy People 2010* targets. Larger reductions might occur earlier under a high-impact scenario, but this scenario implies an unprecedented rate of change in smoking that is far less likely to be attained.

APPENDIX 2.1: SIMSMOKE MODEL DETAILS

This appendix provides additional detail about the SimSmoke model, including a discussion of the population and smoking modules, two of the policy modules, and the construction of the average quantity and PCC measures. Table 2.7 provides information on data sources for the model.

TABLE 2.7 Data Used in SimSmoke Model

VARIABLE	SOURCE	SPECIFICATIONS
I. Population model		
A. Population	2002 Current Population Survey	Breakdowns by age and gender
B. Fertility rates	U.S. Census Vital Rate Inputs Tables, 2002	Breakdowns by age
C. Mortality rates	2001 Multiple Cause-of-Death File, NCHS	Breakdowns by age and gender, 2001
II. Smoking model		
A. Baseline prevalence rates for current and ex-smokers	Tobacco Use Supplement of the CPS (2001/2002) for ages 15+, and 1993 Teenage Attitudes and Practices Survey for <age 15	Based on 100+ cigarettes lifetime and distinction between current and ex-smokers. Ex-smokers by years quit (<1, 1–2, 3–5, 6–10, 11–14, 15+ years), breakdowns by age and gender
B. Initiation rates	Change in smoking prevalence between contiguous age groups	Breakdowns by age and gender
C. First-year quit rates	Tobacco Use Supplement of the CPS (2001/2002) for ages 24+	Breakdowns by age and gender
D. Relapse rates	Gilpin, Pierce, and Farkas (1997); McWhorter, Boyd, and Mattson (1990); U.S. DHHS (1989, 1990); and COMMIT data	Breakdowns by age
E. Relative death risks of smokers and ex-smokers	Cancer Prevention Study II	Breakdowns by age and gender
F. Average quantity smoked per smoker	Tobacco Use Supplement of the CPS (2001/2002) for ages 15+	Breakdowns by age and gender, with corrections for someday smokers (see text)
G. Per capita consumption	U.S. Department of Agriculture's *Tobacco Outlook* (2005), http://usda.mannlib.cornell.edu/MannUsda/viewDocumentInfo.do?documentID=1392	Complete census of tax paid sales in the US, measured as per capita (adult ages 18+) sales (in packs of cigarettes), and adjusted to include inventory changes, taxable removals, miscellaneous shipments, and imports

TABLE 2.7 *(Continued)*

VARIABLE	SOURCE	SPECIFICATIONS
III. Policy Modules (data for 2002–2005)		
A. Taxes	Tobacco Institute, Tobacco freekids.org; www.bls.gov/cpi/home.htm	Prices, consumer price index, and taxes
B. Clean air laws	http://apps.nccd.cdc.gov/StateSystem/stateSystem.aspx?selectedTopic=600&selected Measure=999&dir=leg_report&ucName=UCLegSmkFree Summary&year=&excel= htmlTable;slati.lungusa.org/search-form.asp (National Cancer Institute 2000)	Different types of laws and their stringency
C. Media & other educational campaigns	CDC and various state Web sites; Wakefield and Chaloupka (2000); Farrelly, Pechacek, and Chaloupka (2003)	Expenditures per capita and audience (adult and youth or youth only)
D. Cessation Treatment Policies	Coverage rates at McPhillips-Tangum et al (2002) and www.cdc.gov/tobacco/educational materials/ essation/page1.html; insurance coverage rates at ferrer.bls.census.gov/macro/032002/health/h02_001.htm. Quitlines at www.cdc.gov/tobacco/quit/Quitlines/Appendix.pdf	Mandated cessation treatments, brief interventions, quitlines (reactive or proactive, with or without NRT, extent of publicity)
E. School Education/Community Media	IOM panel; see media references above	Existence of comprehensive, well-designed school education programs and community media campaign
F. Youth access	CDC at apps.nccd.cdc.gov/StateSystem/stateSystem.aspx?, SAMHSA at prevention.samhsa.gov/tobacco/01synartable.asp	Enforcement checks, penalties, community campaigns, self-service and vending machine bans

POPULATION MODULE

SimSmoke begins with a demographic module. The module starts with the population, distinguished by age, starting in the year 2002. The population evolves over time through fertility and mortality using a discrete first-order Markov process. Mathematically, the total population (Pop) is distinguished by time period t and age a (and is further distinguished in the model by gender). Mortality rates ($Mort$) are distinguished by age and gender. The number of newborns depends on fertility rates ($Fert$) of females by age, assuming an equal birth ratio of males to females and equal first-year death rates. Births, or $Pop_{t,0}$ through the first year (age 0) for each gender, are:

$$Pop_{t,0} = 0.5 * \Sigma^a \, (Pop_{t,a,1} * Fert_a) * (1 - Mort_0),$$

where $t = 1, \ldots, 20$; $a = 14, \ldots, 49$. After the first year, $a = 1, \ldots,$ the population evolves as:

$$Pop_{t,a} = Pop_{t-1,a-1} * (1 - Mort_a).$$

Population data are obtained from the 2000 Census of Population and projected forward to 2002. Fertility rates are from the U.S. Census Vital Rate Inputs Tables for the year 2002. Mortality rates are from the 2001 Multiple Cause-of-Death File compiled from death certificates, compiled by the National Center for Health Statistics available (www.nchs.gov). The file includes information on all deaths in the United States in 2001.

SMOKING PREVALENCE MODULE

SimSmoke models the prevalence of established smokers using the standard definition: established smokers are individuals who have smoked more than 100 cigarettes in their lifetime and are currently smoking. Never smokers are individuals who have not smoked 100 cigarettes in their lifetime. Ex-smokers are those who have smoked more than 100 cigarettes in their lifetime but are not currently smoking (i.e., have not smoked in the past 30 days). The model distinguishes 16 categories of ex-smokers ($n = 1, \ldots, 16+$), corresponding to years since last smoking. By these definitions the population is divided into the different smoking groups in the base year. Over time the smoking population, in the absence of policy changes, evolves based on initiation, cessation, and relapse rates based on a first-order discrete Markov process.

After the base year, individuals are classified as never smokers (**ns**) from birth until they initiate smoking or die, according to:

$$Neversmokers_{t,a} = Neversmokers_{t-1,a-1} * (1 - MortRate_{a,ns}) * (1 - Initiation\ Rate_a)$$

Once a smoker, an individual cannot return to never-smoking status but could become an ex-smoker if he or she quit smoking.

Because smoking rates typically level off by age 24 (U.S. Department of Health and Human Services 1994), initiation in the module occurs until age 24. Because of empirical challenges in measuring initiation, quitting, and relapse before age 24 (when there is a greater degree of experimentation), and to ensure stability and internal consistency of the model, initiation rates at each age are measured net of quitting. Specifically, net initiation is measured as the difference between the smoking rate at a given age and that same rate at the previous age. Because the duration of smoking is not considered, we do not track the specific year when individuals initiate in this population-level model. Through age 24, the number of smokers (s) is tracked as:

$$Smokers_{t,a} = Smokers_{t-1,a-1} * (1 - MortRate_{a,s})$$
$$+ Neversmokers_{t-1,a-1} * (1 - MortRate_{a,ns}) * Initiation\ Rate_a$$

Cessation is tracked from age 24 because the relative risks of mortality from smoking are not discernable for those who stop smoking before that age (U.S. Department of Health and Human Services 1990, 2004a). Cessation rates in the first year are distinguished by age and gender, but relapse rates in later years are only distinguished by years since quitting (i.e., are assumed invariant to the age or gender of the ex-smoker).

Once a smoker, an individual continues in that category until he/she quits, dies, or reenters the group through relapse. After age 24, smokers are tracked as:

$$Smokers_{t-a} = Smokers_{t-1,a-1} * (1 - MortRate_{t,a,s}) * (1 - Cessation\ Rate_a)$$
$$+ \Sigma_{n=1}^{16}\ Ex\text{-}smokers_{t-1,a-1,n} * (1 - MortRate_{t,a,n}) * (Relapse\ Rate_{a,n})$$

The number of first-year ex-smokers is determined by the first-year cessation rate applied to surviving smokers in the previous year:

$$Ex\text{-}smokers_{t,a,1} = Smokers_{t-1,a-1,1} * (1 - MortRate_{t,a,s}) * (Cessation\ Rate_a)$$

The number of individuals who have been ex-smokers for more than one year (n = 2, . . . 16+) is calculated as:

$$Ex\text{-}smokers_{t,a,n} = Ex\text{-}smokers_{t-1,a-1,n-1} * (1 - MortRate_{a,n})$$
$$* (1 - Relapse\ Rate_{a,n-1})$$

For those who have ceased smoking for more than 15 years, we add to the above equation the ex-smokers from the previous year who had remained abstinent for more than 15 years and did not die or relapse in the previous year.

The primary source of baseline data on smoking habits by age and gender is the Current Population Survey—Tobacco Use Supplements (CPS-TUS), a sample of approximately 475,000 respondents conducted in June 2001, November 2001, and February 2002. This survey is the largest nationally representative data set for the United States that measures smoking behavior. Data collection was conducted primarily by telephone, but about 30 percent of interviews were conducted in person in the household. Response rates are generally above 80 percent. Smoking may begin before age 15, but the TUS only asks individuals age 15 and older about their smoking status. For those younger than age 15, we use data from the 1993 Teenage Attitudes and Practices Survey (TAPS). To correct for a slight discrepancy in rates, we scale those data by the ratio of the TAPS 15- to 17-year-old smoking rate to the U.S. 15- to 17-year-old smoking rate.

For our purposes, the data are obtained by single age from 15 to 24 and then by 10-year age groups through age 85. Smoking rates are multiplied by the relevant 2002 population to determine the number of smokers and ex-smokers by demographic group. In the smoking module, we assign the prevalence value for the age bracket to the midpoint age of the bracket and interpolate between that bracket and the midpoint value in the previous age bracket.

POLICY MODULES

TAXES For the period 2002–2005, prices are averaged over states with weights based on tobacco sales and are adjusted for inflation using the U.S. Bureau of Labor Statistics consumer price index. Data on retail prices and taxes were obtained for 2002 and 2003 from Orzechowski and Walker (2003) and for 2004 and 2005 from tobaccofreekids.org/research/factsheets/pdf/0212.pdf (accessed March 7, 2005). The retail price is measured by a price index that includes generic cigarettes weighted by their proportionate sales. Inflation-adjusted prices increased slightly from $3.75 to $4.20 between 2002 and 2005, and the average state tax in 2005 was $1.23.

From 2005 we assume that cigarette prices relative to inflation stay constant (i.e., we assume that taxes adjust upward to reflect general price inflation). To model the effect of additional tax changes, we assume that change in prices equals change in the average state plus federal tax on cigarettes, based on studies reported in Jha and Chaloupka (2000).

CESSATION TREATMENT Although some recent evidence suggests a decline in the effectiveness of pharmacotherapy (Pierce and Gilpin 2002; Thorndike, Biener, and Rigotti 2002), new pharmacotherapies and other forms of therapy targeted to specific populations could improve treatment effectiveness in the future. Brief physician advice is reported to have increased six-month quit rates by 30 percent (Fiore et al. 2000), although a recent review indicated a larger effect (Lancaster and Stead 2004). Proactive quitlines with follow-up, as recommended by the IOM, doubled the quit success rate of state quitlines (Zhu et al. 2002), consistent with previous studies (Hopkins et al. 2001). We will assume that effectiveness ranges for each of these treatments can vary between 50 and 125 percent of the values above.

THE EFFECTS OF POLICIES ON SMOKING PREVALENCE

The effects of tobacco control policies on smoking prevalence are calculated as percentage reductions (PR) relative to the initial rates (i.e., PR = [postpolicy rate − initial rate]/initial rate, where PR < 0). For most policies, their greatest effect is in the first years in which the policy is in effect. These are modeled as a permanent additive effect on smoking prevalence (i.e., $Smokers_{t,a} * [1 + PR_{i,t,a}]$) for policy i at time period t and which may vary by age a. Although the effect may be spread over several years, we model the effects as occurring in the first year that the policy is implemented.

If the policy affects initiation, the effects of the policy are sustained through lower initiation rates. After the first year that the policy is in effect, the percentage reduction lowers the initiation rate (as $Initiation\ Rate_a * [1 + PR_i]$) as long as policy i is in effect. The effects of policy i may also be augmented over the same time period through increases in the first-year cessation rate (as $Cessation\ Rate_a * [1 - PR_i]$) in future years. Higher future cessation rates arise from the higher propensity to quit among individuals who smoke less (Hughes 2000; Hymowitz et al. 1991, 1997) and other (e.g., economic and informational) factors. We assume that the proportion of individuals who relapse increases in direct proportion with any changes in first-year cessation, which is to say that the rates of relapse are unaffected by policy changes.

When more than one policy is in effect, the percentage reductions are multiplicatively applied (i.e., $[1 + PR_i] * [1 + PR_j]$ for policies i and j), which implies that the relative effect is independent of other policies but the absolute effect is smaller when another policy is in effect. Some specific synergies between policies are built into the model.

AVERAGE QUANTITY SMOKED

As with prevalence (Levy, Nikolayev, and Mumford 2005a), trends in quantity have two components: (1) status quo changes that would have otherwise occurred in the absence of policy change and (2) policy-induced changes. We begin with quantity data in the 2002 base year broken down by age. We then apply the equation:

$$QS_{t,a,g} = QS_{t-1, \ldots a}(1 + percent\Delta Quantity_{t.a, \, stat \, quo} + percent\Delta Quantity_{t.a, \, pol})$$

where QS is quantity smoked, $percent\Delta Quantity_{t.a, \, stat \, quo}$ is the status quo percentage change, and $percent\Delta Quantity_{t.a, \, pol}$ is the policy-induced percentage change. The extant literature provides little guidance on these two components, but there is some basis for considering the effect of taxes, clean air laws, and media/comprehensive campaigns. Based on studies that consider the effect of policies on quantity smoked, quantity changes were found to be similar in percentage terms to (i.e., 100 percent of) the effects on prevalence. Therefore, $percent\Delta Quantity_{t.a, \, pol}$ is set equal to 1* the overall effect of policy on prevalence by age. Based on empirical work by the authors and fit of the model (Levy and Mumford 2007), we estimated a long-term downward trend of −0.5 percent per year after adjusting for policies. Thus, policy effects differ by age, but we assume the same downward status quo trend in quantity, implying common effects over different cohorts.

To develop quantity estimates by age and gender and to validate the model for selected subgroups, we used survey data collected from the CPS-TUS, the same source used for smoking prevalence. Current everyday smokers were asked how many cigarettes they smoked on the average day (CPD), and someday smokers were asked how many days they had smoked in the last month and the CPD on the days that they smoked. The CPD by someday smokers was calculated as the number of days they had smoked in the last month multiplied by the CPD on the days that they smoked and divided by the average number of days per month (30.4). The average quantity smoked by everyday and someday smokers was then calculated by multiplying the average CPD for each age and gender group by their respective percentages in the smoking population.

PER-CAPITA CONSUMPTION

Because PCC equals smoking prevalence multiplied by the average quantity smoked per smoker, we decomposed changes in PCC into quantity and prevalence changes using the relation:

$$Percent\Delta PCC = percent\Delta Prevalence + percent\Delta Quantity$$

The model begins with the level of PCC in the base year, 2002. The percentage change in prevalence is derived from the model. As above, we decomposed quantity into status quo changes and policy-induced changes using the parameters above: percentΔQuantity$_{\text{t.a, stat quo}}$ equals -0.5 percent annually, and percentΔQuantity$_{\text{t.a, pol}}$ equals 1 times the overall effect of policy on prevalence by age. Because it is based on a census of all sales, PCC does not distinguish by age or gender. Since the effects of policy on prevalence differ by age in SimSmoke, we weight the age-specific policy parameters by the proportion of smokers in each age group, ages 18 and older, to obtain a policy adjuster (reflecting the effect of policies on quantity or PCC) for all adults.

PCC data for 2002 are from the United States Department of Agriculture's *Trade Outlook* (2005, www.ers.usda.gov/Publications/so/view.asp?f=specialty/tbs-bb/), and reflect a complete census of tax-paid sales in the United States. PCC is measured as per-capita (adults aged 18+) sales (in packs of cigarettes) and is adjusted to include inventory changes, taxable removals, miscellaneous shipments, and imports.

PART 1

ECONOMY

3

ECONOMIC IMPLICATIONS FOR U.S. TOBACCO FARMERS OF MEASURES TO REDUCE TOBACCO CONSUMPTION IN THE UNITED STATES

DANIEL A. SUMNER AND JULIAN M. ALSTON

Tobacco control measures in the United States affect tobacco farmers by reducing the demand for consumer products that use tobacco and thereby reducing the demand for leaf tobacco. This chapter describes the current leaf tobacco industry in the United States and considers the economic implications for tobacco growers of measures to reduce cigarette consumption. Under these tobacco control measures, individual growers will face a lower market price for their tobacco, and the overall quantity demanded will be lower as well. The result will be a smaller crop produced and less total revenue earned from growing tobacco. The magnitudes of these impacts and the responses by growers will depend on many factors, including the role of international trade and the supply response to lower market prices.

The chapter proceeds through several steps to assess the impacts of tobacco control measures on growers. First, we characterize the leaf tobacco production industry in the United States, including regional distribution, numbers of growers, and cost of production. We also discuss industry trends in prices, quantities, and revenues, including the role of international trade in tobacco products. Second, we summarize leaf tobacco policies, especially the major changes in policy that first took effect in the 2005–2006 marketing year. Third, we discuss the implications for tobacco leaf supply of changes in cigarette demand and simulate the impacts of two tobacco control policy scenarios on market price, leaf quantity produced, total revenue, net revenue, and related economic variables.

THE LEAF TOBACCO INDUSTRY IN THE UNITED STATES

The U.S. tobacco industry has played a significant role in the agricultural economy of the Southeastern and Appalachian region for many decades. Starting with the Jamestown colony, tobacco was a significant cash and export crop for growers who produced other products for home consumption and local use.

PRODUCTION

Tobacco is produced in 16 states, but it is heavily concentrated: in 2005, 42 percent of tobacco acreage was in North Carolina and 27 percent was in Kentucky. Georgia, South Carolina, Tennessee, and Virginia each accounted for between 5 and 8 percent of acreage. There are six significant classes of tobacco including flue-cured, air-cured (including Burley tobacco), fire-cured, cigar filler, cigar binder, and cigar wrapper. Flue-cured tobacco accounts for more than 60 percent, and Burley tobacco for about 30 percent, of the tobacco grown in the United States. Flue-cured tobacco is grown mainly in North Carolina, Virginia, South Carolina, and Georgia, whereas Burley is grown mainly in Kentucky and Tennessee. These two major types comprise more than 98 percent of the domestic tobacco used in domestic cigarettes. They also account for almost all U.S. tobacco exports.

From the 1930s to 2005, tobacco farming was governed by strict supply controls and a federal price support program (Sumner and Alston 1984). The government set minimum prices at which it acquired tobacco of each major type and quality, and limited tobacco marketing to those who held production acreage allotments or, later, poundage quotas. The amount of tobacco allowed on the market was adjusted from year to year by adjusting the marketing allotments or quotas of individual growers. The aim of the marketing restrictions was to limit supply so that the market price remained above the government-set minimum price and to minimize the amount of tobacco entering government stockpiles. In general, the program severely limited U.S. tobacco production and kept U.S. tobacco prices substantially above where they would otherwise have been (Sumner and Alston 1984).

Under this program, the production of tobacco in the United States declined gradually over more than 50 years (figure 3.1). More rapid declines in production and acreage have occurred over the past decade with changes in leaf tobacco policy, changes in the environment for the domestic cigarette industry, and changes in international trade patterns. Trends in acreage and yields differ for flue-cured and Burley tobacco, however (Gale, Foreman, and Capehart 2000).

Acreage of flue-cured tobacco peaked in 1952 with about 1.11 million acres. With rapid yield increases and stagnant demand, acreage allotments were progressively reduced, and acreage declined rapidly to about 0.56 million acres in 1965. At that point the federal supply control policy shifted from acreage allot-

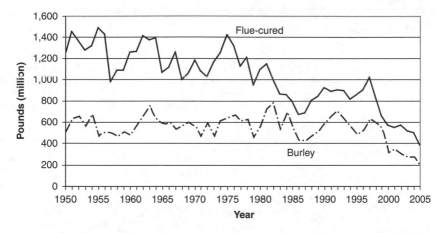

FIGURE 3.1 Production of Flue-Cured and Burley Tobacco in the United States

Data Source: Economic Research Service, U.S. Department of Agriculture, *Tobacco Yearbook*, http://usda.mannlib.cornell.edu/MannUsda/viewDocumentInfo.do?documentID–1392, tables 16 and 17.

ments to poundage quotas, causing yields to stabilize and allowing acreage to rise in the early 1970s before declining again to about 0.31 million acres in 1985. Acreage grew to 0.46 million acres in 1997 and then dropped steeply to 0.18 million acres by 2005.

Burley tobacco acreage peaked at 0.46 million acres in 1952 and followed a pattern of periodic rapid declines over the subsequent five decades. Acreage had risen from a previous low of about 0.21 million acres in 1986 to a recent high of 0.34 million acres in 1997. Similar to flue-cured tobacco acreage, Burley acreage fell by half from 1997 to 2004 and then fell another 50 percent to just 0.11 million acres in 2005.

The number of farms that grow tobacco has declined even more rapidly than has the total acreage. Table 3.1 shows that acreage per farm rose from about 3 acres per farm in 1954 to about 7.5 acres per farm in 2002. Most tobacco operations in 2002 remained part-time enterprises, either on larger full-time farms with most acreage devoted to other crops or on small part-time farms whose operators were retired or worked primarily off the farm. An average eight-acre tobacco enterprise generated about 16,000 pounds of tobacco; with an average price of about $1.90 per pound, the total gross revenue of the operation was about $30,000.

Figure 3.2 shows that despite rapid declines in size of the industry, in 2002–2004 tobacco still represented a large share of agriculture in Kentucky, accounting for about 37 percent of cash crop receipts, and was also significant in North Carolina, with about 20 percent of crop receipts. Both states have sizable

TABLE 3.1 Number of Farms Growing Tobacco and Average Tobacco Acreage per Farm, 1954–2002

YEAR	FARMS (THOUSANDS)	ACRES (THOUSANDS)	AVERAGE ACREAGE PER TOBACCO FARM
1954	512	1,547	3.0
1959	417	1,108	2.7
1964	331	1,025	3.1
1969	276	877	3.2
1974	198	877	4.4
1978	189	963	5.1
1982	179	932	5.2
1987	137	633	4.6
1992	124	831	6.7
1997	94	837	9.0
2002	57	429	7.5

Source: Capehart (2004).

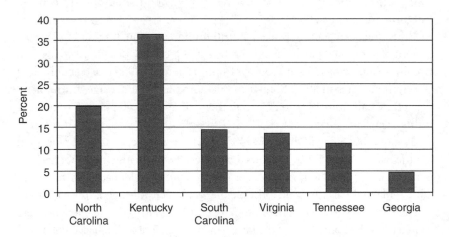

FIGURE 3.2 Tobacco Cash Receipts as a Share of Total Cash Crop Receipts by State, 2002–2004 Average

Data Source: Economic Research Service, U.S. Department of Agriculture, *Tobacco Year-book*, http://usda.mannlib.cornell.edu/MannUsda/viewDocumentInfo.do?documentID=1392, table 31.

TABLE 3.2 Cost of Production per Hundredweight for Flue-Cured Tobacco and Burley Tobacco, 2004

ITEM	FLUE-CURED	BURLEY
Gross value of production	184.4	198.6
Cash expenses		
Seed and plant bed	3.4	5.9
Fertilizer	14.9	18.3
Chemicals	9.6	5.1
Custom operations	0.4	0.7
Fuel, lube, and electricity	4.6	5.7
Curing fuel	26.8	
Repairs	5.6	4.3
Hired labor	32.0	32.1
Marketing expenses	7.2	2.9
Other variable cash expenses	0.2	1.2
Total, variable cash expenses	104.6	76.4
General farm overhead	9.2	12.0
Taxes and insurance	6.8	2.5
Interest	7.2	3.8
Total, fixed cash expenses	23.2	18.3
Total, cash expenses	127.8	94.7
Gross value of production less cash expenses	56.6	103.9
Price (dollars/cwt.)	184.4	198.6
Yield (cwt./acre)	22.7	19.5

Source: Economic Research Service, "Commodity Costs and Returns Data," http://www.ers.usda.gov/Data/CostsAndReturns/TestPick.htm, Cost of Production.

livestock enterprises, so the share of tobacco in total, crops and livestock, agricultural receipts was only 13 percent in Kentucky and 8.5 percent in North Carolina. Tobacco comprised a smaller share in the other states. All of these shares fell in 2005, with large declines in market price and in production.

Table 3.2 shows the costs of production for flue-cured and Burley tobacco production in 2004. Cash expenses are distributed across a wide range of items.

Hired labor is a major expense for both crops, with curing fuel particularly important for flue-cured tobacco and fertilizer more important for Burley tobacco. Cost of acquiring quota is not represented in these cash expenses. A major share of revenue was accounted for by the value of production minus cash expenses—mainly returns to unpaid labor, management, owned land, and quota. For the many growers who leased quota, however, quota rent was an additional cash cost that accounted for a significant share of the returns, so that returns to unpaid labor, management, and owned land were very small or negative in some cases. With removal of the quota program in 2005, revenue per pound declined by about 25 percent for both 2005 and 2006, consistent with the rental rate typically paid for marketing quota (Brown, Rucker, and Thurman 2007).

INTERNATIONAL TRADE

International trade has long been an important feature of the industry. Leaf tobacco exports are as old as tobacco farming itself, and the cigarette industry has been importing leaf tobacco for a century. Cigarette exports have also long been important. International trade plays a crucial role in determining how policies aimed at domestic cigarette consumption affect the leaf tobacco industry.

Figure 3.3 shows the share of total disappearance—that is, tobacco removed from warehouses—that is exported for the two main types of tobacco. For flue-

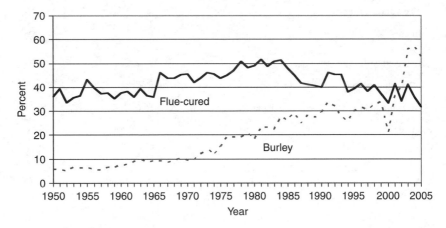

FIGURE 3.3 Exports as a Share of Total Disappearance, Flue-Cured Tobacco and Burley Tobacco, 1950–2005

Data Source: Economic Research Service, U.S. Department of Agriculture, *Tobacco Yearbook*, http://usda.mannlib.cornell.edu/MannUsda/viewDocumentInfo.do?documentID=1392, tables 16 and 17.

cured tobacco, the share exported rose from about 35 percent in the early 1950s to about 50 percent in the late 1970s and early 1980s, then dropped back more recently to the 35 to 40 percent range. For Burley tobacco, the share of leaf exports grew gradually from less than 6 percent of disappearance in the early 1950s to more than 30 percent by the end of the 1990s and then jumped to more than 50 percent in the years 2003 through 2005.

Leaf tobacco imports are also important. In general, the United States has imported types of tobaccos not grown here (Turkish tobacco) as well as lower-quality leaf, which the United States could not produce competitively under the quota program. Imports have increased steadily and gained in importance in the manufacture of cigarettes in the United States. Even as total tobacco per cigarette declined, the amount of imported tobacco grew steadily from about 0.16 pounds per 1,000 cigarettes in 1950 to about 0.9 pounds in recent years. Imported leaf now comprises about half of the tobacco content of U.S.-made cigarettes.

Cigarette exports are the third important element of international tobacco trade. The quantity of cigarette exports has declined steadily. About 25 percent of cigarettes produced in the United States are exported, compared to about one-third in the 1980s. When cigarette exports are combined with leaf tobacco exports, the United States remains a net exporter of tobacco, although the net export margin has declined markedly (Capehart 2005a).

DOMESTIC CONSUMPTION AND PRICES

Domestic consumption of U.S. tobacco has fallen dramatically since 1950, dropping more steeply over the past two decades. There are three reasons for this decline. First, total tobacco per cigarette fell from about 2.7 pounds per 1,000 cigarettes in the early 1950s to about 1.7 pounds in recent years. Second, as discussed earlier, the use of imported tobacco in U.S.-made cigarettes has grown steadily. Third, since 1981 total cigarette consumption in the United States has fallen from 640 billion to less than 400 billion cigarettes per year (figure 3.4), even as the size of the adult population has grown.

The price of tobacco rose in nominal terms as the government-set price support ratcheted up over time. In nominal terms, this price stopped rising after the early 1980s (Capehart 2005a). Adjusted for inflation, the prices of Burley and flue-cured tobacco held steady between 1950 and the early 1980s, ranging between about $2.50 and $3.00 per pound in 2004 dollars. Since then, real prices have declined significantly, falling to less than $2.00 per pound in 2004. Prices fell another 25 percent from 2004 to 2005, when the price support program was removed, and remained relatively low for several years afterwards (Dohlman, Foreman, and Da Pra 2009).

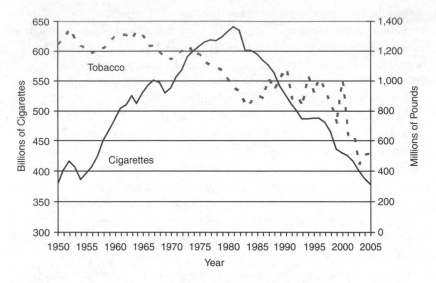

FIGURE 3.4 U.S. Cigarette Consumption and Disappearance of Domestic Flue-Cured Tobacco and Burley Tobacco, 1950–2005

Data Source: Economic Research Service, U.S. Department of Agriculture, *Tobacco Yearbook*, http://usda.mannlib.cornell.edu/MannUsda/viewDocumentInfo.do?documentID=1392, table 1.

LEAF TOBACCO POLICY

Many of the trends described above were caused in part by the farm program for U.S. tobacco, as consequences of long-run dynamic responses in both domestic and international markets. The farm program held the U.S. tobacco price above the world market price, leading to substantial economizing responses by tobacco producers and users around the world, with serious consequences for the U.S. industry. By keeping the price of domestic leaf high, the policy encouraged cigarette manufacturers in the United States and overseas to substitute other tobacco for U.S. tobacco and nontobacco inputs for tobacco. As a result, U.S.-made cigarettes included less tobacco overall and a smaller share of U.S.-grown tobacco; the U.S. share of the world's tobacco production also fell. The same policies encouraged the U.S. industry to specialize in higher-quality tobaccos (Babcock and Foster 1991). As the domestic and foreign industries responded to the U.S. policy, the policy itself had to adapt, progressively ratcheting down the total U.S. quota quantity to accommodate the declining demand that reflected the dynamic response to the policy itself.

Because marketing rights could not be shifted across county lines—or in minor cases, state lines—the program also kept the industry frozen in place geographically. Evidence from differences in quota lease rates across regions suggested that production costs relative to quality varied considerably and that tobacco production would have moved substantially if restrictions had been lifted (Brown, Rucker, and Thurman 2007; Rucker, Thurman, and Sumner 1995). In general, the low-cost region for flue-cured tobacco was in the coastal plain of North Carolina, and the low-cost region for Burley tobacco was in the central regions of Kentucky.

Two major changes in tobacco policy that directly impact tobacco growers have taken place over the past decade. The Master Settlement Agreement of 1998 (MSA) between the state attorneys general and the cigarette manufacturers required manufacturers to make payments of $206 billion over 25 years. In return for the payments, state tobacco health litigation was curtailed (Bulow and Klemperer 1999). As part of the Agreement, $5.15 billion was allocated to aid tobacco growers who were expected to suffer losses because of declining consumption. Following the MSA, cigarette prices rose rapidly and by much more than the direct cost of the Agreement on a per-unit basis (Ciliberto and Kuminoff 2010).

The second major change was the elimination of the price support and tobacco quota program system described above. The Fair and Equitable Tobacco Reform Act of 2004 (P.L. 108-357, Title VI) provided for compensation of quota owners and growers for the capital value of quota held at the time of the Act. Quota owners are being paid about $7 per pound of quota, and growers receive an additional $3 per pound. The total cost of the buyout is about $9.6 billion, funded by an assessment on the tobacco product industry (Brown, Rucker, and Thurman 2007; Womach 2005).

About 440,000 quota owners and about 57,000 growers are receiving payments. Prior to the buyout the rental rate for quota varied substantially from region to region with average values of about $0.50 per pound typical in many regions. The capital value of tobacco quota averaged about $2.00 per pound in 2004—only four times the rental rate—because of the risk of holding quota in a declining industry where the asset value hinged on continued government support of the program. The buyout paid substantially more than the previous market value of the asset. Quota owners are receiving about 14 times the previous rental value and, in some high-cost regions, an even higher ratio. Curiously, growers also receive payment even though, for them, the end of the quota program caused a reduction in their costs of operation.

In addition to paying for a quota buyout, the 2004 Act allocated funds, estimated to be about $5.0 billion, to cover losses on the government-held stocks. With removal of the price support program, the price of tobacco has fallen, and the government must liquidate its stocks at market prices well below the acquisition prices (Capehart 2005b).

The market prices for flue-cured and Burley tobacco fell by about 25 percent from 2004 to 2005. In addition, because of the large government-held stocks and the elimination of the requirement that the government buy any unsold leaf, tobacco production declined by about 23 percent for flue-cured tobacco and by about 30 percent for Burley tobacco. Beginning during the early 2000s, even before the end of the price support and quota system, most tobacco has been grown under annual marketing contracts. Evidently, buyers, aware that large stocks would become available with the end of the price support program, cut back on contracted quantities, at least in the short run. In North Carolina, flue-cured tobacco production rose back to its 2004 level in 2006, but the other regions of flue-cured tobacco and overall Burley tobacco production have not recovered.

With the elimination of marketing quotas and price supports, economists and industry experts expect exports to grow absolutely and as a share of production. That did not occur during 2005, nor did production expand immediately. This may be a function of the transition and the fact that large stocks had accumulated as the quota and price support programs were ending (Brown, Rucker, and Thurman 2007).

Other shifts in 2005 included a geographic movement of the industry: Burley tobacco concentrated in central or western Kentucky, and flue-cured tobacco moved to the coastal plain (Snell 2005). Further, some tobacco, such as Burley tobacco in coastal North Carolina and Pennsylvania, was grown outside its traditional regions. The geographic shift in tobacco production was accompanied by a substantial decline in the number of growers, which fell by 56 percent among Burley growers and 63 percent among growers of flue-cured tobacco (Dohlman, Foreman, and Da Pra 2009). Many very small growers had operated in the outlying high-cost regions, where production declined most steeply. Ending the quota support seems to have reduced the number of small tobacco operations in these fringe regions, and the current size distribution of farms is likely less skewed than it was in 2002 (Brown, Rucker, and Thurman 2007; Capehart 2005a; Snell 2005; Tiller, Snell, and Brown 2007). This shift also reflected consolidation and expansion of larger full-time tobacco growers. Finally, for the first time in more than a century, some minor tobacco types, including Northern Wisconsin cigar binder and Virginia sun-cured, were not produced in 2005 (Capehart 2006).

EFFECTS OF TOBACCO CONTROL POLICY ON THE LEAF TOBACCO INDUSTRY: A SIMULATION

As domestic cigarette consumption in the United States has grown and then declined, the domestic leaf tobacco industry has followed course. However, as figure 3.4 shows, the linkage between U.S. cigarette use and the fortunes of the domestic tobacco industry is less direct than one might presume. This is because the domestic leaf industry sells leaf tobacco to foreign manufacturers and to foreign consumers in the form of exported cigarettes. Furthermore, even in the domestic cigarette market, the amount of tobacco per cigarette has fallen over time, and domestic tobacco competes with imported tobacco in domestic cigarette production.

In any market, reductions in demand must be absorbed through reductions in quantity demanded, price, or both. These market parameters were involved in the past but were conditioned by government policy. Under the farm program for U.S. tobacco, the government determined how growers would respond to reductions in demand by setting price supports and by controlling supply through acreage allotments and, more recently, poundage quotas. The federal price support for tobacco was set by formulas that derived from legislation and changed only occasionally. The Department of Agriculture (USDA) adjusted quotas annually depending on anticipated demand but also on government stocks and other data. Thus, shifts in cigarette use affected leaf tobacco quantities and prices largely though government program responses that attempted to reflect market realities. This suggests a long-run relationship between consumption and leaf tobacco production, with relatively little immediate impact of changes in smoking rates on the demand for tobacco.

Now that the farm program for tobacco has ended, market mechanisms will determine the degree to which tobacco control measures affect quantity grown or price. We use a simulation approach to model the effects of tobacco control policies on growers. This simulation model formally links domestic tobacco prices and quantities to domestic cigarette use. The model is based on the work of Sumner and Wohlgenant (1985), which considered the impacts of an increase in the federal wholesale tax on cigarettes. The model they developed was later applied to the potential impacts of mandates for fire-safe cigarettes by Sumner (1987) and to a tax increase again by Brown (1995).

MODEL EQUATIONS AND PARAMETERS

The model consists of a supply equation and a demand equation for domestic leaf tobacco, with the latter derived from export and domestic demands for U.S. cigarettes. Demand for domestic leaf depends on the demand for cigarettes, which is affected by taxes and other tobacco control policies. The formal model is specified as a system of linear logarithmic differential equations, which can be solved for approximate percentage, or proportional, changes in endogenous prices and quantities in response to exogenous changes in demand or taxes. The details of the model, along with additional background on the parameter values and their interpretations, are reported in appendix 3.1. Here we describe the logic of the model and the results of simulations for the leaf tobacco industry.

The exogenous tobacco policy changes that drive the simulations are derived from the SimSmoke model, which projects total cigarette consumption under a status quo scenario and two alternative policy scenarios. The status quo scenario holds the policy environment of 2005 constant over the next 20 years; under this scenario, as discussed in chapter 2, demand for cigarettes declines because of projected demographic changes and in response to tobacco policy measures enacted before 2005. The first alternative policy scenario is based on the IOM best-case policies, which include a $2.00 tax increase per pack as well as other tobacco control measures. SimSmoke projects changes in cigarette consumption resulting from these policy changes. The high-impact scenario assumes more stringent tobacco control measures and derives lower cigarette use figures over the 20-year horizon. We calculate the implied percentage changes in key variables, relative to the status quo, for each policy alternative for each of the five years in the horizon. Policies are assumed to be implemented in 2006, with the effects playing out over the following 20 years. We present impacts for the years 2010, 2015, 2020, and 2025.

Table 3.3 summarizes the parameter definitions and values or value ranges used in our simulation. The simulations use an elasticity of supply for leaf tobacco of 4.0, meaning that marginal cost of production of leaf tobacco falls by 2.5 percent for each 10 percent reduction in quantity produced. Sumner and Alston (1984) and Rucker, Thurman, and Sumner (1995) provide estimates of this elasticity that are in the range of 2.0 to 5.0. The analysis of McDonald and Sumner (2003) suggests relatively large supply elasticities when the growers are unencumbered by government marketing restrictions and is consistent with a supply elasticity of 4.0. An alternative would be to assume the supply elasticity is very large in the long run—almost infinite. In that case, there would be only transitional losses and almost no effect on the price of tobacco, which would be determined solely by the almost constant marginal cost of production. Even with up to 20 years for adjustment, however, we expect the supply function to be less than infinitely elastic. We also assume that returns to scale are constant in cigarette manufacturing and that the prices of other inputs, such as paper, taxes, additives, labor, and promotion services, do not fall when their use by the U.S. cigarette industry declines. Given that the cost of U.S. tobacco represents only about 2 percent of the cost of cigarette manufacturing at wholesale, including the excise tax, the implicit elasticity of supply of U.S. cigarettes is very high, and the marginal cost function for cigarettes is almost horizontal.

Another key parameter assumption of the model is that demand for U.S. tobacco in the world market is elastic; we use a demand elasticity of −2.5 based on Sumner and Alston (1987), Beghin and Hu (1995), and Rezitis, Brown, and Foster (1998). This means that as the price of U.S. tobacco falls relative to tobacco grown in other countries, U.S. tobacco exports will rise substantially,

TABLE 3.3 Parameters Used in the Simulation Analysis

PARAMETER DEFINITION	VALUE OR RANGE
Elasticity of demand for cigarettes in the United States	−0.24 to −0.30
Elasticity of demand for cigarette exports	−3.0
Elasticity of demand for leaf tobacco exports	−2.5
Elasticity of supply of leaf tobacco	4.0
Share of U.S. leaf tobacco exported	0.49 to 0.42
Share of U.S. cigarettes exported	0.24
Share of U.S. tobacco in cost of production of cigarettes	0.02
Own elasticity of substitution for tobacco used in U.S. cigarettes	2.2
Initial ad valorem equivalent cigarette tax	0.27
Implied demand shift due to tobacco control measures	0.27 to 0.61
Tax increase as a share of initial price	0.54

Source: Author. Simulation model input values based on data and estimates cited and discussed in the text.

offsetting the impact of reductions in demand from U.S. manufacturers. We also note that tobacco imports comprise about half of the tobacco used in a U.S. cigarette, and the model allows for significant substitution between imported and domestic tobacco. Therefore, when the price of U.S. tobacco declines, cigarette manufacturers will use more domestic leaf. The model also allows for increase in cigarette exports (demand elasticity −3.0) when the cost of production declines slightly, but this effect has very small impacts on the leaf tobacco industry. Finally, we use a cigarette demand elasticity between −0.22 and −0.31 over the 20-year horizon, based on a large econometric literature. A few representative early papers in this literature include Lewit, Coate, and Grossman (1981), Baltagi and Levin (1986), and Wasserman et al. (1991). Chaloupka (1991) and Becker, Grossman, and Murphy (1994) applied the theory of rational addition to study cigarette smoking behavior.

SIMULATION RESULTS

Results from the simulation are shown in table 3.4, which displays the impact of tobacco control policy measures on leaf tobacco prices, quantities, and revenues. We begin with a discussion of the IOM scenario results. The first row of table 3.4, taken from the estimates in chapter 2, shows that under this scenario,

TABLE 3.4 Relative Effects of Cigarette Control Scenarios on Leaf Tobacco Prices, Quantities, and Revenues Relative to Status Quo Path of Cigarette Use

ENDOGENOUS VARIABLE	2010	2015	2020	2025
IOM Scenario				
Quantity of cigarettes consumed in the United States	−0.40	−0.44	−0.47	−0.50
Quantity of cigarettes produced in the United States	−0.33	−0.35	−0.37	−0.38
Price of U.S. tobacco	−0.031	−0.040	−0.042	−0.043
Quantity of U.S. tobacco used in U.S. cigarettes	−0.33	−0.35	−0.37	−0.38
Quantity of U.S. tobacco exported	0.11	0.15	0.16	0.17
Total quantity of U.S. tobacco produced	−0.13	−0.16	−0.17	−0.17
Total tobacco revenue	−0.16	−0.20	−0.21	−0.22
Change in producer net returns (producer surplus) (millions)	−$24	−$29	−$29	−$29
High-Impact Scenario				
Quantity of cigarettes consumed in the United States	−0.75	−0.75	−0.76	−0.77
Quantity of cigarettes produced in the United States	−0.60	−0.59	−0.59	−0.59
Price of U.S. tobacco	−0.058	−0.067	−0.067	−0.067
Quantity of U.S. tobacco used in U.S. cigarettes	−0.59	−0.59	−0.58	−0.58
Quantity of U.S. tobacco exported	0.15	0.17	0.17	0.17
Total quantity of U.S. tobacco produced	−0.23	−0.27	−0.27	−0.27
Total tobacco revenue	−0.29	−0.34	−0.34	−0.34
Change in producer net returns (producer surplus) (millions)	−$43	−$46	−$44	−$41

Source: Author, based on simulation model results.

the percentage decline in the quantity of cigarettes consumed in the United States rises from −40 percent in 2010 to −50 percent in 2025 after the various measures have had many years to influence consumption. As the second row shows, we project that U.S. cigarette production would fall by less because exports would expand.

The next set of rows details the implications for tobacco growers. In response to the cigarette demand shocks, the real, inflation-adjusted, price of leaf tobacco is expected to be 3.1 percent lower in 2010 and 4.3 percent lower in 2025 than in the status quo scenario. The quantity of leaf tobacco used by domestic cigarette manufacturers is 33 to 38 percent lower than in the status quo—less than the decline in domestic cigarette consumption because exports of cigarettes are maintained and because more domestic leaf is used per cigarette. In addition, between 11 percent and 17 percent more U.S. leaf is exported as foreign buyers respond to the lower price of U.S. tobacco. The overall quantity of U.S. leaf produced falls between 13 percent and 17 percent. The percentage change in total revenue approximately equals the sum of the percentage changes in price and quantity. Compared with the status quo, farmers' total revenue from tobacco is 16 percent lower in 2010 and 22 percent lower by 2025. This loss in total revenue affects payments to input suppliers, land rent, and compensation for farmer-supplied inputs such as family labor and management. The final row under the IOM scenario shows that the net economic return to producers falls by about $24 million in 2010 and $29 million by 2025. To put these losses in perspective, about 300,000 acres of Burley and flue-cured tobacco were harvested in 2005, so the loss in producer net returns would amount to about $80 per acre in 2010. For a full-time tobacco farm with 100 acres under cultivation, this loss is about $8,000 in net returns.

The bottom panel of table 3.4 considers the effects of the high-impact scenario, under which the U.S. consumption of cigarettes falls by about three-quarters. The impact of this scenario on tobacco prices, quantities, and revenues is more severe, with most of the losses about 50 percent larger than under the IOM scenario. Total revenue losses range from about 29 to 34 percent relative to the status quo scenario. Losses of producer net revenue are in the range of $41 million to about $46 million for all the years considered. In 2010, for a full-time tobacco farm with 100 acres under cultivation, the loss would be about $14,300 in net returns.

LIMITATIONS

We note two limitations of this model. First, it does not account for the likely effects of tobacco taxes on the quality of cigarettes. An excise tax increase, because it taxes each unit by the same amount regardless of the price net of the tax, creates an incentive to increase the quality and thus raise the net revenue per taxable unit. For cigarettes that would imply an incentive to put more and higher-quality tobacco in each cigarette, all else remaining equal. Our analysis does not take this effect into account, and for that reason may overstate the negative effect of a cigarette excise tax on tobacco use. Although this effect is clear in theory, we expect its impact to be relatively small (Sobel and Garrett 1987).

Second, the model does not incorporate imperfect competition by manufacturers. Market power by cigarette companies may affect both the purchase of leaf tobacco and the sale of cigarettes (Ciliberto and Kuminoff 2010; Sullivan 1985; Sumner 1981). Under oligopsony power in the purchase of tobacco—in other words, because the cigarette manufacturers are very large firms with oligopoly power—the price of U.S. leaf tobacco is lower than it would otherwise be, and producers sell less tobacco to U.S. buyers than under a competitive market. The same would be true if there is oligopoly power in the market for cigarettes; that is, the price of leaf tobacco would be lower and the quantity purchased would be smaller because fewer cigarettes would be sold. To our knowledge, researchers have not considered this point in detail. Although market power may have significant implications for the level of prices and quantities, we expect it to have relatively small effects on the impacts of retail tobacco control measures on tobacco producers.

CONCLUSIONS

Tobacco production remains a significant crop industry in parts of the southeastern United States, especially in Kentucky and North Carolina. However, the gradual decline in tobacco production and prices and growth in other industries has diminished the importance of tobacco to farm incomes in these regions. More vigorous tobacco control policies would lead to further decline. Our simulation model, based on the model developed by Sumner and Wohlgenant (1985), projects how two alternative scenarios to reduce cigarette demand would affect leaf tobacco prices, quantities, and revenues. We find that international trade in tobacco and cigarettes is likely to insulate the domestic leaf tobacco industry from the full impact of declining cigarette consumption in the United States. Nonetheless, in the high-impact scenario, if cigarette use fell by about three-quarters, tobacco producer revenue would fall by about one-third.

Projection of the impact of measures to discourage smoking is complicated by the recent termination of the tobacco farm program. For many years the federal tobacco program kept production lower and prices higher than would otherwise have occurred. This policy led manufacturers to reduce the amount of tobacco per cigarette and to substitute imported for domestic leaf in U.S.-made cigarettes. It also reduced leaf tobacco exports. The tobacco quota program raised the costs of operation for tobacco growers by transferring benefits to owners of tobacco quota, most of whom did not produce tobacco themselves. It also kept tobacco production fixed in the locations in which it had been established in the early part of the twentieth century.

The U.S. farm program for tobacco ended with the 2005 crop, but the influence of the program continued to suppress production for a few more years as government-owned stocks were liquidated. The liquidation of government stocks at reduced prices is expected to cost about $5 billion. In 2005 we saw the beginnings of the new era for tobacco as prices declined and production began to consolidate in low-cost regions and on low-cost farms. As compensation for termination of the price support and quota program, tobacco growers and quota owners are receiving about $10 billion over a 10-year period. Quota owners will receive $7.00 per pound of quota owned. This payment compares favorably to the approximately $2.00 per pound that was a typical market price for quota prior to the buyout program. Despite the fact that quota represented a cost rather than a benefit to growers, they too received compensation at the rate of $3.00 per pound of quota used in their operations. This tobacco program buyout, which was financed by tobacco manufacturers, has substantially increased the wealth of tobacco growers and quota owners.

APPENDIX 3.1: DETAILS ON MODELING THE EFFECTS ON THE U.S. LEAF TOBACCO INDUSTRY OF CIGARETTE TAX INCREASES AND OTHER POLICY-INDUCED REDUCTION IN CIGARETTE DEMAND

DERIVATION OF THE MODEL STRUCTURE

The model presented here is designed to simulate the effects of tax changes and shifts in U.S. demand for cigarettes on the U.S. tobacco farm sector and closely follows the model developed by Sumner and Wohlgenant (1985) for a similar purpose. In the model, domestic and foreign markets for cigarettes and tobacco are represented by nine equations in linear, logarithmic differential form. The model maintains the same kinds of simplifying assumptions as used by Sumner and Wohlgenant but is specified using recent values for prices, quantities, and policy in a context in which leaf tobacco marketing quotas are no longer applicable. The variables and parameters of the model are listed and defined in tables 3.5 and 3.6.

The equations developed here use the notation defined there.

TABLE 3.5 Definition of Price and Quantity Variables

SYMBOL	DEFINITION
Q_{cd}	Quantity of cigarettes sold in domestic markets by U.S. manufacturers
P_{cd}	U.S. retail price of cigarettes
Q_{ce}	Quantity of cigarettes sold in foreign markets by U.S. manufacturers
P_{ce}	Export wholesale price of U.S. cigarettes
Q_c	Total U.S. cigarette production
P_{td}	Market price of domestically produced tobacco (weighed average of flue-cured and Burley market prices)
T	Federal tax on cigarettes
δ	Policy-induced reduction in U.S. cigarette demand as a proportion or quantity
Q_{td}	Quantity of U.S. tobacco purchased by U.S. manufacturers
Q_{te}	Quantity of U.S. tobacco exported
Q_t	Total domestic production of tobacco
R_t	Total domestic leaf tobacco revenue $(P_{td})(Q_t)$
ΔS_t	Change in total domestic tobacco producer surplus

First, a demand function for domestic cigarettes relates the quantity of cigarettes consumed domestically, Q_{cd}, to their domestic retail price, P_{cd}, and a demand shift, which represents the effect of policy measures other than taxes on consumer preferences for smoking. This last term is represented by ΔQ_{policy} in the following equation:

$$Q_{cd} = f(P_{cd}) - \Delta Q_{policy} \qquad (1)$$

The policy-induced demand shift ΔQ_{policy} is used to incorporate the results from the SimSmoke simulations of consumption under different policy scenarios in the tobacco-sector model.

Export demands for cigarettes and leaf tobacco can be written in similar general form as:

$$Q_{ce} = f_{ce}(P_{ce}) \qquad (2)$$

$$Q_{te} = f_{td}(P_{td}), \qquad (3)$$

TABLE 3.6 Definition and Values of Share and Elasticities Parameters

SYMBOL	DEFINITION	SOURCE OR COMMENT	VALUE(S)
η_{cd}	Domestic retail price elasticity of demand for cigarettes (absolute value)	SimSmoke (implied from tax effect on quantity consumed)	0.22–0.30
η_{ce}	Export price elasticity of demand for cigarettes (absolute value)	N/A	4.0
η_{te}	U.S. export price elasticity of demand for tobacco (absolute value)	Sumner and Wohlgenant (1985)	2.5
ε	Elasticity of supply of U.S. leaf tobacco with respect to price	Two values are simulated for a long run to check for the sensitivity of the results	2.0 or 4.0
β_{td}	Quantity share of domestic tobacco used by U.S. cigarette manufacturers	Economic Research Service (2006)	0.51–0.58
β_{cd}	Quantity share of U.S. cigarette sold in the domestic market	Capehart (2005a)	0.76
α_{td}	Domestic tobacco share of domestic wholesale cigarette costs	Other costs include imported tobacco and other inputs	0.02
σ_{dd}	Own-elasticity of substitution for domestic tobacco	Includes especially substitution with imported tobacco	2.2
α_T	Tax share of domestic cigarette cost	Capehart (2005a) (average pack price = $3.715)	0.27

along with the domestic supply of leaf tobacco

$$Q_t = h_{td}(P_{td}). \tag{4}$$

In these equations, Q_{ce} and P_{ce} are the quantity and price of U.S. cigarette exports, Q_{te} and P_{td} are the quantity and price of U.S. leaf tobacco exports, and Q_t and P_{td} are the U.S. production and market price of domestically produced tobacco. These equations do not include policy shifters because the only policy effects in the model are the change in cigarette tax at retail, which is incorporated explicitly in our model, and the effects of other policy instruments such as information campaigns on domestic demand for cigarettes, represented by ΔQ_{policy} with values taken from the SimSmoke simulations.

In addition to these four explicit supply and demand function equations, three equations describe the behavior of cigarette manufacturers and traders. First, we assume competitive behavior by cigarette manufacturers. This assumption, combined with assumptions about the cigarette manufacturing process, implies the following market-clearing condition:

$$P_{cd} = P_{td} + T + P_{\text{other inputs}} \tag{5}$$

where T is the tax per unit of cigarettes sold domestically, and $P_{\text{other inputs}}$ is the price of inputs other than tobacco used to make cigarettes. The prices in this expression are given in dollars per unit of cigarette output, defined by the proportions of tobacco and other inputs in one unit of cigarette output. To account for the tax that applies to the domestic cigarette market but not to the export market we can write:

$$P_{ce} = P_{cd} - T = P_{td} + P_{\text{other inputs}} \tag{6}$$

This last behavioral equation implies that in equilibrium, no opportunities remain for profitable arbitrage between the domestic and export markets for U.S. cigarettes.

Further, we assume cost-minimizing behavior by cigarette manufacturers. A convenient way to represent the behavior of the cigarette manufacturers, and to link the markets for cigarettes and tobacco, is to use the tobacco demand function that stems from the minimization of costs to produce level Q_c of output. This implicit tobacco factor demand is a function of input prices and the output quantity:

$$Q_{td} = g(P_{td}, P_{\text{other inputs}}, Q_c) \tag{7}$$

We assume a perfectly elastic supply of inputs other than tobacco used for cigarette production and thus have an exogenous fixed price, $P_{\text{other inputs}}$.

Finally, the model is closed by a quantity market-clearing condition: for both cigarettes and tobacco, the quantities demanded in foreign and domestic markets add up to the quantity produced, which implies:

$$Q_c = Q_{cd} + Q_{ce} \tag{8}$$

$$Q_t = Q_{td} + Q_{te} \tag{9}$$

To use the model to evaluate policy effects, we transform its nine equations into expressions with proportional changes in prices and quantities as a function of exogenous policy shifts and elasticities. First, totally differentiating equation 1 yields:

$$dQ_{cd} = (\partial f/\partial P_{cd})dP_{cd} - d(\Delta Q_{policy}). \tag{10}$$

Then, dividing throughout by Q_{cd} and gathering terms in a demand elasticity η_{cd} (in absolute magnitude form) yields an expression in which the proportional change in quantity demanded is a function of proportional changes in the price and an exogenous policy-induced proportional demand shift:

$$EQ_{cd} = -\eta_{cd} EP_{cd} - \delta \tag{11}$$

where $E(x)$ is the proportional change operator or logarithmic differential $(E(x) = dx/x \approx d\ln x)$ and δ represents the reduction in demand expressed as a proportion of the initial quantity. Because we are comparing alternative policy scenarios against a no-policy base, ΔQ_{policy} is actually the entire demand shift due to the policy, and thus, $\delta = \Delta Q_{policy}/Q_c$. Further, since the effective supply of U.S. cigarettes is highly elastic (given a very small cost share of tobacco and perfectly elastic supply of other inputs in equation 5, a 100δ percent reduction in demand will imply, approximately, a 100δ percent reduction in quantity demanded. Thus, the SimSmoke simulations of market-equilibrium changes in cigarette consumption quantities can be used as estimates of ΔQ_{policy} and thus of δ.

The other eight equations can be differentiated in the same way to obtain their counterparts in proportional change terms. For all of the equations except 7, we omit these derivation steps here because they follow exactly what is done above for equation 1. Export demands for tobacco and cigarettes expressed in logarithmic differential terms are derived from equations 2 and 3 and are given by:

$$EQ_{ce} = -\eta_{cc} EP_{cc} \tag{12}$$

$$EQ_{te} = -\eta_{te} EP_{td} \tag{13}$$

The domestic supply for tobacco is:

$$EQ_t = \varepsilon EP_{td} \tag{14}$$

Assuming that other input prices are constant in equation 5, changes in the domestic price of cigarettes reflect changes in tobacco price (weighted by its share in the cost share of cigarettes, $\alpha_{td} = P_{td}/P_{cd}$) and changes in tax represented by ET (weighted by the share of taxes in the cost of cigarettes, $\alpha_T = T/P_{cd}$). Therefore,

$$EP_{cd} = \alpha_{td} \, EP_{td} + \alpha_T \, ET \tag{15}$$

A tax change affects the relation between domestic and foreign prices, since only domestic sales are taxed:

$$EP_{ce} = \alpha_{td} \, EP_{td} = (EP_{cd} - \alpha_T \, ET)/(1 - \alpha_T). \tag{16}$$

The quantity market-clearing conditions can be expressed using the shares of domestic tobacco and cigarettes:

$$EQ_c = \beta_{cd} \, EQ_{cd} + (1 - \beta_{cd}) \, EQ_{ce} \tag{17}$$

$$EQ_t = \beta_{td} \, EQ_{td} + (1 - \beta_{td}) \, EQ_{te} \tag{18}$$

To express equation 6 in proportional change terms requires some additional assumptions. First, as noted, we have assumed that inputs other than tobacco are supplied perfectly elastically to the cigarette industry, such that the prices of other inputs are exogenous and fixed. Differentiating equation 6 yields therefore:

$$dQ_{td} = (\partial g/\partial P_{td})dP_{cd} + (\partial g/\partial Q_c)dQ_c. \tag{19}$$

Thus, the proportional changes in quantities of domestic tobacco used can be divided in a substitution term and a scale term:

$$EQ_{td} = -\alpha_{td} \, \sigma_{dd} \, EP_{td} + \varepsilon_{scale}.EQ_c \tag{20}$$

where σ_{dd} is the absolute value of the own elasticity of substitution for tobacco used in the production of cigarettes, and ε_{scale} is the elasticity of demand for domestic tobacco with respect to changes in the scale of cigarette output. Both terms warrant some further explanation. The term $-\alpha_{td} \, \sigma_{dd}$ is equal to the Hicksian or output constant own-price elasticity of demand for domestic tobacco by cigarette manufacturers (i.e., $\eta_{dd}^H = -\alpha_{td} \, \sigma_{dd}$). Given the homogeneity condition, we can define $-\alpha_{td} \, \sigma_{dd} = -(1 - \alpha_{td})\sigma_{do}$, where $\sigma_{do} > 0$ is the elasticity of substitution between domestic tobacco and all other inputs used in cigarette manufacturing. We assume $\varepsilon_{scale} = 1$, as implied by constant returns to scale at the industry level, which is consistent with the assumption of competitive behavior among cigarette manufacturers. Thus:

$$EQ_{td} = -\alpha_{td} \, \sigma_{dd} \, EP_{td} + EQ_c. \tag{21}$$

These nine linear equations in proportional change terms relate our nine variables of interest to the exogenous changes in demand and taxes, using some baseline prices and quantities (and thus shares) and elasticities of supply and demand, and we can solve for the effects of interest using linear algebra methods. Once the changes in prices and quantities have been simulated, the corresponding changes in tobacco industry revenue can be calculated as the sum of proportional changes in price and quantity:

$$ER_t = E(P_{td} Q_t) = EP_{td} + EQ_t \tag{22}$$

The net effect on producers may be represented as the change in producer surplus (expressed in dollars, not percentage changes). Assuming approximately linear supply over the range of the simulated changes, the change in producer surplus is equal to:

$$\Delta S_t = (Q_t^0 + Q_t^f)/2 * dP_{td} = Q_t^0\, P_{dt}^0 (1 + 0.5\, EQ_t)\, EP_{dt} \tag{23}$$

where the superscripts represent the values before and after demand and tax shocks (0 for initial, f for final).

PARAMETER VALUES

The next step in the simulation is to determine reasonable values for the parameters used in the equations above. The period of simulation runs from 2010 to 2025, and to each simulated point corresponds a set of parameter values, which are listed in table 3.6 along with their sources. Some parameters are inherent characteristics of the cigarette industry and are held constant. Others are specific to the scenario simulated.

Our simulations for 2010 to 2025 of the tobacco industry use results of consumption of cigarettes under different scenarios from SimSmoke. The projected quantities in millions of packs are presented in table 3.7. The simulations for cigarette consumption give quantities consumed under a status quo situation, a $2 per pack tax only situation, and a $2 tax implemented along with campaigns aimed at reducing cigarette consumption in the United States. These are referred to as the IOM scenario and the high-impact scenario. The difference between the quantities consumed in the status quo scenario and the $2 tax allows us to calculate an implied demand elasticity η_{cd}, whereas the comparison with the projection where campaigns are implemented provides the estimate of the implied demand function shift. The demand elasticity implied by these projections is consistent with elasticities used by Sumner and Wohlgenant (1985), which are based on previous literature, and with the more recent econometric evidence.

TABLE 3.7 Total Consumption (Both Genders, Ages 18 and Above Only) from SimSmoke Simulations (millions of packs)

	2010	2015	2020	2025
Status quo	18,909.77	18,270.98	17,458.65	16,770.19
$2.00 tax increase	16,460.84	15,666.46	14,765.37	14,002.8
IOM recommendation: All w/$2.00	11,417.6	10,248.99	9,184.092	8,356.127
High-impact case $2.00	4,669.118	4,481.062	4,121.85	3,815.4

Source: Author. Simulation model input values based on data and estimates cited and discussed in the text.

TABLE 3.8 Common Simulation Parameters

PARAMETER	2010	2015	2020	2025
η_{cd}	0.24	0.26	0.28	0.30
η_{ce}	4.0	4.0	4.0	4.0
η_{te}	2.5	2.5	2.5	2.5
β_{td}	0.51	0.582	0.582	0.582
β_{cd}	0.76	0.76	0.76	0.76
α_{td}	0.02	0.02	0.02	0.02
σ_{dd}	2.2	2.2	2.2	2.2
α_{T}	0.27	0.27	0.27	0.27

Note: Parameters common to all simulations.
Source: Author, based on simulation model results.

The quantity share of domestic tobacco used by U.S. cigarette manufacturers, β_{td}, changes over time using projections on imports and exports from USDA Agricultural Baseline Projection Tables 2006. Whenever data were available for flue-cured and Burley tobacco separately, a quantity-share weighted average was used. For the estimated changes in producer surplus and total revenue, initial prices and quantities for domestic tobacco were derived from the SimSmoke cigarette quantities. Details on parameters are presented in table 3.8.

TABLE 3.9 Simulation Results Under Alternative Supply Elasticities and Scenarios

	2010	2015	2020	2025
	Simulations for $\varepsilon = 2$			
Demand shift α in IOM scenario (relative decrease of consumption)	0.27	0.30	0.32	0.34
EQ_{cd}	−0.395	−0.438	−0.473	−0.501
EQ_{ce}	0.005	0.007	0.007	0.007
EQ_c	−0.326	−0.348	−0.366	−0.379
EP_{cd}	0.537	0.537	0.536	0.536
EP_{ce}	−0.001	−0.001	−0.001	−0.001
EP_{td}	−0.051	−0.066	−0.069	−0.071
EQ_{td}	−0.324	−0.345	−0.363	−0.375
EQ_{te}	0.128	0.165	0.173	0.179
EQ_t	−0.102	−0.132	−0.138	−0.143
Q_{c_0} (million packs)	18,909.77	18,270.98	17,458.65	16,770.19
Q_{t_0} (million lbs)	539	521	497	478
P_{t_0} ($/lb)	1.54	1.53	1.51	1.50
Revenue_0 ($ million)	827	785	734	691
ERevenue (proportion)	−0.153	−0.198	−0.207	−0.214
ΔSurplus ($ million)	−40	−48	−47	−46
Demand shift α in high-impact scenario (relative decrease of consumption)	0.62	0.61	0.61	0.61
EQ_{cd}	−0.752	−0.754	−0.763	−0.771
EQ_{ce}	0.01	0.012	0.012	0.012
EQ_c	−0.596	−0.587	−0.585	−0.583
EP_{cd}	0.536	0.536	0.536	0.536
EP_{ce}	−0.002	−0.003	−0.003	−0.003
EP_{td}	−0.093	−0.111	−0.11	−0.11
EQ_{td}	−0.592	−0.582	−0.58	−0.578

TABLE 3.9 *(Continued)*

	2010	2015	2020	2025
EQ_{te}	0.234	0.278	0.277	0.276
EQ_t	−0.187	−0.222	−0.221	−0.221
Q_{c_0} (million packs)	18,909.77	18,270.98	17,458.65	16,770.19
Q_{t_0} (million lbs)	539	521	498	478
P_{t_0} ($/lb)	1.54	1.53	1.51	1.50
Revenue_0 ($ million)	827	786	734	691
ERevenue (proportion)	−0.28	−0.333	−0.331	−0.331
ΔSurplus ($ million)	−70	−78	−72	−68
	Simulations for $\varepsilon = 4$			
Demand shift α in IOM scenario (relative decrease of consumption)	0.27	0.30	0.32	0.34
EQ_{cd}	−0.395	−0.438	−0.473	−0.501
EQ_{ce}	0.003	0.004	0.004	0.004
EQ_c	−0.327	−0.349	−0.367	−0.379
EP_{cd}	0.537	0.537	0.537	0.537
EP_{ce}	0	−0.001	−0.001	−0.001
EP_{td}	−0.031	−0.04	−0.042	−0.043
EQ_{td}	−0.325	−0.347	−0.365	−0.378
EQ_{te}	0.079	0.1	0.105	0.109
EQ_t	−0.127	−0.16	−0.168	−0.174
Q_{c_0} (million packs)	18,909.77	18,270.98	17,458.65	16,770.19
Q_{t_0} (million lbs)	539	521	497	478
P_{t_0} ($/lbs)	1.54	1.53	1.51	1.50
Revenue_0 ($ million)	831	796	753	716
ERevenue (proportion)	−0.158	−0.2	−0.21	−0.217
ΔSurplus ($ million)	−24	−29	−29	−28
Demand shift α in high-impact scenario (relative decrease of consumption)	0.62	0.61	0.61	0.61

TABLE 3.9 *(Continued)*

	2010	2015	2020	2025
EQ_{cd}	−0.752	−0.754	−0.763	−0.771
EQ_{ce}	0.006	0.007	0.007	0.007
EQ_c	−0.597	−0.588	−0.586	−0.585
EP_{cd}	0.537	0.537	0.537	0.537
EP_{ce}	−0.001	−0.001	−0.001	−0.001
EP_{td}	−0.058	−0.067	−0.067	−0.067
EQ_{td}	−0.594	−0.585	−0.583	−0.582
EQ_{te}	0.145	0.168	0.168	0.167
EQ_t	−0.232	−0.27	−0.269	−0.268
Q_{c_0} (million packs)	18,909.77	18,270.98	17,458.65	16,770.19
Q_{t_0} (million lbs)	539	521	498	478
P_{t_0} ($/lb)	1.54	1.53	1.51	1.50
Revenue_0 ($ million)	832	797	753	716
ERevenue (proportion)	−0.29	−0.337	−0.336	−0.335
ΔSurplus ($ million)	−43	−16	44	41

Source: Author, based on simulation model results.

SUMMARY OF RESULTS

Table 3.9 shows changes in prices and quantities as well as changes in domestic tobacco revenue and surplus from an additional $2 per pack tax plus two alternative anti-tobacco campaigns. The simulations for each campaign scenario are shown for two values of the long-run price elasticity of domestic tobacco supply (2.0 and 4.0). In the text we present the results for the supply elasticity of 4.0, which is more consistent with a long-run adjustment in quantity supplied.

4

FALLING CONSUMPTION AND WORKER DISPLACEMENT IN THE CIGARETTE MANUFACTURING INDUSTRY

JAVIER ESPINOSA AND WILLIAM N. EVANS

Domestic cigarette consumption peaked in 1981 at 640 billion cigarettes per year, but since that time consumption has fallen by more than 40 percent. Not surprisingly, employment of production workers in the cigarette manufacturing industry has fallen by more than 55 percent over the same period. A large part of the drop in employment in this sector is due to falling consumption of cigarettes, but that is not the entire story. Rising labor productivity, changing export markets, and the changing cost of labor have also altered the demand for workers in this industry.

In this chapter we estimate the impact of declining domestic cigarette consumption on the employment of production workers in cigarette manufacturing. Combining these estimates with projections about the future path of exports, wages, and worker productivity, we simulate the number of production workers employed by cigarette manufacturers through the year 2025 under alternative policy scenarios. Our simulations suggest that adoption of the Institute of Medicine's (IOM) recommended tobacco control policies, which would lower domestic cigarette consumption by 36 percent by 2010, would reduce employment of production workers by roughly 3,600 workers—about 29 percent of the baseline employment we would expect under status quo policy conditions. In the high-impact scenario, in which cigarette consumption is cut by 74 percent within five years, we estimate that by 2010, employment of production workers in the cigarette industry would fall by over 7,500 workers, or roughly 60 percent of baseline employment.

We also examine the impact of job displacement on production workers in the cigarette manufacturing industry. As we show, production workers in cigarette manufacturing are paid very well compared with other manufacturing workers. With statistical controlling for characteristics such as age and education, workers in this industry earn 41 percent more per week than the average production worker in manufacturing. Because the earnings loss from displacement tends to be larger for workers in high-wage industries, workers displaced from cigarette manufacturing are likely to have a larger earnings loss than the average displaced worker. We estimate the impact of displacement for production workers in high-earnings manufacturing industries. In this group of displaced workers, we find that 17 percent are still unemployed 3 years after losing their jobs. Among those who have found employment, weekly earnings are 24 percent lower than before displacement.

The first section of this chapter discusses trends in cigarette manufacturing employment and models the relationship between cigarette consumption and manufacturing employment. The second section presents results of our simulation of manufacturing employment through 2005 under alternative policy scenarios, and the third discusses the impacts on displaced workers.

CIGARETTE CONSUMPTION AND MANUFACTURING EMPLOYMENT

In this section we examine the relationship between cigarette consumption and cigarette manufacturing employment. This section highlights key factors determining the level of employment in this industry and provides some background information to motivate the econometric and simulation models we construct below. Data are drawn from the Bureau of Labor Statistics Current Employment Statistics (CES) survey, a monthly survey of payroll records for over 160,000 businesses. The industry classification system used in the CES survey changed recently, making it impossible to present consistent trend data for tobacco manufacturing after 2000. In addition, the new system groups tobacco-processing plants with cigarette manufacturing. Whenever possible, therefore, we examine data using the older Standard Industrial Classification (SIC) system.

Figure 4.1 presents trends in average monthly employment of production and nonproduction workers in the cigarette manufacturing sector from 1970 through 2002.[1] Employment of production workers peaked in 1976 and has fallen almost every year since then except during the late 1970s and early 1980s. By 2002 employment had fallen by a total of 52 percent, to 16,600. The time series for nonproduction workers such as managers and administrative staff followed a different pattern: the number of nonproduction employees rose between 1973 and 1985 and then fell until 1994, when employment levels stabilized. Compared

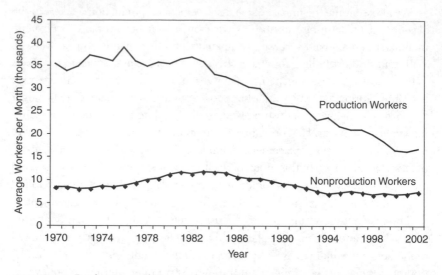

FIGURE 4.1 Production and Nonproduction Workers in Cigarette Manufacturing

Source: Bureau of Labor Statistics, Current Employment Statistics, www.bls.gov/ces/.

with the change in production employment, the change in nonproduction employment was far less dramatic, with the 2002 levels only 7 percent lower than in 1973. Over this time the fraction of all cigarette manufacturing employees who were production workers fell from 82 to 69 percent.

Trends in domestic cigarette production were driven both by domestic consumption and by the export market. Consumption of cigarettes in the U.S. has been declining since 1981, but until recently the growth in the export market offset the decline in domestic consumption. In figure 4.2 we present trends in domestic production, domestic consumption, and nondomestic consumption between 1970 and 2005. Nondomestic consumption includes exports, changes in inventories, and shipments to Puerto Rico and other U.S. territories. In the later years almost all nondomestic consumption has been exports.[2] The fraction of cigarettes that are exported has changed considerably over time. Between 1971 and 1996 the number of U.S.-made cigarettes that were exported increased from 21 billion to over 268 billion per year. Recently, however, the size of the export market has dropped sharply, with exports falling 62 percent between 1996 and 2005. According to Thomas Capehart, a tobacco industry analyst at the USDA, this decline in exports is caused by a number of factors including a shift by U.S. manufacturers toward overseas production, poor economic performance in some Asian countries that had been heavy consumers of U.S. cigarettes, and declining consumption of cigarettes in European countries.[3]

Because the domestic cigarette industry produces for export as well as for the domestic market, the economic impact of a drop in domestic demand is affected

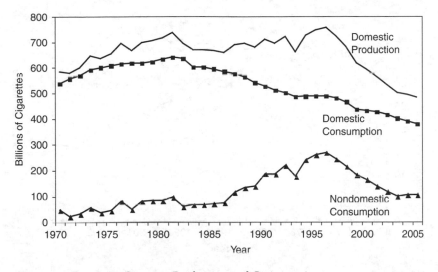

FIGURE 4.2 Domestic Cigarette Production and Consumption

Source: Capehart (2005).

by the size of the export market. For example, suppose that labor demand fell by 10 percent for every 10 percent drop in production. If all cigarettes produced domestically were consumed within the United States, then a 10 percent reduction in cigarette demand would lead to a 10 percent reduction in production worker employment. In contrast, if the domestic market represented only 75 percent of cigarette production, and the export market remained constant, the same 10 percent reduction in demand would reduce employment by only 7.5 percent. Therefore, our analysis proceeds in two steps. First, we examine the impact of domestic production on employment. Then, we examine how much changes in domestic consumption will alter domestic production.

In figure 4.3 we graph trends in domestic cigarette production and manufacturing employment. The left vertical axis measures average monthly employment of production workers while the right shows annual domestic production. Note that the decline in employment has been steeper than that in production. The number of production workers in cigarette manufacturing has fallen steadily since 1976. In contrast, cigarette production remained at or above 1970 levels until 1996, when it dropped by 30 percent. Between 1976 and 2002 employment of production workers dropped by 55 percent while cigarette production fell by only 17 percent.

One reason employment fell faster than production is rising labor productivity. Data from the Bureau of Labor Statistics indicate that output per worker in manufacturing increased by 74 percent between 1987 and 2004. Cigarette manufacturing experienced similar although less spectacular gains in productivity.

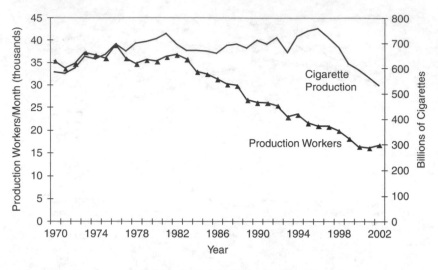

FIGURE 4.3 Employment and Production in Cigarette Manufacturing

Sources: Capehart (2005); Bureau of Labor Statistics, Current Employment Statistics, www.bls.gov/ces/.

Figure 4.4 displays trends in three measures of productivity, all scaled so that the index is equal to 100 in 1987. The first is from the Bureau of Labor Statistics,[4] graphed as a solid line.[5] The other two use cigarette output data from the USDA and employment data from the BLS; one represents output per production worker, and the other is simply output per worker. All three indexes track reasonably well.[6] Between 1987 and 2000, the BLS series indicates that output per worker increased by 51 percent while the constructed output per production worker and output per worker series show 58 and 50 percent increases, respectively. If output had remained constant, the demand for labor would still have fallen by more than 33 percent simply because of productivity gains.

Although employment in cigarette manufacturing has declined, those production workers still employed in the industry are earning higher wages than before. Real (inflation-adjusted) earnings of cigarette manufacturing workers have increased over the last several decades. Figure 4.5 compares the weekly earnings in constant 2004 dollars of production workers in cigarette manufacturing and all manufacturing. For the manufacturing sector as a whole, real earnings have been flat for nearly 30 years. Between 1970 and 2002, weekly earnings for all production rose by only 1.2 percent, while earnings of production workers in cigarette manufacturing have increased 91 percent over the same period, from $655 to $1,252.

To examine wage differences across industries in more detail, we used a sample of workers from the 2000 Census public use microdata samples (www.ipums.org).

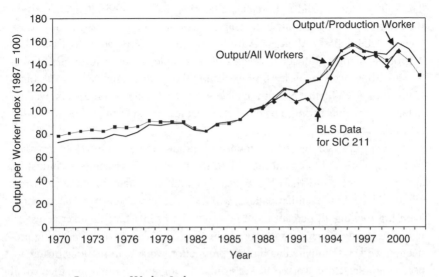

FIGURE 4.4 Output per Worker Indexes

Source: Bureau of Labor Statistics, Productivity and Cost Data, www.bls.gov/lpc/.

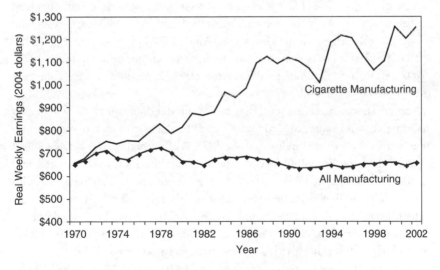

FIGURE 4.5 Real Weekly Earnings of Production Workers

Source: Bureau of Labor Statistics, Current Employment Statistics, www.bls.gov/ces/.

The 2000 Census provides annual labor earnings data for 1999. The table reports the average weekly earnings from employment and the estimated hourly wage, both in 2004 dollars.[7] All averages in the table are constructed using Public Use Microdata Sample individual weights. The sample includes full-time/full-year workers (those working at least 39 weeks in 1999 with a usual work week of 30 hours or more). The first column in table 4.1 presents data for production workers in tobacco manufacturing. The other three columns allow comparison with other categories of workers.

As the numbers in table 4.1 demonstrate, production workers in tobacco manufacturing earned 10 percent more than the typical worker across all industries and 38 percent more than the typical production worker in manufacturing. Hourly wages show a similar pattern, with production workers in tobacco manufacturing making 18 percent more per hour than the average worker across all industries, and 45 percent more per hour than the average manufacturing production worker. Compared with other production workers in manufacturing, tobacco manufacturing workers have a similar demographic profile, and their small educational advantage is not enough to explain such a large gap in earnings.[8]

There are a number of potential reasons why production workers in cigarette manufacturing are paid so well. In cigarette manufacturing, wages have tracked productivity well. Between 1970 and 2000, output per worker in the cigarette industry increased by 93 percent while real weekly earnings over this period increased by 91 percent. The tobacco industry has several characteristics that tend to be associated with higher wages: high profitability (Blanchflower, Oswald, and Sanfey 1996),[9] large firm size (Brown and Medoff 1989; Troske 1999), concentration of production in large firms,[10] and higher rates of unionization. In the 1995–2004 period, among production workers in cigarette manufacturing, 32 percent were covered by unions.[11]

Some simple algebra shows that falling production combined with rising productivity and wages can explain most of the decline in employment of production workers in this industry since 1973. As outlined above, between 1973 and 2002, domestic output in cigarette manufacturing fell by 17 percent, and productivity increased by 50 percent. As a result of these two changes, and with the assumption that cigarette manufacturing has constant returns to scale (i.e., when inputs double, outputs should double as well), employment would be expected to fall by 45 percent.[12] The actual decline in employment over this period was 55 percent. It is likely that cigarette manufacturers responded to the 73 percent increase in wages between 1973 and 2002 by trimming employment. A modest elasticity of demand for labor (the percent decrease in employment for every 1 percent increase in wages) of only −0.14 would explain the remaining decline.

To verify these conjectures we use a simple regression model to examine changes in cigarette manufacturing employment between 1973 and 2002; this

TABLE 4.1 Characteristics of Production Workers in Tobacco Workers Ages 18–64 Years Old, 2000 Census 5-Percent Public Use Microdata Sample

VARIABLE	PRODUCTION WORKERS IN TOBACCO MANUFACTURING	WORKERS IN ALL INDUSTRIES	PRODUCTION WORKERS IN MANUFACTURING	PRODUCTION WORKERS IN HIGH-EARNINGS MANUFACTURING INDUSTRIES
Weekly earnings	$1028.86	$932.59	$743.61	$934.82
Hourly earnings	$24.60	$20.82	$16.94	$20.91
% Male	74.1	58.5	75.2	82.8
Age	44.8	40.1	40.4	41.5
Education				
% <High school	12.9	7.3	17.1	10.0
% High school	49.7	29.6	51.5	50.5
% Some college	28.3	32.5	26.9	33.6
% College	9.1	30.6	4.6	5.9
Race/Ethnicity				
% White, non-Hispanic	63.2	74.9	70.4	76.6
% Black, non-Hispanic	30.4	9.9	11.0	12.2
% Other race, non-Hispanic	2.5	5.7	5.5	3.5
% Hispanic	3.8	9.4	13.1	7.7
% Married	69.6	61.2	62.7	67.4
Observations	784	4,090,495	460,782	114,251

Note: Dollar values are in constant 2004 dollars.
Source: 2000 Census 5-Percent Public Use Microdata Sample.

model is discussed in more detail in appendix 4.1. We regressed cigarette manufacturing production employment on a linear time trend, representing technological progress that raises labor productivity and other factors affecting the demand for labor. We find the demand for labor fell by 2.9 percent per year. The elasticity of demand was −0.15; in other words, demand for labor fell by 0.15 percent for every 1 percent increase in wages—although this parameter was not statistically significant. Results of this regression were used to project employment between 2006 and 2025 under the three tobacco control policy scenarios.

SIMULATING THE CHANGE IN EMPLOYMENT OF PRODUCTION WORKERS OVER TIME

Our next step is to estimate the impact of declining domestic consumption of cigarettes on the demand for production workers in the cigarette manufacturing sector under alternative policy scenarios. Here we use the results from the previous section as well as the SimSmoke estimates of domestic cigarette consumption from chapter 2 to simulate these numbers. This section presents a general discussion of the model; more details are available in appendix 4.1.

Our model estimates labor demand as a function of domestic cigarette consumption. We make several simplifying assumptions. We assume that the rental price of capital will not change, that productivity (output per worker) will continue to grow at 2.8 percent per year, and that real wages will continue to grow at a rate of 2.1 percent per year. These assumptions about the rental price of capital, productivity, and real wages are based on time series that have been relatively smooth over time. Because the demand for domestic production of cigarettes is driven partly by the export market, we must also make assumptions about trends in exports between 2006 and 2025. The time series in exports has been far more uneven, making these projections a more uncertain exercise. For now we assume that exports will fall by 2 percent per year. Later, we show how the results vary if we alter these assumptions about exports as well as other key parameters of the model.

The results of the baseline simulations are presented in table 4.2. In the first row of the table we present the SimSmoke model predictions for the consumption of cigarettes in millions of packs under the status quo or current policy conditions. In the next row is our estimate of the employment of production workers in cigarette manufacturing under this scenario. Between 2005 and 2025, SimSmoke predicts that annual domestic consumption will fall by 13.5 percent, from 19.4 billion to 16.8 billion packs, and we estimate that employment of production workers will fall by 55.5 percent, from 15,161 to 6,753 workers. The three factors driving the fall in demand for labor are increases in labor productivity, increases in the real wage of labor, and declining demand for cigarettes.

TABLE 4.2 Simulated Impact of Falling Demand for Cigarettes on Employment of Production Workers in Cigarette Manufacturing Through 2025

				YEAR		
VARIABLE	**2002**	**2005**	**2010**	**2015**	**2020**	**2025**
	Baseline Estimates					
(1) Domestic consumption[a]	20,003	19,377	18,910	18,271	17,459	16,770
(2) Production workers	16,625	15,161	12,490	10,216	8,286	6,753
			IOM Scenario			
(3) Domestic consumption[a]	20,003	19,377	11,418	10,249	9,184	8,356
(4) Δ in domestic cons. from (1)	0	0	-7,492	-8,022	-8,275	-8,414
(5) % Δ in domestic cons. from (1)	0%	0%	-39.6%	-43.9%	-47.4%	-50.2%
(6) Employed production workers	16,625	15,161	8,526	6,576	5,067	3,946
(7) Δ in employment from (2)	0	0	-3,964	-3,640	-3,220	-2,808
(8) % Δ in employment from (2)	0%	0%	-31.7%	-35.6%	-38.9%	-41.6%
			High-Impact Scenario			
(9) Domestic consumption[a]	20,003	15,377	4,669	4,481	4,122	3,815

TABLE 4.2 (Continued)

VARIABLE	YEAR					
	2002	2005	2010	2015	2020	2025
(10) Δ in domestic cons. from (1)	0	0	−14,241	−13,790	−13,337	−12,955
(11) % Δ in domestic cons. from (1)	0%	0%	−75.3%	−75.5%	−76.4%	−77.3%
(12) Employed production workers	16,626	15,161	4,955	3,959	3,097	2,430
(13) Δ in employment from (2)	0	0	−7,535	−6,257	−5,190	−4,323
(14) % Δ in employment from (2)	0%	0%	−60.3%	−61.2%	−62.6%	−64.0%

[a] Domestic consumption is measured in millions of packs.
Source: Authors; calculations; Bureau of Labor Statistics, Current Employment Statistics; U.S. Department of Agriculture, *Tobacco Situation and Outlook Yearbook* (annual).

In the middle third of the table we report the SimSmoke projections for total cigarette consumption if the IOM's recommendations for tobacco control policies are adopted. Row 3 shows the projected consumption of cigarettes, and rows 4 and 5 show the absolute and percent difference in consumption between the status quo and IOM scenarios. In row 6 we report our predictions for the demand for production workers under this scenario. In lines 7 and 8 we report the predicted drop in employment and the percentage change from baseline levels, respectively. Notice that by 2010, SimSmoke predicts that adopting the IOM's recommendations will reduce baseline cigarette consumption from 19,377 million packs to 11,418 million packs, a 40 percent reduction. Under this scenario, employment of production workers would be lower by 3,964, a drop of 32 percent. By 2025, SimSmoke estimates that adopting the IOM recommendations would reduce domestic consumption of cigarettes by 50 percent; we estimate that the number of jobs lost would be smaller but would represent a larger share—41.6 percent—of the baseline workforce. The actual number of workers displaced is smaller in 2025 than in 2010 because increases in labor productivity and real wages are expected to drive down baseline employment between 2010 and 2025, outweighing the further decline in cigarette consumption over that time.

In the final block of results we simulate the high-impact scenario outlined earlier. In this scenario, the SimSmoke model assumes that prevalence is cut in half, there is no initiation until age 18, and quit rates for those under 40 years of age double. Under the high-impact scenario, cigarette consumption is projected to fall by 75 percent by year 2010 and 77 percent by year 2025. In row 12 our model predicts that by 2010, employment of production workers would fall by 7,535, about 60 percent of baseline employment (row 13). By 2025, job loss due to tobacco control policy would be only 4,323 workers because baseline employment is expected to have fallen by that time as a result of increases in labor productivity and real wages. The policy-induced job loss represents 64 percent of predicted baseline employment in that year.

In table 4.3 we report the sensitivity of our simulation results through 2010 when we change a number of key assumptions in our analysis. For comparison, column 1 repeats results from table 4.2. In column 2 we reduce the annual growth rates of real wages and productivity to 1 and 1.5 percent, respectively. These estimates are lower than historical averages but may be more in line with more recent time periods. Given the way we structured the model, altering these parameters impacts the baseline and policy-produced employment totals in proportional values; therefore, changing these numbers will not alter our estimate of the percentage of workers displaced. However, if we assume slower growth rates for wages and productivity, our estimate of the number of people displaced because of the IOM policies rises by 483 workers (column 2). The

TABLE 4.3 Sensitivity of Simulation Estimates in 2010 to Model Parameters

VARIABLE	RESULTS FROM TABLE 4.2 (1)	WAGES GROW AT 1%, PRODUCTION AT 1.5% (2)	EXPORTS GROW AT 2% (3)	ELASTICITY OF LABOR DEMAND IS −0.56 (4)	ASSUMPTIONS IN COLUMNS 2, 3, AND 4
(1) Production workers	12,490	14,010	13,040	11,667	14,157
			IOM Scenario		
(2) Employed production workers	8,526	9,563	9,076	7,964	9,854
(3) Δ in employment from (1)	−3,964	−4,447	−3,964	−3,703	−4,303
(4) %Δ in employment from (1)	−31.7%	−31.7%	−30.4%	−31.7%	−30.4%
			High-Impact Scenario		
(5) Employed production workers	4,955	5,558	5,505	4,629	5,977
(6) Δ in employment from (1)	−7,535	−8,452	−7,535	−7,038	−8,180
(7) %Δ in employment from (1)	−60.3%	−60.3%	−57.8%	−60.3%	−57.8%

Source: Authors' calculations.

numbers are higher because wages and productivity grow at lower rates; as a result, baseline employment does not drop as quickly.

We also consider the sensitivity of our results to assumptions about cigarette exports. As noted earlier, it is difficult to project exports based on previous trends. Unlike productivity and wages, which increased continuously between 1970 and 2002, exports varied widely over this period; thus it is more difficult to predict whether exports will increase or decrease over the next 20 years. In the baseline simulations we assumed exports will fall at 2 percent per year. In column 3 of table 4.3 we assume the opposite and allow exports to grow at 2 percent per year. Changing the growth rate of exports does not alter the predicted number of workers displaced due to tobacco control policies, but it does alter the estimated percentage of workers displaced. As column 3 shows, if exports grew rather than declined, a slightly smaller percentage of workers would be displaced.

Our estimated elasticity of demand for labor is small (−0.15), but this value is estimated with a great deal of imprecision. In column 4 we use an elasticity of −0.56, which is at the lower end of a 95 percent confidence interval; this more negative elasticity means that employment falls more as wages rise. Altering the elasticity of demand alters the predicted number of workers displaced but not the fraction of workers displaced. A large increase in the elasticity of demand reduces the estimated number of workers displaced under the IOM scenario by only 261 workers.

In columns 2 to 4 we change key assumptions one at a time. In column 5 we change all three key assumptions at once. In this case the predicted change in baseline employment is slightly higher than the original estimates shown in column 1, and the estimated fraction displaced falls by only 1.3 percentage points. Rows 5–7 of table 4.3 carry out the same exercise for the high-impact scenario. The findings are similar. Changing our assumptions about trends in wages and productivity, cigarette exports, or the effect of wage increases on the demand for labor has little effect on our projections of either the number or the proportion of workers displaced as a result of changing tobacco control policies.

THE EMPLOYMENT AND WAGE LOSS ASSOCIATED WITH DISPLACEMENT

In the previous section we estimated the number of production workers who would be displaced from their jobs in cigarette manufacturing under different policy scenarios. In this portion of the chapter we provide some evidence about the costs associated with displacement for these workers.

A number of authors have estimated the wage and employment costs of job displacement. Although these studies vary in design and data, the results suggest that the displacements due to demand shocks can be severe and long-lived. For example, using data from unemployment insurance systems in different states, Jacobson, Lalonde, and Sullivan (1993) find that workers who lose their jobs to a mass layoff are earning 25 percent less per quarter six years after displacement. Stevens (1997), using data from the Panel Study of Income Dynamics (PSID) and restricting her attention to displaced workers who were able to find work, finds that income falls by 30 percent the year of displacement and is still almost 10 percent lower six or more years after displacement. Using data from the PSID from an earlier period, Ruhm (1991) finds that three years after displacement, wages of the reemployed are 16 percent lower than they would have been otherwise. Finally, Farber (2005), using data from the 2004 Displaced Worker Survey (DWS) supplement to the Current Population Survey (CPS), finds that 35 percent of workers displaced within the previous three years were not employed at the time of the survey, and those displaced workers who did find employment were earning 17 percent less than they would otherwise have earned in the absence of displacement.

The economic impact on cigarette manufacturing workers may be more severe than these studies suggest, however. Production workers in cigarette manufacturing are among the highest-paid workers in the manufacturing sector, and previous research shows that the economic costs of displacement tend to be greater for high-wage workers. For example, Jacobson, Lalonde, and Sullivan (1993) found that the earnings losses of displacement are greater for workers displaced from union jobs, from larger establishments, and from high-wage industries such as mining, construction, primary metals, and transportation. To estimate the costs of displacement for workers in cigarette manufacturing, therefore, we use a sample of high-earnings production workers.

The data we use for this section are from periodic DWS supplements to the CPS. The CPS is a monthly survey of 60,000 households and roughly 180,000 adults, and the survey is designed to provide data on key labor market indicators such as the monthly unemployment rate. The DWS has been fielded every two years since 1984 in either January or February. For recently displaced workers the survey includes current labor market status as well as questions about the job from which they were displaced, including industry and occupation, wages, timing of displacement, and the reason for job loss. These data have been used in the past by authors such as Kletzer (1993), Card (1997), and Farber (2001, 2005) to examine the impact of displacement. To provide large enough sample sizes and at the same time generate results that are relevant for today's workers in cigarette manufacturing, we restrict our attention to the DWS supplements from 1996, 1998, 2000, 2002, and 2004. These surveys asked respondents about jobs lost in the past three years.

The five DWS supplements used for this analysis include 5,000 to 7,000 respondents per survey who were displaced within the previous three years. Given the small size of the cigarette manufacturing industry, it is no surprise that only four respondents across the five surveys were displaced from this industry. To generate estimates of displacement for high-earnings production workers, we used a sample of displaced production workers who work in other high-earnings manufacturing industries as a proxy sample. Our procedure for identifying these high-earnings workers is detailed in appendix 4.1.

The high-earnings industries are listed in table 4.4. There are few surprises here: the industries include petroleum refining, aerospace products, chemicals, pulp and paper, aircraft and motor vehicles, and, of course, tobacco

TABLE 4.4 High-Earnings Manufacturing Industries Among Full-Time/Full-Year Production Workers Aged 18–64, 2000 Census 5-Percent Public Use Microdata Sample

RANK	INDUSTRY NAME	DIFFERENCE BETWEEN AVERAGE RESIDUAL LOG EARNING IN THE INDUSTRY AND THE AVERAGE LOG EARNINGS FOR MANUFACTURING
1	Petroleum refining	48.1
2	Tobacco manufacturing	41.9
3	Aerospace products and parts	35.9
4	Industrial and misc. chemicals	34.8
5	Pulp, paper, and paperboard mills	34.1
6	Aircraft and parts	33.1
7	Motor vehicles and motor vehicle equipment	30.6
8	Pharmaceuticals and medicine	29.2
9	Iron and steel mills and steel products	28.1
10	Tires	28.1
11	Engines, turbines, and power transmission equipment	23.6
12	Resin, synthetic rubber, and fibers and filaments	23.4
13	Beverages	22.7
14	Construction, mining, and oil field machinery	21.9
15	Aluminum production and processing	21.9

Source: 2000 Census 5-Percent Public Use Microdata Sample.

manufacturing. In the table we also report the difference between the industry effect and the average log earnings in manufacturing—roughly equivalent to the percentage difference in earnings. After adjustment for demographic characteristics, for instance, workers in petroleum refining earn roughly 48 percent more than the average worker. Workers in tobacco manufacturing have the second highest difference, with weekly earnings that are almost 42 percent higher than the average.[13] Table 4.1, discussed in the first section of this chapter, shows that production workers from high-earnings manufacturing industries earn roughly 26 percent more per week than the average production worker in manufacturing but 10 percent less than a typical production worker in tobacco manufacturing.

THE PROBABILITY OF REEMPLOYMENT AFTER DISPLACEMENT

Using this pooled DWS sample, we estimate the fraction of workers who remain unemployed three years after displacement. We use Farber's (2005) definition of displacement. The numerator in the fraction displaced includes those who report losing a job in the past three years because of a plant closing, insufficient work, their position being abolished, or some other reason.[14] Those at risk of being displaced (in other words, the denominator) include those with a job at the time of the survey as well as those displaced in the previous three years.

In the first two rows of table 4.5 we report the number at risk of being displaced and the fraction displaced over the past three years for four different samples: all workers, workers in manufacturing, production workers in manufacturing, and production workers from high-wage manufacturing industries. Displacement rates were slightly higher for production workers than for all manufacturing workers and 2.6 percentage points higher than for the entire economy. In contrast, the risk of displacement was much lower for production workers in high-earnings manufacturing industries.

In the middle portion of the table we estimate the fraction of workers still unemployed one, two, and three years after displacement. Although displacement rates are very different across the samples, there is little difference in the fraction still unemployed. Among production workers in high-earnings industries, nearly 60 percent of workers were unemployed one year after displacement. This number fell to 23 percent two years after displacement and to nearly 18 percent three years after displacement. In the final sample there are only 127 displaced workers from high-earnings industries, so these estimates are less precise than estimates for the larger samples of other workers.

The DWS also asked displaced respondents whether they have health insurance. Because nearly all workers currently employed in high-earnings manufacturing industries have health insurance, any change in insurance status for workers displaced from those industries is likely due to displacement. Here, too,

TABLE 4.5 Frequency of Displacement and Unemployment After Displacement for Various Samples

	ALL WORKERS	MANUFACTURING WORKERS	PRODUCTION WORKERS IN MANUFACTURING	PRODUCTION WORKERS IN HIGH-WAGE MANUFACTURING INDUSTRIES
Observations (n)	213,654	36,084	20,875	4,242
% displaced in previous 3 years	0.064 (0.0005)	0.083 (0.0014)	0.090 (0.0020)	0.030 (0.0026)
% still unemployed	0.365 (0.0042)	0.440 (0.0091)	0.467 (0.0116)	0.614 (0.042)
1 year after	0.598 (0.0070)	0.585 (0.0134)	0.603 (0.0163)	0.594 (0.0526)
2 years after	0.225 (0.0059)	0.225 (0.0114)	0.227 (0.0140)	0.230 (0.0451)
3 years after	0.177 (0.0054)	0.191 (0.0107)	0.170 (0.0125)	0.176 (0.0408)
% displaced without health insurance	0.375 (0.0042)	0.342 (0.0087)	0.417 (0.0114)	0.486 (0.0433)
1 year after	0.554 (0.0071)	0.553 (0.0156)	0.559 (0.0178)	0.527 (0.0619)
2 years after	0.261 (0.0063)	0.251 (0.0136)	0.250 (0.0155)	0.279 (0.056)
3 years after	0.185 (0.0055)	0.196 (0.0124)	0.191 (0.0141)	0.194 (0.0490)

Note: Standard errors are in parentheses.
Source: Pooled CPS Displaced Worker Surveys from 1996, 1998, 2000, 2002, and 2004.

the numbers are similar across the different categories of workers. More than half lacked health insurance a year after displacement, and almost 20 percent still lacked health insurance three years after displacement.

If the recent experience of high-earnings displaced workers is a reasonable basis for projecting outcomes for cigarette manufacturing workers, we would expect that 17.6 percent of production workers displaced from the cigarette man-ufacturing industry would still be unemployed three years after displacement.

EARNINGS LOSS AMONG REEMPLOYED DISPLACED WORKERS

We also used the DWS samples to examine the impact of job loss on earnings among displaced workers who find employment. In this analysis, we used the difference-in-difference model outlined in Farber (2005). In this model the treat-ment group includes displaced workers who are reemployed within three years af-ter displacement. Because we measure weekly earnings before (period 0) and after (period 1) displacement, we could simply generate an estimate of how displace-ment impacts earnings directly. This comparison of earnings before and after dis-placement, however, would understate the economic impact of job loss because earnings usually rise over time for workers who remain in their jobs. To estimate earnings loss we construct a comparison sample of workers who were not dis-placed over the previous three years. Details of this procedure are in appendix 4.1.

Table 4.6 shows our estimates of the change in earnings over three years for displaced workers (row 1) and nondisplaced workers (row 2); row 3 pres-ents estimates of the total earnings loss from job displacement. The first column in table 4.6 shows results for all full-time workers. In this sample we estimate that displaced workers earned 14.8 percent less as a result of their displacement. Most of this difference is because of a fall in earnings after reem-ployment (9.7 percentage points), but a little over a third of the loss (5.1 per-centage points) is related to the fact that wages for the comparison group rose over time. If the displaced workers had remained employed, their wages are likely to have risen as well. Columns 2 and 3 show estimates of the impact of displacement for all manufacturing workers and for production workers in manufacturing. In these samples, the estimates of earnings loss are larger than in the all-workers sample, and this difference was entirely due to earnings change after displacement.

Column 4 reports estimates of the earnings loss associated with displacement for production workers in high-earnings manufacturing industries such as to-bacco. As expected, the estimated earnings loss is much larger for these workers. For full-time workers displaced in the previous three years, weekly earnings of those reemployed are estimated to be nearly 24 percent lower than they otherwise

TABLE 4.6 Estimated Impact of Displacement on Wage Rates of the Reemployed

MEASURE	ALL WORKERS	MANUFACTURING WORKERS	PRODUCTION WORKERS IN MANUFACTURING	PRODUCTION WORKERS IN HIGH-WAGE MANUFACTURING INDUSTRIES
Change in earnings for displaced workers	−0.097 (0.0067)	−0.134 (0.0126)	−0.120 (0.0152)	−0.200 (0.0394)
Change in earnings for nondisplaced workers	0.051 (0.0027)	0.045 (0.0058)	0.049 (0.0069)	0.039 (0.016)
Estimated earnings loss due to displacement	−0.148 (0.0079)	−0.179 (0.0154)	−0.169 (0.0186)	−0.239 (0.0442)

Note: Standard errors are in parentheses.
Source: Pooled CPS Displaced Worker Surveys.

would have been. In this case, 3.9 percentage points of the decline is because real wages would have risen had the workers stayed employed, and 20 percentage points of the decline is due to the drop in earnings after displacement.

Combining these results with those in table 4.2, we can estimate the lost earnings expected among production workers in cigarette manufacturing due to more vigorous tobacco control policies. If the reemployment and earnings patterns of displaced cigarette manufacturing workers match those of high-wage industries more generally, we expect that 17.6 percent of those displaced will still be unemployed three years after displacement. Those who find work can expect to earn 23.9 percent less. Taking into account both unemployment and the drop in wage rates among those reemployed, the earnings of workers displaced from cigarette manufacturing are likely to be 37.3 percent lower over-all. Adopting the IOM's recommended tobacco control policies would reduce employment by 29 percent over baseline estimates. If we assume that these workers were displaced in the same year and that the earnings of those not displaced did not change, then this reduction in employment would reduce aggregate labor earnings by 10.8 percent (0.373×0.291) compared to the baseline under status quo conditions. This is admittedly an oversimplification—we would not anticipate that all workers would be laid off immediately. However, this calculation illustrates the magnitude of the potential income loss associated with reduced demand for cigarettes.

JOB TURNOVER AND DISPLACEMENT IN
CIGARETTE MANUFACTURING

In this section we consider whether the decline in cigarette manufacturing employment could be accommodated through normal turnover. If a displaced worker leaves the labor market to retire, return to school, or take care of children, he or she would not be counted as unemployed. Movement out of the labor force is not uncommon among displaced workers. We estimate that roughly 16 percent of production workers displaced from high-wage industries exit the labor market. For workers who do so, wage and salary income would obviously fall to zero, but they would not be considered unemployed in the numbers in table 4.5.

Some of the job loss in the cigarette industry generated by policy-induced changes in demand considered above could be absorbed by the normal attrition. Suppose a firm normally has 100 workers and loses 5 each month to turnover. Because of a drop in demand for its products, the firm is forced to reduce the size of the permanent workforce by 10 workers. The firm can reach the desired workforce size by laying off 10 workers, not hiring workers over the next two months, or a combination of the two.

Job turnover is common in the U.S. economy. Shimer (2005) estimates that between 2000 and 2004, almost 5.8 percent of workers left their jobs in any given month, with roughly 1 percent quitting to take another job, 1.8 percent becoming unemployed, and another 3 percent leaving the labor force.[15] Using data from the monthly CPS for the same period, we can estimate job turnover rates in the tobacco industry.[16] On average, 1.2 percent of cigarette production workers become unemployed each month, another 0.9 percent leave the labor force, and 1.7 percent shift from cigarette manufacturing to another industry.[17] Although we cannot determine how much of this turnover is normal and how much represents layoffs due to declining demand, it is clear that cigarette manufacturing employees overall have a relatively low turnover rate: 3.8 percent per month compared with 5.8 percent for the economy as a whole. Thus, the cigarette industry is less able than most industries to deal with declining demand through normal turnover.

It is also unlikely that reduction in employment could be achieved through retirement of older workers. Although cigarette manufacturing workers are five years older, on average, than other workers, analysis of the DWS survey indicates that most people displaced from high-wage industries are not elderly workers: only 12 percent of production workers displaced from high-wage industries were aged 55 and above, and 51 percent of displaced workers were aged 41 and below. In addition, although production workers in cigarette manufacturing are older on average than the typical worker, few are near retirement age. In the 2000 Census, only 4.3 percent of full-time/full-year production workers in cigarette manufacturing were aged 60 and above.

CONCLUSION

Adoption of the IOM's recommended tobacco control policies is projected to reduce domestic consumption of cigarettes 40 percent by 2010 and 50 percent by 2025 over baseline levels. Although exports are a large portion of the current business, most of the cigarettes produced in this country are destined for the domestic market; thus, the export market, which has continued to weaken, can buffer only some of this loss. We project that adoption of the IOM's recommendations would lead to the displacement of 3,964 workers by 2010 and 2,808 workers by 2025. These figures represent 32 and 42 percent of those we estimate would be employed in the absence of these policy changes. The corresponding figures for the high-impact scenario are 7,535 workers in 2010 and 4,323 workers in 2025.

The decline in cigarette consumption caused by anti-smoking policies would clearly be a blow to workers in the cigarette manufacturing industry. Given the high wages in this industry, workers would find it difficult to replace their current income in another sector of the economy. In recent years, 17.6 percent of workers displaced from high-earnings manufacturing industries were still unemployed three years after displacement. For those who do find employment, weekly earnings after displacement were almost 24 percent lower on average. Therefore, average earnings of those displaced would be about 37 percent lower three years after displacement.

It is important to keep in mind, however, that the number of workers affected would be small. In 2002 there were only about 16,600 production workers in the industry. As the later chapter by Ribisl, Evans, and Feighery (chapter 6) shows, more people are employed selling cigarettes in specialized tobacco shops than are employed in U.S. factories manufacturing cigarettes for the entire domestic and export market. In addition, even under the status quo scenario—in the absence of further changes in tobacco control policy—productivity growth and declines in sales would still reduce employment in the industry by more than half, an estimated 8,408 workers in 20 years. In tobacco manufacturing it is relatively simple to identify workers impacted by tobacco control policies—more so than in retail, advertising, or other sectors that might be affected by a drop in cigarette consumption. In manufacturing, some of the economic dislocation generated by tobacco control policies could be mitigated through industry-specific worker retraining and/or extended jobless benefits.

This chapter did not consider the impact plant closings might have on the local community. As noted above, cigarette manufacturing plants are larger than most manufacturing establishments and are concentrated in a few states. Data from the 2000 Census indicate that most production workers in cigarette manufacturing live in North Carolina and Virginia. The diversification of these states' economies over the past several decades may help protect the local communities from the loss of cigarette manufacturing jobs. Although these two states have strong historic ties to tobacco production and cigarette manufacturing, production workers in cigarette manufacturing are now less than 0.5 percent of all full-time/full-year workers in these two states. The next chapter examines tobacco-dependent communities in more detail.

APPENDIX 4.1

DATA SOURCES

Time-series data on employment, hours, and earnings of production workers are available for detailed industries and the nation as a whole from the Bureau of Labor Statistics (BLS) as part of their CES survey, which is a monthly survey of payroll records for over 160,000 businesses representing 400,000 establishments. Data on total number of workers, production workers, weekly earnings, as well as other variables, are downloadable from the BLS Web site.[18] Current data are reported by industries using the National American Industry Classification System (NAICS), which replaced the Standard Industrial Classification (SIC) system in 2000. Unfortunately, the data using NAICS codes go back only a few years. More importantly, the publicly available data only provide information for NAICS industry 3122, which is defined as Tobacco Manufacturing. Although the majority of workers in this industry are in cigarette manufacturing, this larger industry grouping does contain data for workers outside the scope of this chapter. However, archived monthly data through March 2003 are available for SIC industry code 2110, which is defined as Cigarette Manufacturing Plants. Subsequently, when possible, we examine CES data reported by SIC rather than NAICS codes.

Data on domestic cigarette production are available from the United States Department of Agriculture's (USDA) Economic Research Service as part of its annual *Tobacco Situation and Outlook Yearbook*.[19] The data report annual production, taxable removals from warehouses, exports, and shipments to U.S. territories. The *Yearbook* uses the taxable removals and data on inventory changes to estimate annual domestic consumption.

MODELING THE DEMAND FOR LABOR

We used a simple regression model to estimate the relationship between cigarette consumption and the demand for labor over the period between 1973 and 2002. A cost-minimizing firm is interested in producing a given quantity of output (Q) at the lowest possible cost. For simplicity, assume manufacturers have two inputs, capital (K) and labor (L), and real per-unit prices of these inputs are given as r and W, respectively. Given the desired level of output, the firms have a demand for factor inputs that is conditional on output and input prices. Assume that the conditional factor demand for production workers in the cigarette manufacturing industry can be approximated by the following model:

$$\ln(L_t) = \beta_0 + \beta_1 \ln(W_t) + \beta_2 \ln(r_t) + \beta_3 \ln(Q_t) + \beta_4 TIME_t + \varepsilon_t \tag{1}$$

where observations are annual aggregates, time is a linear time trend, and ε_t is an autocorrelated error. We include the time trend to capture technological progress, which impacts labor productivity; that is, holding all else constant, we would expect the demand for labor to have declined as firms became more efficient over time.[20] We expect the coefficient on β_1 to be negative, reflecting downward sloping demand for labor,[21] and β_2 can be either positive or negative, depending on whether capital and labor are substitutes or complements, respectively. The coefficient β_3 indicates the scale of production. If β_3 is less than 1, equal to 1, or greater than 1, the production technology is decreasing returns to scale, constant returns to scale, or increasing returns to scale, respectively.

We estimate equation 1 using annual data from the 1970 through 2002 period. Data on L, Q, and W were introduced above. We obtained unpublished data on the nominal rental prices for all capital assets for the tobacco manufacturing sector from the BLS over the 1970–2002 period.[22] We constructed a real rental price (in 2004 dollars) by dividing by the producer price index.

Estimates of equation 1 that allow for first-order autocorrelation in the errors are reported below. The asymptotic standard errors are reported in parentheses below the parameter values.

$$\ln(L_t) = 0.938 - 0.147 \ln(W_t) - 0.098 \ln(r_t) + 0.967 \ln(Q_t) - 0.029 \ TIME_t$$
$$(1.315) \qquad (0.206) \qquad\quad (0.053) \qquad\quad (0.201) \qquad\quad (0.005) \qquad (2)$$

The R^2 from this regression is 0.953, and we estimate the first-order autocorrelation coefficient (standard error) to be 0.472 (0.170). In this regression, the output-constant elasticity of demand for labor is −0.15, but the coefficient is statistically insignificant. The negative coefficient on the real rental price for capital suggests that capital and production workers are complements in the production process, but again, this estimate is statistically insignificant. If other factors are held constant, the model predicts that demand should fall by a statistically significant 2.9 percent per year due to persistent factors such as technological progress. Finally, the coefficient on log output is a statistically significant 0.97, and we cannot reject the null hypothesis that the parameter is equal to 1. The proximity of the coefficient to 1 suggests that the production technology in cigarette manufacturing exhibits constant returns to scale.

SIMULATING THE CHANGE IN CIGARETTE MANUFACTURING EMPLOYMENT

We used the following model in our simulation of employment change in cigarette manufacturing. Let L_t be the demand for production workers in cigarette
manufacturing at some point in some year in the future t. A labor demand curve
that corresponds to equation 2 above is

$$L_t = \alpha \, \theta_t \, W_t^{\beta_1} r_t^{\beta_2} Q_t^{\beta_3} \tag{3}$$

where α is a constant, θ_t is some measure of technological progress, and β_1 is the
elasticity of labor demand. We began our simulations in 2002, the last year for
which we have measured values of all inputs. The ratio of labor in year t to the
baseline year is therefore

$$L_t/L_{02} = (\theta_t/\theta_{02})(W_t/W_{02})^{\beta_1}(r_t/r_{02})^{\beta_2}(Q_t/Q_{02})^{\beta_3} \tag{4}$$

For simplicity, we assume that real rental prices for capital will not increase in the
future, and therefore r_t/r_{02} is assumed to equal 1. Given the estimates from equa-
tion 2 above, $\beta_3 = 1$. The ratios W_t/W_{02}, Q_t/Q_{02}, and θ_t/θ_{02} are indexes that equal 1
in 2002 and can rise or fall over time. A value of W_t/W_{02} that equals 1.5 means that
real wages have rise by 50 percent by year t over 2002 values. Let the first two indexes be represented by w_t and q_t, respectively. We capture the productivity index
as one over an output per worker index γ_t. If we substitute these values into equation 4 and solve for L_t, the demand for production workers in year t is therefore

$$L_t = L_{02}[w_t^{\beta_1}][q_t]/\gamma_t \tag{5}$$

Given the actual value of employment in 2002, the estimated elasticity of
labor demand from equation 2, plus assumed growth rates in wages, output,
and productivity after 2002, we can then predict what labor demand will be in
year t.[23] The basic structure of this model allows for simulations that are easy to
construct. Holding all else equal, if output increases by 20 percent, labor demand will increase by 20 percent as well. Likewise, if output per worker increases by 50 percent, then labor demand will fall by a factor of 1/1.5, which is
33 percent, holding all else constant.

During the 20 years ending in 2002, output per worker increased at an annual
average rate of 2.8 percent per year, and real wages increased at a rate of 2.1 percent per year. Therefore, w_t is estimated to equal $(1.021)^t$, and productivity in
year t equals $(1.028)^t$.[24] We also begin by assuming the elasticity of demand for
production workers (β_1) equals -0.15.

Production in any given year is destined for either domestic consumption (C_t) or nondomestic consumption, which we refer to as exports (X_t). The results from the SimSmoke model provided us with estimates of C_t, but to calculate q_t, we must know the future value of exports. Let x_t represent an index that measures the growth in exports compared to the base year 2002. In any given year the production index q_t would then equal $q_t = [C_t + X_{02}x_t]/Q_{02}$; so we must make assumptions about the annual growth rate of exports. Unlike the time series for productivity and wages, which have been relatively smooth over time, exports increased rapidly in the early 1990s and fell just as quickly after 1996. As a first pass we assumed that exports will fall by 2 percent per year.[25]

IDENTIFYING HIGH-EARNINGS INDUSTRIES

To choose these industries, we use the following regression-based procedure. Using data on 18- to 64-year-old full-time/full-year production workers from the 2000 Census 5-Percent Public Use Microdata Sample, we estimate a standard human-capital earnings function of the form

$$\ln(W_{ij}) = X_{ij}\beta + \mu_j + \varepsilon_{ij} \tag{6}$$

where W_{ij} is weekly earnings for worker i in industry j, X is a vector of individual characteristics, μ_j is a complete set of industry fixed effects, and ε_{ij} is an idiosyncratic error. The individual characteristics included in X are a complete set of dummy variables for age, education, marital status, and four race/ethnicity variables.[26] The industry fixed effects represent persistent differences in earnings across workers within an industry conditional on X, so we select workers based on estimates of $\hat{\mu}_j$. Ordering $\hat{\mu}_j$ from highest to lowest, we take as our proxy sample production workers from the industries with the largest industry effects that represent 25 percent of all production workers in manufacturing. We refer to this sample as production workers from high-earnings industries.

MEASURING EARNINGS LOSS AMONG REEMPLOYED DISPLACED WORKERS

Because we measure weekly earnings before (period 0) and after (period 1) displacement, we can generate an estimate of how displacement impacts earnings directly. We label this value Δ_t. This value, however, understates the true value of earnings loss because, in most cases, earnings would have risen in the absence of displacement. To estimate this value, labeled Δ_c, we constructed a comparison sample and produced estimates of the real wage changes that occurred in the absence of displacement. The difference-in-difference of the earnings loss of displacement after reemployment is therefore $\Delta\Delta = \Delta_t - \Delta_c$.

Constructing the comparison sample was not straightforward. For the postdisplacement period, Farber selects all full-time workers surveyed at the time of the DWS who were not displaced in the previous three years but answered questions about weekly earnings as part of the Outgoing Rotation Group (ORG) for that month.[27] For the comparison sample in the predisplacement period, Farber selects a random sample of full-time workers from the Merged ORG in years (MORG) $t-1$, $t-2$, and $t-3$. The MORG contains responses from all people who answer ORG question in a particular year. This sample must be comparable in size to the posttreatment samples of nondisplaced workers, and it must be comparable in distribution to the time when people in the treatment group were displaced. For displaced workers surveyed in year t, let p_{jt} represent the fraction displaced in year j where $j = t-1$, $t-2$, and $t-3$ and note that $p_{t-1,t} + p_{t-2,t} + p_{t-3,t} = 1$. Recognizing that the posttreatment group of nondisplaced workers is roughly one-twelfth the size of a MORG, Farber picks a random sample that represents $p_{jt}/12$ of the original sample in year j.

The difference-in-difference model of Farber (2005) is of the form

$$\ln(W_{is}) = X_{is}\beta + \gamma_1 T_s + \gamma_2 D_i + \gamma_3 T_s D_i + \varepsilon_{is} \tag{6}$$

where W_{is} is the wages observed for individual i in year s (where $s = 1$ for postdisplacement and $s = 0$ for predisplacement), X is a vector of characteristics, T_s is a dummy that equals 1 in the postdisplacement period, and D_i is a dummy that equals 1 if the respondent is part of the treatment sample.

In this model, because we have a synthetic panel of respondents in the comparison group panel rather than a longitudinal data set, our control sample is contaminated in that some of the respondents will eventually be displaced. If θ is the fraction displaced in the entire sample, the difference-in-difference estimates will be too low by a fraction of $1-\theta$, the fraction of workers in the comparison sample who will not be displaced in the next three years. The sum $\Delta_t = \gamma_1 + \gamma_3$ represents the change in earnings over time for workers displaced. Since the comparison sample is contaminated with people who may eventually be displaced, Farber shows that the growth in earnings between the pre- and postdisplacement periods for people not displaced equals $\Delta_c = \gamma_1 - \theta\,\gamma_3(1-\theta)$.[28] Therefore, the difference-in-difference estimate is $\Delta\Delta = \Delta_t - \Delta_c = \gamma_3/(1-\theta)$. If the comparison sample were not contaminated by workers who would eventually be displaced, then the difference-in-difference estimate would equal the coefficient γ_3.

In table 4.7 we report estimates for the four different categories of workers used in the previous table. In the first row, we report the fraction displaced (θ), calculated from table 4.5. Rows 2 and 3 provide parameter estimates for γ_1 and γ_3, from ordinary

TABLE 4.7 Difference-in-Difference Estimates, Impact of Displacement on Wage Rates of the Reemployed, and Pooled CPS Displaced Worker Survey Estimates

PARAMETER	ALL WORKERS	MANUFACTURING WORKERS	PRODUCTION WORKERS IN MANUFACTURING	PRODUCTION WORKERS IN HIGH-WAGE MANUFACTURING INDUSTRIES
θ	0.064 (0.0005)	0.083 (0.0014)	0.090 (0.0020)	0.030 (0.0026)
γ_1	0.039 (0.0028)	0.030 (0.0062)	0.034 (0.0075)	0.032 (0.0168)
γ_3	−0.136 (0.0073)	−0.164 (0.0141)	−0.154 (0.0169)	−0.232 (0.0430)
Δ_t	−0.097 (0.0067)	−0.134 (0.0126)	−0.120 (0.0152)	−0.200 (0.0394)
Δ_c	0.051 (0.0027)	0.045 (0.0058)	0.049 (0.0069)	0.039 (0.016)
$\Delta\Delta$	−0.148 (0.0079)	−0.179 (0.0154)	−0.169 (0.0186)	−0.239 (0.0442)

Note: Standard errors are in parentheses
Source: Pooled CPS Displaced Worker Surveys.

least squares estimates of equation 6. In the final three rows, we report the change in earnings for displaced workers before and after displacement (Δ_t), the average time-series change in earnings of nondisplaced workers over the same period (Δ_c), and the difference-in-difference estimate of the earnings loss due to displacement ($\Delta\Delta$).[29]

NOTES

1. In this figure we calculate a simple average of monthly values within a year.
2. For example, in 2005, domestic production was 481.9 billion pieces, domestic consumption was 378.0 billion, and therefore, nondomestic consumption was 103.9 billion. Only 2.8 billion pieces were shipped to U.S. territories, but 109.2 billion units were exported, with the difference being additions to inventories.
3. http://www.ers.usda.gov/publications/tbs/oct01/tbs250-01/tbs250-01.pdf.
4. ftp://ftp.bls.gov/pub/special.requests/opt/dipts/iprsicdata.txt.
5. Comparable data for cigarette manufacturing are available only from 1987 through 2000.
6. Over the 1987–2000 period the correlation coefficient between the two constructed series is 0.99, while the correlation coefficient between the BLS series and constructed output per production worker and output per work series over the same period are 0.95 and 0.93, respectively.
7. Weekly earnings are constructed by dividing annual earnings reported by weeks worked in the previous year. Hourly wage rates are constructed by dividing weekly earnings by usual hours worked per week. Because of reporting inconsistencies in hours, earnings, or weeks worked, we generate some very high and low values of hourly

wages. We delete the outliers from the sample by dropping observations with the top and bottom 1 percent of hourly wages.

8. Given the availability of multiple race codes in the 2000 Census, we define whites as those reporting white only, blacks as those responding black with any other race.

9. In 2005 Philip Morris reported domestic revenues from cigarette sales of $18.1 billion and operating income of $4.6 billion (http://www.altria.com/AnnualReport/ar2005/2005ar_03_0100.aspx). That same year R. J. Reynolds reported domestic revenues of $8.3 billion, producing $1 billion in operating income (http://www.reynolds american.com/common/ViewDoc.asp?postID=1104&DocType=PDF).

10. www.census.gov/prod/ec02/ec0231i312221t.pdf; www.census.gov/prod/ec02/ec0231sglt .pdf.

11. The information in this paragraph is constructed with data from the Merged Outgoing Rotation Samples of the CPS, a data set discussed in more detail in the final section of the chapter.

12. The demand for workers should fall by a factor equal to $[(1-0.17)/1.5] = 0.55$ or 55 percent of the 1973 levels, which is a 45 percent reduction in labor demand.

13. This difference is slightly larger than the unconditional difference in earnings we calculated in table 4.1. This is no surprise. Although production workers in tobacco manufacturing earn more than the average worker in manufacturing, the average tobacco worker tends to have observed characteristics that are associated with lower earnings, such as a higher fraction of low-educated, women, and nonwhite workers. Once we control for these differences, the difference in earnings conditional on observed characteristics should increase.

14. Farber (2001) notes that because of wording changes in the question that identifies the reason for displacement, the fraction of people citing "some other reason" increased dramatically after 1991. Comparing the time series in this number of time, Farber argues that the true fraction displaced in the post-1991 period for "some other reason" should be discounted by 74.8 percent, which is the procedure we follow here.

15. These data are available at home.uchicago.edu/~shimer/data/flows.

16. We use data for 2000 to 2004 and look at month-to-month transitions in employment status; the data for this period include 388 tobacco industry employees. Respondents in the monthly CPS are in the sample for the same four months in two contiguous years (e.g., April through July of 2001 and 2002). Using data from the January 2000 through December 2004 CPS, we match respondents in one month to the next and follow their employment transitions. This month-to-month matching generates a sample of about 3.5 million transitions over this period, and 388 of these observations are for production workers in the cigarette industry.

17. This procedure will understate job-to-job transitions if the movement is intra-industry. This would be a problem if the movement we need to measure were between two retail establishments, but, given the geographic dispersion of cigarette manufacturing plants and the fact that there are few locations with multiple plants, this should be a good estimate in this case.

18. http://www.bls.gov/ces/home.htm.

19. http://www.ers.usda.gov/publications/so/view.asp?f=specialty/tbs-bb/.

20. Some have suggested that we directly add a measure of productivity (output per work) as a control variable to measure the impact of changing productivity on demand. However, this variable is, by construction, mechanically related to the dependent variable, making the coefficient subject to an omitted variables bias. Although

productivity has not advanced in a linear fashion throughout the entire period, we felt using the linear trend was the lesser of two evils.

21. This model assumes firms are price takers in the labor market; that is, wages are not altered by the number of workers hired by tobacco firms. The growing disparity between wages of production workers in cigarette manufacturing and the rest of the manufacturing sector, however, calls this assumption into question (figure 4.3). To adequately address this issue in a statistical model would require that we use a two-stage least-squares procedure. In this model, we must identify an "instrument" that is correlated with wages but has no direct impact on employment in the sector. We initially thought that wages in other industries, such as malt beverages or soft drinks, could be used in this fashion, but these wage series were not sufficiently correlated with wages in cigarette manufacturing to be used as instruments. Subsequently, we maintain the assumption that wages are exogenous in these models.

22. We thank Larry Rosenblum of the BLS for providing us with these data and answering our numerous questions about the series.

23. For this model we have obviously made a number of simplifying assumptions, such as that there are only two inputs into the production process and that there is no real change in the price of capital. There are, however, a number of assumptions that are not so transparent. For example, we implicitly assume that an exogenous drop in the demand for cigarettes will not alter the time path of wages paid to workers.

24. We attempted using coefficients from regressions with higher-order polynomials to predict wages and productivity over time, but these predictions had unattractive out-of-sample properties. Although the models predicted well within sample (e.g., the models had high R^2s), odd-ordered polynomials tended to predict incredibly low levels of wages and productivity 15 years or more out of sample, and even-numbered polynomials predicted incredibly high values in the late years of the simulations. This is not uncommon when one attempts to make time-series predictions with higher-order polynomials this far out of sample.

25. Our assumption concerning exports is consistent with those of Sumner and Alston in chapter 3. In that chapter, the authors assume that the ratio of exports to total production is a constant 24 percent over time. Therefore, their model assumes exports will fall by 11.4 percent between 2005 and 2025 under the status quo or by 53 percent if the IOM's recommendations are adopted. Our assumption means that exports will fall by 33 percent between 2005 and 2025 in all three scenarios. As we demonstrate later in this section, the results do not change qualitatively when we assume exports rise by a modest amount over time.

26. The four race/ethnicity groups we consider are white non-Hispanics, black non-Hispanics, other race but non-Hispanic, and Hispanics.

27. Respondents in the CPS are interviewed during the same four months (e.g., January through April) in two adjacent years, and one-quarter of the sample exits temporarily or permanently each month. In their fourth and eighth months in the survey, respondents are asked detailed questions about their current job including weekly earnings.

28. Wage growth is γ_1, but the contaminated sample contains a fraction θ of people who will eventually be displaced. Each of these workers will lose $\gamma_3/(1-\theta)$ if displaced, so $\Delta_c = \gamma_1 - \theta \gamma_3(1-\theta)$. Note that if the comparison sample is not contaminated and $\theta = 0$, then $\Delta_c = \gamma_1$.

29. To calculate the standard errors on these final three values, we use the "delta" method and assume that the covariance between θ and the two regression parameters is zero.

5

TOBACCO-DEPENDENT COMMUNITIES AND TOBACCO CONTROL POLICY

KATHRYN M. NECKERMAN AND CHRISTOPHER C. WEISS

A decline in smoking could have its most severe economic impact on the southeastern region of the United States, where domestic tobacco growing and cigarette manufacturing have historically been concentrated. As public health advocates seek to reduce smoking rates, there is concern that stronger tobacco control policies could lead to hardship in economically vulnerable southeastern communities. Although a few case studies have described how communities have changed as tobacco farming has declined (Markley et al. 2001; Stull 2000), we have little systematic information about the economic role of tobacco in the region and thus about the potential economic consequences of efforts to curb tobacco use.

This chapter examines the changing economic role of tobacco in seven southeastern states: Florida, Georgia, Kentucky, North Carolina, South Carolina, Tennessee, and Virginia. We show how tobacco-dependent counties have fared between 1982 and 2002, a time of significant change in the regional economy as well as in tobacco production, and we describe patterns of economic adaptation in counties where tobacco income has declined. Based on this assessment, we consider the economic prospects for tobacco-dependent communities.

Two caveats are important to mention. First, whereas chapters 3 and 4 examined the consequences of tobacco control policy for individual farmers and manufacturing workers, our focus here is on the economic well-being of communities (defined here as counties). The rationale for such an approach is that community-wide economic disruption makes it more difficult for individual tobacco farmers or manufacturing workers to adapt to new economic conditions because a decline in the local economy makes it more difficult to find alternative opportunities and because the loss of local tax revenue may weaken social services. The broader impact of such economic decline is magnified by the fact that tobacco-related farming and manufacturing employment have historically been well paid compared with other opportunities available in the area. Second, although our focus in this chapter is on economic and demographic change, it is important to keep in mind that the decline in tobacco production, like other structural economic changes, might also disrupt the social fabric of a community (Stull 2000). Although such social disruption is beyond the scope of this chapter, it merits attention from those concerned with the future prospects of the region.

TOBACCO FARMING AND MANUFACTURING IN THE SOUTHEAST

Tobacco is grown in a number of U.S. states, and some varieties, such as cigar tobacco, are grown largely outside the Southeast. However, most U.S. tobacco is grown in the Southeast, and two varieties represent most of this production. The first, flue-cured tobacco, is relatively high in sugar; because it is vulnerable to rot, it must be heated while it is cured, In flue-curing, furnace-heated air is piped through the barns where tobacco is "cured," or dried. Flue-curing became widely used after the Civil War; it reduced the risk of fire and produced a milder tasting tobacco (Brandt 2007). Flue-cured tobacco is grown mostly in the coastal southeastern states, with North Carolina the biggest producer. The other variety, Burley tobacco, can be air-cured; it is light in color and absorbs flavors readily. Burley tobacco is grown mostly in Kentucky, Tennessee, and western parts of Virginia and the Carolinas; Burley farms tend to be smaller than farms growing flue-cured tobacco. Between 1938 and 2004, as chapter 3 describes, tobacco was regulated by marketing quotas that were assigned to counties; although quotas could be rented or purchased, in most cases they could not be transferred across county lines. Because of this marketing quota program, which provided price supports, the geographic distribution of tobacco farming was very stable during the years this tobacco program was in effect.

Traditional methods of tobacco cultivation were highly labor intensive, but these methods have changed in recent decades. In flue-cured production, mechanized harvesting and bulk curing (in which leaves are packed in a crate and stacked in a curing barn) became widespread during the 1970s. Equipment for mechanized harvesting of Burley tobacco became available more recently, and its use is not economical on many smaller farms (van Willigen and Eastwood 1998). With increasing mechanization, tobacco farm operations grew larger, with some farmers buying or leasing quota in order to expand their operations while others stopped growing tobacco altogether. This consolidation has occurred particularly in the farming of flue-cured tobacco; in North Carolina, where production of flue-cured tobacco is centered, the number of tobacco farmers dropped by almost three-quarters between 1982 and 2002 (Capehart 2004). The decline in the number of farmers in Burley-growing areas such as Kentucky was not as steep, in part because the production of Burley tobacco has been slower to mechanize.

Between 1982 and 2002, inflation-adjusted tobacco sales in the Southeast fell by more than two-thirds. This decline in tobacco farm income reflects several trends, as the chapter by Sumner and Alston describes. The production of tobacco leaf fell because of a decline in leaf exports, a decline in domestic consumption of cigarettes, and an increase in the use of imported tobacco in U.S. cigarettes; imports of tobacco leaf have increased, with foreign tobacco comprising 38 percent of U.S.-manufactured cigarettes in 1995 and 60 percent in 2004 (Dohlman, Foreman, and Da Pra 2009). In addition, the real (inflation-adjusted) price of tobacco leaf has fallen by a third since the early 1980s. The end of the tobacco program and the rise of contracting are expected to lead to further downward pressure on prices. In the past tobacco was sold at auction, with a minimum price guaranteed by the tobacco program. After the quota program ended, the cigarette manufacturers increasingly contracted directly with growers, bypassing the auction system.

Mass production of cigarettes began in the late nineteenth century with the invention of automated cigarette-rolling machines. The industry quickly became concentrated as entrepreneurs such as the Duke family and R. J. Reynolds bought up smaller manufacturers. In 1890 the five largest firms joined together in the American Tobacco Company, accounting for 90 percent of cigarette sales in the U.S. The Department of Justice brought suit under the Sherman Anti-Trust Act, and in 1911 the "tobacco trust" was divided into four companies, the American Tobacco Company, Liggett & Myers, R. J. Reynolds, and P. Lorillard. These four companies, later joined by Philip Morris and Brown & Williamson, continued to dominate the cigarette market (Brandt 2007). Over the past 15 years the industry has become more concentrated. The American Tobacco Company (under a new name, American Brands) sold its cigarette brands to Brown & Williamson. Liggett & Myers sold its most prominent brands to Philip Morris. R. J. Reynolds and Brown & Williamson merged, forming Reynolds American. In 2008 Philip Morris, Reynolds American, and Lorillard accounted for more than 85 percent of the U.S. market.

Like tobacco farming, U.S. cigarette manufacturing is concentrated in the Southeast. Winston-Salem, North Carolina, and Richmond, Virginia, are well known for cigarette production, but cigarettes have been manufactured in other locations as well. The past several decades have seen a number of changes in the location of cigarette production with the expansion and contraction of business, corporate mergers, and the search for lower production costs. In addition to its Richmond facilities, Philip Morris operated a facility in Louisville, Kentucky, for five decades, shutting it down in 2000. Another Philip Morris plant, in Concord, North Carolina, opened in 1983 and closed in 2009. Brown & Williamson made cigarettes in Petersburg, Virginia, until the company closed that plant in 1985 and shifted operations to Macon, Georgia. Both the Macon factory and an older Louisville plant were shut in 2004 when Brown & Williamson merged with R. J. Reynolds. Although Lorillard bills itself as the oldest cigarette company in the United States, it has made cigarettes in Greensboro only since 1956, when the company moved its operations from Jersey City, New Jersey. The decline and eventual sale of the American Tobacco Company closed factories in Richmond, Virginia and in Durham and Reidsville, North Carolina.

The tobacco manufacturing industry includes stemming and redrying operations as well as cigarette manufacturing. After tobacco leaves are dried in curing barns on the farm, they are sent to stemming and redrying plants where stems are removed and the leaves are sorted and dried to the buyer's specifications. Most such plants are small and located close to the growers. In recent years, ownership of these operations became more concentrated, and some plants were closed, reducing tobacco manufacturing employment in some rural counties.

Tobacco production has been economically important in the Southeast in part because it offered a relatively high and stable income in a region where economic development has lagged behind the rest of the country. For farmers, tobacco provided much higher receipts per acre than they could earn from other agricultural commodities. In the mid-1990s, for instance, the net return (gross value of production minus cash expenses) for tobacco was about $2,000 per acre, compared with $267 for cotton, $174 for corn, and $89 for soybeans (Gale, Foreman, and Capehart 2000). Many cigarette manufacturing workers have union representation (the Bakery, Confectionery, Tobacco Workers and Grain Millers International Union, BCTGM); regardless of their union status, these employees earn higher wages than most other blue-collar workers, as chapter 4 documents. As tobacco declines, these high farm receipts and wages may be difficult to replace without strategic investments in building a new infrastructure that supports production and distribution of new on-farm enterprises. The adjustment is likely to be more difficult in locations where tobacco represents a larger share of local economic activity, including farm counties as well as towns or cities with a concentration of tobacco-related manufacturing jobs.

MEASURING TOBACCO DEPENDENCE

Measures of "tobacco dependence" quantify how much of the local economy is tied to tobacco production. Gale, Foreman, and Capehart (2000) measured tobacco dependence in farm counties with a ratio of tobacco leaf sales to local personal income. In a study of North Carolina counties, Markley et al. (2001) compiled multiple measures of both tobacco farming and manufacturing. Building on their work, we constructed county-level measures of tobacco dependence that take into account both agriculture and manufacturing. Our measures include three components, all measured at the county level: farm income from sales of tobacco leaf, earnings from tobacco manufacturing, and total earnings. As Gale (1999, p. 40) notes, gross sales of tobacco provide a good measure of the role of tobacco in the local economy because "an important share of the expenditures made by farmers stay within the local economy: payments to local hired labor, repair shops, warehouse fees, interest paid to local banks, and rental payments to owners of land or quotas. Although gross receipts overstate the income received by farmers, they may be the best estimate of the amount of tobacco income circulating within a local economy." We used data on gross sales of tobacco leaf collected by the Census of Agriculture, which is conducted in years ending in 2 and 7. For measures of annual earnings from tobacco manufacturing and of total annual earnings, we relied on the Bureau of Economic Analysis Regional Economic Information Service (REIS), which provides annual estimates of earnings at the county level. Both measures come from the CA05 SIC data series; they include earnings by workers and proprietors but exclude other sources of income such as income transfer payments (Social Security) and dividends. (Note that payments to nonresident quota owners cannot be identified in the REIS data; such payments to nonresident owners are unlikely to be sufficiently large and spatially concentrated to make a county tobacco dependent.)

To compare tobacco earnings to total earnings in a county, we constructed a *tobacco dependence ratio,* which equals the sum of tobacco leaf sales and tobacco manufacturing earnings divided by the sum of labor and proprietor earnings in the county. Counties in which that ratio was at least 0.05 were categorized as "tobacco dependent."[1] We also constructed separate measures for tobacco farming and tobacco manufacturing. "Tobacco-farm-dependent" counties were those in which the ratio of tobacco leaf sales to total earnings was at least 0.05. Similarly, "tobacco-manufacturing-dependent" counties were those in which the ratio of tobacco manufacturing earnings to total earnings was at least 0.05. We constructed tobacco dependence measures for 1982, 1987, 1992, 1997, and 2002, corresponding to years in which the Census of Agriculture was conducted. The time period begins at about the peak of cigarette consumption in the United States and ends at a time when cigarette consumption had fallen by about a third. All income and sales figures are expressed in 2002 dollars.

Both total and tobacco manufacturing earnings figures are based on "earnings by place of work"; in other words, they include all labor and proprietor income earned within the county by both residents and nonresidents. REIS industry-specific earnings data are available only by place of work; for consistency, we used the same type of measure for total earnings. In counties with cigarette or other to-bacco manufacturing plants, our tobacco dependence measures are likely to over-state the economic importance of tobacco in the county where the plant is located and understate its importance in nearby counties because some tobacco manufac-turing employees work in one county and live in another. In addition, our tobacco dependence measures are likely to overstate the economic importance of tobacco in counties where many people commute to jobs outside the county; the denomi-nator does not include the earnings of these commuters. This bias is more likely to affect rural counties, where more residents cross county lines to go to work.

We constructed tobacco dependence measures for a total of 692 counties. Virginia has a number of "independent cities" that are not part of any county; we followed the Bureau of Economic Analysis practice of combining smaller inde-pendent cities with neighboring counties. The larger independent cities, such as Richmond, remained separate, and we refer to them as counties in this chapter. Appendix 5.1 discusses our measures in more detail and describes procedures for handling missing data.

TRENDS IN TOBACCO DEPENDENCE

In 1982, 163 southeastern counties—nearly one in four—were classified as to-bacco dependent. Most of these "tobacco counties" were tobacco-farm depen-dent. In Kentucky 55.0 percent of counties were tobacco dependent, and in North Carolina 37.0 percent were; together these two states accounted for nearly two out of three of such counties in the region. As measured by the tobacco dependence ratio, the economic importance of tobacco varied widely. In more than a third of these counties, the dependence ratio was less than 0.10, while a small fraction of counties had ratios of 0.25 or higher. The highest ratio, in Robertson County, Kentucky, was 0.73.

Between 1982 and 2002, tobacco income (including tobacco leaf sales and tobacco manufacturing earnings) in the region's tobacco-dependent counties fell by an average of 67.2 percent (see table 5.1). As figure 5.1 illustrates, the proportion of tobacco-dependent counties fell sharply between 1982 and 2002, from 23.6 percent to 4.2 percent. Because of the tobacco program, the contrac-tion in tobacco farming was distributed more or less evenly; when quotas were reduced, tobacco leaf production dropped everywhere by a similar proportion. Table 5.1 displays the numbers and proportions of tobacco-dependent counties by state in 1982 and 2002. Because tobacco dependence ratios were higher in

TABLE 5.1 Tobacco-Dependent Counties by State, 1982 and 2002

	NUMBER OF TOBACCO-DEPENDENT COUNTIES (PERCENTAGE OF ALL COUNTIES)		MEAN TOBACCO DEPENDENCE RATIO (TOBACCO-DEPENDENT COUNTIES ONLY)		MEAN PERCENTAGE CHANGE IN TOBACCO INCOME (COUNTIES THAT WERE TOBACCO DEPENDENT IN 1982)
	1982	2002	1982	2002	
Southeastern states	163 (23.6%)	29 (4.2%)	.150	.085	−67.2%
Florida	4 (6.0)	0 (0.0)	.086	—	−75.4%
Georgia	24 (15.1)	1 (0.6)	.100	.079	−60.3%
Kentucky	66 (55.0)	17 (14.2)	.189	.088	−71.5%
North Carolina	37 (37.0)	6 (6.0)	.144	.087	−64.7%
South Carolina	6 (13.0)	0 (0.0)	.108	—	−69.5%
Tennessee	14 (14.7)	3 (3.2)	.109	.075	−62.7%
Virginia	12 (11.0)	2 (1.9)	.143	.063	−66.3%

Note: Tobacco income refers to the sum of tobacco leaf sales and tobacco manufacturing earnings. The tobacco dependence ratio is the ratio of tobacco income in a county to the sum of labor and proprietor income earned in that county.
Source: Authors' calculations (see appendix 5.1 for data sources).

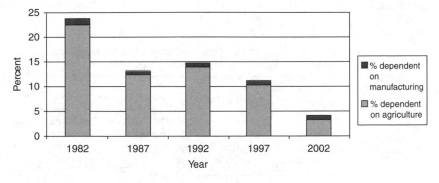

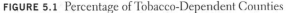

FIGURE 5.1 Percentage of Tobacco-Dependent Counties

Source: Author's calculations (see appendix 5.1 for data sources).

Kentucky than in other states, more Kentucky counties remained classified as tobacco dependent even as tobacco income declined.

Table 5.2 describes changes in the 156 counties that were tobacco-farm dependent in 1982. In general, farming was in decline between 1982 and 2002. The average number of farms per county dropped by about a quarter, and an average of 12,000 acres per county were converted to nonagricultural use. Of the counties that were tobacco-farm dependent in 1982, only 14.7 percent were so classified 20 years later. The proportion of farms growing tobacco fell from 61.6 percent to 29.3 percent, while the mean acreage on farms growing tobacco increased from 8.6 to 16.3. As table 5.2 suggests, changes in farming patterns were more pronounced in the eastern states; in the Burley-growing states of Kentucky and Tennessee, a larger share of farmers continued to grow tobacco, and tobacco farming remained a smaller-scale enterprise.

Between 1982 and 2002, tobacco manufacturing earnings in the region fell by less than a third. Only eight counties in 1982 and five in 2002 were classified as tobacco-manufacturing dependent. Over the two decades, cigarette factories closed in Durham and in Petersburg, Virginia, and opened in Cabarrus County, North Carolina; in addition, small-scale tobacco manufacturing operations declined or closed in Lunenburg County, Virginia, and Stokes County, North Carolina. Four counties—Bibb County (Macon), Georgia, Richmond, Virginia, and Forsythe and Rockingham Counties in North Carolina—remained tobacco-manufacturing dependent throughout the entire period.

Tobacco-dependent counties did not account for all tobacco production in the region. In 1982 more than half of all southeastern counties grew at least some tobacco, and 1 in 12 counties reported some earnings from tobacco-related manufacturing. A county with a large and diversified economy can produce a significant amount of tobacco and still not be classified as tobacco dependent.

TABLE 5.2 Farm Indicators for Counties That Were Tobacco-Farm Dependent in 1982

| | COUNTIES THAT WERE TOBACCO-FARM DEPENDENT IN 1982 | | | | | |
| | TOTAL | | COUNTIES IN KENTUCKY AND TENNESSEE | | COUNTIES IN OTHER SOUTHEASTERN STATES | |
	1982	2002	1982	2002	1982	2002
Mean total number of farms	938.0	711.8	1,055.8	887.4	814.0	526.9
% Counties that were tobacco-farm dependent	100.0	14.7	100.0	23.8	100.0	5.3
% Farms that grew tobacco	61.6	29.3	79.4	38.6	42.9	19.4
Mean tobacco acreage per county	3,819.5	1,919.5	2,843.6	1,301.7	4,846.7	2,596.6
Mean tobacco acreage on farms growing tobacco	8.6	16.3	3.5	4.1	14.4	29.7
Number of counties that were tobacco-farm dependent in 1982	156		80		76	

Note: The tobacco farm dependence ratio is the ratio of tobacco income (the sum of tobacco leaf sales and tobacco manufacturing earnings) in a county to the sum of labor and proprietor income earned in that county. In tobacco-farm-dependent counties, nearly all tobacco income was derived from farming. *Source*: Authors' calculations (see appendix 5.1 for data sources).

For instance, Jefferson County (Louisville), Kentucky, and Guilford County (Greensboro), North Carolina, were both home to cigarette factories, but neither county was tobacco dependent in 1982.

ECONOMIC CHANGE IN TOBACCO-DEPENDENT COUNTIES

To provide an initial look at economic change in tobacco-dependent counties, we compared trends in population and per capita income in counties that were and were not tobacco dependent in 1982 (table 5.3). Because metropolitan areas

TABLE 5.3 Mean Percentage Change in County Population and Per-Capita Income by Tobacco Dependence and Metropolitan Status, 1982–2002

	TOBACCO DEPENDENT IN 1982	NOT TOBACCO DEPENDENT IN 1982
Percentage change in population		
Metropolitan counties	25.8%	58.9%
Counties adjacent to metropolitan areas	27.8%	35.7%
Other nonmetropolitan counties	16.6%	17.3%
Percentage change in per-capita income (inflation-adjusted)		
Metropolitan counties	43.2%	43.9%
Counties adjacent to metropolitan areas	40.7%	44.6%
Other nonmetropolitan counties	41.8%	45.8%

Source: Authors' calculations (see appendix 5.1 for data sources).

grew more rapidly during this time, we reported separate figures for counties that were in metropolitan areas, adjacent to metropolitan areas, and neither in nor adjacent to metropolitan areas. Compared with other counties, tobacco-dependent counties tended to have slower population growth between 1982 and 2002; this difference was most evident among metropolitan counties. Nonmetropolitan tobacco counties tended to have slower growth in per-capita income, although the differences were small. It is important to keep in mind that this slower growth in population and income may not be due to trends in tobacco alone. Economic and demographic trends in these counties are affected by a wide range of factors including the decline in other traditional industries such as textiles and furniture.

The decline in tobacco income did not affect all counties in the same way. The southeastern region is internally very diverse, with some counties better positioned than others to find economic alternatives when an existing industry declines. Factors likely to affect economic change include state government policies and programs, proximity to metropolitan areas, transportation and communication infrastructure, and natural resources such as fertile soil or terrain favorable to agriculture. To explore how tobacco counties fared as tobacco-related income declined in the 1980s and 1990s, we constructed indicators of several kinds of economic development, including a shift to other agricultural commodities, nonfarm employment, and suburban or metropolitan development. We also examined indicators of economic growth and decline. This section briefly discusses the indicators we selected and then describes patterns of economic change in tobacco-dependent counties.

MEASURES OF ECONOMIC CHANGE

CHANGE IN SALES OF AGRICULTURAL COMMODITIES OTHER THAN TOBACCO
In part because of the importance of crop rotation to maintain the productivity of the soil, most tobacco farmers do not grow tobacco exclusively; in the mid-1990s, some 56 percent of Burley farms and 82 percent of flue-cured farms also sold other commodities (Gale, Foreman, and Capehart 2000). As tobacco income has declined, some agricultural extension agencies, with mixed success, have promoted alternatives with a relatively high value per acre, such as fruits and vegetables, industrial hemp, and even ostriches (Reaves 1999). A number of farm counties have shifted from tobacco to poultry and hog production, often in confined animal feeding operations (CAFOs) (Stull 2000). We used data from the Census of Agriculture to compare trends in tobacco leaf sales to sales of other agricultural commodities, including livestock (e.g., hogs, poultry, beef cattle, dairy products, and eggs) and nontobacco crops. We also identified counties in which sales of nontobacco commodities increased enough to offset the decline in tobacco sales.

NONFARM EMPLOYMENT Many farm households supplement farm income with earnings from nonfarm employment. Opportunities for rural nonfarm employment grew over the 1980s and 1990s as some manufacturers relocated their production facilities from the "rustbelt" to the "sunbelt," where labor and other production costs tended to be lower. The auto industry is a prime example; employment in automobile and auto parts manufacturing expanded in the South after 1980. Growth in service-sector employment also helped offset the decline of traditional industries such as mining, textiles, apparel, and furniture. We created two county-level indicators of growth in nonfarm employment. First, using figures from the REIS, we identified counties in which the absolute change in nonfarm employment was larger (more positive) than the absolute change in population between 1982 and 2002. Second, using figures from the 1980 and 2000 U.S. Censuses, we identified counties in which percentage of workers with a commute time of at least 45 minutes increased by more than 5 percentage points; this measure is intended to capture the long commutes to cities or towns that members of farm households may face as they take nonfarm jobs.

SUBURBAN/METROPOLITAN GROWTH Most tobacco is produced in counties that are in or adjacent to metropolitan areas (Gale et al. 2000). During the

1980s and 1990s, metropolitan areas in the Southeast grew rapidly, with sprawl-style suburban development extending into counties adjacent to or near large cities. This new suburban development provided an alternative use for farmland and is likely to have brought new retail and service jobs to the area. To chart the rise of this suburban development, we identified counties that became classified as metropolitan between 1983 and 2003. In addition, we used two alternative measures of suburban growth outside metropolitan areas. First, we identified nonmetropolitan counties that were not adjacent to metropolitan areas in 1983 and became adjacent by 2003. In addition, we defined "new bedroom communities" as counties that were nonmetropolitan in 1983 and 2003 and had above-the-median growth in population, in the proportion of workers with long commutes, and in the decline in farm acreage.

ECONOMIC DECLINE AND INCOME TRANSFERS Some tobacco-dependent counties had relatively few opportunities to replace tobacco income they had lost. Poor soil quality or hilly terrain may have limited the substitution of other farm commodities for tobacco, while low educational levels, inadequate transportation and communications infrastructure, and distance from metropolitan areas may have limited opportunities for nonfarm employment or suburban development. Such counties may have experienced economic decline as income from tobacco fell. To index economic decline, we identified counties where poverty rates increased between 1979 and 1999 (from the 1980 and 2000 decennial censuses) and those where population fell between 1982 and 2002; we also report the average change in inflation-adjusted per-capita income.

Residents of tobacco-dependent counties might offset the loss of tobacco income by turning to public income transfers such as family assistance (e.g., Aid to Families with Dependent Children, now Temporary Assistance for Needy Families); Supplemental Security Income, or SSI (for low-income elderly or disabled persons); food stamps; or unemployment benefits. Studies of Kentucky coal counties found that SSI enrollment increased when energy prices fell and coal mining employment declined (Black, McKinnish, and Sanders 2003); we might expect the decline in tobacco to have similar consequences. Using county-level estimates from the REIS, we calculated the average percentage change in per-capita income transfer receipt between 1982 and 2002.

ECONOMIC CHANGE IN TOBACCO-DEPENDENT COUNTIES

Table 5.4 displays our measures of economic change for counties that were tobacco dependent in 1982. As the first column shows, these counties changed in a variety of ways. On average, sales of other agricultural commodities did not offset the decline in tobacco leaf sales, although one in five counties did experience an increase in other agricultural sales that was larger than the decline in

TABLE 5.4 Measures of Economic Change Between 1982 and 2002, Tobacco-Dependent Counties in 1982, by Subregion

	ALL TOBACCO-DEPENDENT COUNTIES	FLORIDA, GEORGIA, AND SOUTH CAROLINA	NORTH CAROLINA AND VIRGINIA	KENTUCKY AND TENNESSEE
Trends in sales of tobacco and other agricultural commodities				
Mean change in tobacco leaf sales (in thousands)	–$15,440	–$10,535	–$25,314	–$11,477
Mean change in sales of other agricultural commodities (in thousands)	$7,835	–$1,661	$33,004	–$3,545
Percentage of counties with growth in inflation-adjusted total sales of agricultural commodities	19.6%	26.5%	26.5%	12.5%
Off-farm employment				
% Counties with increase in nonfarm jobs relative to population	45.4%	20.6%	46.9%	55.0%
% Counties with an increase in long (> 45 minute) commutes greater than 5 percentage points	33.7%	38.2%	36.7%	30.0%
Suburban and metropolitan growth				
% Counties that were nonmetropolitan in 1983 and became metropolitan by 2003	21.5%	20.6%	24.5%	20.0%

% Counties that were nonmetropolitan and nonadjacent in 1983 and became adjacent to metropolitan areas by 2003	20.2%	20.6%	18.4%	21.2%
% Counties classified as "new bedroom communities"	6.1%	14.7%	6.1%	2.5%
Economic decline				
% Counties with a decline in population	12.9%	2.9%	20.4%	12.5%
% Counties with an increase in the poverty rate, 1979–1999	8.6%	17.6%	6.1%	6.2%
Average percentage change in per capita income	41.6%	38.2%	44.8%	40.1%
Average percentage change in:				
Per-capita family assistance	−15.5%	−19.6%	−14.3%	−14.6%
Per-capita SSI	49.5%	47.1%	55.4%	46.9%
Per-capita food stamps income	−26.6%	−11.9%	−25.0%	−33.7%
Per-capita unemployment benefits	10.2%	27.7%	33.9%	−11.8%

Note: Comparison is between 1982 and 2002 unless otherwise indicated.
Source: Authors' calculations (see appendix 5.1 for data sources).

tobacco sales. In addition, in almost half of tobacco-dependent counties, the number of nonfarm jobs grew more rapidly than the population increased, and about a third had a substantial increase in long commutes, suggesting a growth in off-farm employment. About one in five tobacco-dependent counties became classified as metropolitan, and another one in five became adjacent to metropolitan areas; 6.1 percent were classified as "new bedroom communities." These changes are likely to provide access to a more diverse set of economic opportunities. Paralleling national trends, most tobacco-dependent counties had an increase in per-capita income between 1982 and 2002, but 8.6 percent had an increase in the rate of poverty and 12.9 percent experienced a decline in population. Per-capita income from Aid to Families with Dependent Children (now TANF) declined, as did food stamp receipt. Per-capita unemployment benefits rose slightly, and per-capita SSI income rose more substantially.

There were striking differences within the region in patterns of economic change. We grouped states into the three categories shown in the last three columns of table 5.4. In the southernmost states—Florida, Georgia, and South Carolina—tobacco played only a small role in the economy in 1982 and continued to decline over the next two decades. Of the 34 counties in these states that were tobacco dependent in 1982, only one county remained so in 2002: Bibb County, Georgia, was home to a Brown & Williamson cigarette factory that closed in 2004. For the most part, the tobacco-dependent counties in these three states did not fare well during the 1980s and 1990s. In one out of four counties, the decline in tobacco leaf sales was more than offset by an increase in sales of other crops or livestock, but job growth relative to population was lower than in other parts of the region, and poverty rose in 17.6 percent of the counties.

In North Carolina and Virginia, the tobacco industry remained economically important, but the number of tobacco-dependent counties fell from 49 to 8. Many rural counties replaced tobacco with other crops or livestock. North Carolina in particular is notable for an expansion of hog and poultry production, often in "factory farms" or CAFOs. This increase in factory farming may be due in part to the state's environmental regulations (Kenyon 1994), which were relatively permissive until the extensive flooding associated with Hurricane Floyd in 1999 prompted the state to curb the growth in CAFOs. In addition to growth in livestock farming, there was substantial growth in both states' metropolitan areas, with one out of four tobacco-dependent counties absorbed into a metropolitan area. Although poverty rose in only a few tobacco-dependent counties, receipt of unemployment benefits increased substantially, and one out of five counties lost population, suggesting that residents may have moved away to areas of greater economic opportunity.

In the Burley-growing states of Kentucky and Tennessee, relatively few counties showed an increase in income from livestock or crops other than tobacco; this limited substitution of other farm commodities for tobacco may in some cases reflect hilly terrain or poor soil quality. However, more than half of tobacco-dependent counties had an increase in nonfarm jobs relative to population. Perhaps because of this economic development, tobacco-dependent counties in these two states saw relatively little growth in poverty or unemployment receipt and a decline in per-capita receipt of unemployment benefits.

Although patterns of economic change differed across the region, most tobacco-dependent counties do not appear to have been severely affected by the loss of tobacco income. In part this is because the decline in tobacco production has been relatively gradual and has to some extent been anticipated by tobacco farmers and others involved in tobacco production. But even when tobacco incomes have dropped abruptly—for instance, when a cigarette factory closed—the impact could be relatively modest. In 1984 the Brown & Williamson cigarette factory in Petersburg, Virginia, accounted for 18 percent of personal income in the city. After the plant closed, however, personal income in the city fell by only 5.4 percent (Gale, Foreman, and Capehart 2000). Although an analysis using the IMPLAN regional economic model predicted a 22 percent decline in income, because of the multiplier effect of tobacco production on the local economy, in fact the impact was far more limited.

FUTURE PROSPECTS

In 2002, 29 southeastern counties remained tobacco dependent, most of them in Kentucky. If smoking rates continue to decline, we may expect a further drop in the number of tobacco-dependent counties, particularly if cigarette manufacturers continue to import a large fraction of the tobacco leaf used in production. To project change in tobacco dependence through 2025, we applied estimates from the previous two chapters to our 2002 county-level figures (see appendix 5.1 for details). We used the same three scenarios that were used in the previous chapters: a status quo scenario in which tobacco control policy does not change between 2006 and 2025, compared with the Institute of Medicine (IOM) and high-impact scenarios, which represent successively larger declines in smoking (see chapter 2). Our projections of the number of tobacco-dependent counties differed little across the three scenarios. In 2025 the status quo scenario left five tobacco-dependent counties (Jones County in North Carolina, and Bracken, Nicholas, Owen, and Robertson Counties in Kentucky), whereas under the IOM and high-impact scenarios there were projected to be two (Nicholas and Robertson).

These projections assume that tobacco production will decline at the same rate across all counties. However, the quota buyout is expected to accelerate the consolidation of tobacco growing into a smaller number of large farms, with production shifting to areas with topography conducive to large-scale mechanized farming, particularly for flue-cured tobacco (Gale, Foreman, and Capehart 2000). This could mean a greater decline in tobacco income in Kentucky and Tennessee; in that case, the remaining tobacco-dependent counties might well be located in North Carolina rather than Kentucky. In addition, state agricultural and economic development programs shape patterns of economic change in tobacco-producing counties. For instance, although North Carolina's Tobacco Trust Fund Commission has spent some resources promoting crop diversification, this fund has also provided substantial resources to support new investments in tobacco farming (Jones et al. 2007).

The projected decline in the number of tobacco-dependent counties between 2002 and 2025 is on a much smaller scale than the transition that occurred between 1982 and 2002. As table 5.5 indicates, the number of counties and the size of the population at risk are both much smaller. In addition, compared with tobacco-dependent counties in 1982, the tobacco-dependent counties of 2002 appear less vulnerable; they were less poor, less dependent on tobacco farming or manufacturing, and more likely to be located in or adjacent to metropolitan areas, giving them a wider range of economic alternatives. Finally, as figure 5.2 shows, in 1982 many tobacco-dependent counties were adjacent to other tobacco-dependent counties, making it more difficult to find new opportunities in nearby areas when tobacco income declined. In 2002, by contrast, tobacco-dependent counties were more spatially isolated from other tobacco-dependent counties (see figure 5.3).

In adjusting to changing economic circumstances, tobacco-dependent counties can draw on programs intended to assist tobacco farmers and the regions affected by the decline in tobacco-related income. Between 1999 and 2004, tobacco farmers and quota holders received payments from the National Tobacco

TABLE 5.5 Tobacco-Dependent Counties in 1982 and 2002

COUNTY CHARACTERISTICS	1982	2002
Number of counties	163	29
Total population	4,534,362	1,187,200
Mean tobacco dependence ratio	.150	.085
Mean poverty rate (in 1979/1999)	22.2%	17.6%
% Metropolitan	12.9%	37.9%
% Adjacent to metropolitan area	36.8%	48.3%
% Other nonmetropolitan	50.3%	13.8%

Source: Authors' calculations (see appendix 5.1 for data sources).

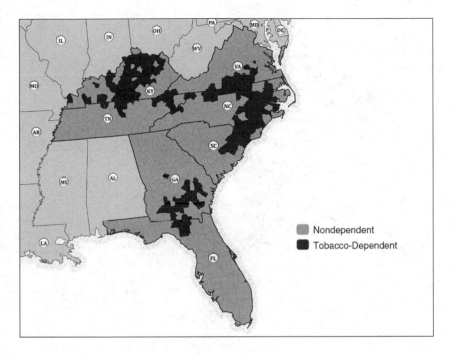

FIGURE 5.2 Tobacco-Dependent Counties, 1982

Source: Map created by James W. Quinn based on authors' calculations.

Growers' Settlement Trust Fund, created by Phase II of the Master Settlement Agreement (MSA) from payments made by the major tobacco companies. In addition, the Tobacco Transition Payment Program (TTPP), established by the Fair and Equitable Tobacco Reform Act of 2004, is making annual transition payments to quota holders and tobacco farmers until 2014. Most tobacco-producing states have used some portion of the MSA funds to support agricultural diversification, vocational education and training, infrastructure improvements, and incentives intended to attract new industry. OneGeorgia Authority has received nearly a third of Georgia's MSA funds, which are spent on economic development in rural counties. Kentucky allocates half of its MSA payments to the state's Agricultural Development Fund. North Carolina's Golden Leaf Foundation usually receives half of the state's MSA funds, spent for economic development; the Tobacco Trust Fund Commission receives one-fourth to promote development in agricultural areas. In Virginia, the Tobacco Indemnification and Community Revitalization Commission supports economic development in tobacco-dependent communities. However, a study of the distribution of MSA funds in North Carolina found that a sizable share of MSA funds was diverted to the state's general fund or used for purposes unrelated to tobacco, such as a

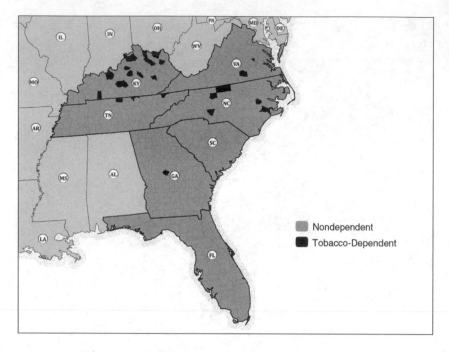

FIGURE 5.3 Tobacco-Dependent Counties, 2002

Source: Map created by James W. Quinn based on authors' calculations.

prescription drug benefit program (Jones et al. 2007). The extent to which MSA-funded programs have aided the communities most affected by structural change in the tobacco industry is unclear.

Despite these resources, it is important to take seriously the challenges that tobacco-dependent counties may face if tobacco production declines still further. During the 1980s and 1990s, the region gained economically as manufacturers shifted operations from higher-cost locations in the Northeast and Midwest, and this new economic development offset the loss of jobs and income from tobacco production. The economic context is different now. Manufacturing in the South is increasingly vulnerable to global competition. Traditional industries such as furniture and apparel face intensifying competition from imports (Bernard, Jensen, and Schott 2005). Between 2002 and 2007, the southeast region faced the steepest drop in manufacturing employment of any region in the country (based on authors' calculations from BEA REIS employment figures).

Over the longer term, researchers may identify alternative uses for the tobacco plant, including applications in the production of food, energy, and plant-made pharmaceuticals (Fisher 1999). Researchers, including those at the University of Kentucky's Tobacco Research and Development Center and the University of

Maryland's Alternative Uses for Tobacco project, are beginning to develop commercially viable applications. Tobacco is attractive for biopharmaceutical use because it grows quickly, produces a large number of seeds per plant, and is relatively easy to engineer genetically. In 2006 the USDA approved production of a vaccine against a poultry disease (Newcastle disease) in genetically engineered tobacco plants. Scientists are developing methods to use tobacco plants in production of vaccines against human papillomavirus, amoebiasis, anthrax, the plague, and even a form of cancer, as well as a therapeutic for Gaucher's disease.

As exciting as this potential may be, biopharmaceutical applications do not represent a near-term solution to the problem of declining demand for domestic tobacco. Despite a promising start, it will take time to address the scientific and regulatory challenges involved in commercial production of biopharmaceuticals. For growers, moreover, producing tobacco for biopharmaceutical use may require additional expenses for equipment and labor as well as changes in methods of cultivation (Nevitt et al. 2003). Ultimately, agricultural economists expect transgenic tobacco to account for a relatively small amount of acreage (Konstandini, Mills, and Norton 2006).

CONCLUSION

During the mid- to late 1990s, as the tobacco industry became increasingly embattled, and as farm policy experts and politicians began to talk about an end to the tobacco quota program, tobacco farmers and public health advocates began a series of meetings to try to reach common ground. The Virginia Tobacco Communities Project, founded in 1994, served as a model for the Southern Tobacco Communities Project, which was established in 1997 with support from the Robert Wood Johnson Foundation. These efforts brought together representatives from tobacco agriculture, state government, economic development organizations, and medicine and health services in a discussion of ways to reconcile public health objectives with protection of the livelihood of farmers. Building on these efforts, in 2000 President Clinton established the President's Commission on Improving Economic Opportunity in Communities Dependent on Tobacco Production While Protecting Public Health, which issued a report in 2001 outlining a series of recommendations.

Yet the ground was shifting even as these initiatives were being organized. Several decades ago, tobacco was at the center of many farm communities and a few cities and towns: it represented an economic foundation and also a shared way of life (Altman et al. 2000). Stable farm incomes anchored rural life in tobacco-producing counties, supporting communities marked by intergenerational continuity and dense social networks (Hamilton 2003; Stull 2000; van Willigen and Eastwood 1998).

By the time President Clinton's commission issued its report, these "tobacco communities" were largely gone. In 2002, fewer than 1 in 20 southeastern counties were classified as tobacco dependent. Certainly, there may be more subtle social costs of the decline of tobacco. As we look forward, however, the tobacco-dependent community is not the best way to conceptualize the economic impact in the region of a decline in smoking. Instead, we should focus on two kinds of costs. First, individual farmers and others involved in tobacco production will face a loss of income if smoking rates decline. As chapters 3 and 4 have discussed, although relatively few people are affected, their income losses may be considerable. Second, there are parts of the region—especially remote rural areas or older industrial towns—that face economic challenges because of the simultaneous decline of a number of traditional industries such as textiles, apparel, and furniture as well as tobacco. Targeting economic development assistance based on a single industry, such as tobacco, may not address the needs of communities that face economic decline in multiple industries.

Readers should keep in mind several limitations of this work. First, the threshold used to categorize counties as tobacco dependent (a tobacco dependence ratio of 0.05 or more) is an arbitrary criterion; some readers may view this threshold as either too high or too low. Second, the measure of tobacco dependence does not account for the costs of tobacco production. For this reason, while the measure indexes the importance of tobacco production in the local economy, it is not a good measure of the economic status of tobacco farmers. If costs of production have increased over time, for instance, the net income of tobacco farmers will have declined more than the measure suggests. Finally, as noted above, the chapter does not address the social disruption of structural economic change. Like the economic costs, these social costs may be compounded by the fact that a number of traditional industries have declined alongside tobacco.

APPENDIX 5.1

The empirical analysis reported here is based on data for the 692 counties or independent cities in seven southeastern states: Florida, Georgia, Kentucky, North Carolina, South Carolina, Tennessee, and Virginia. As discussed above, county-level data were drawn primarily from the BEA REIS, the Census of Agriculture, and the U.S. decennial census. Measures using the REIS and the Census of Agriculture were constructed for 1982, 1987, 1992, 1997, and 2002. Population characteristics such as poverty rates and commuting time were drawn from the 1980 and 2000 U.S. decennial census. Metropolitan status and adjacency to a metropolitan area were based on the rural-urban continuum codes (Beale codes) available from the USDA (http://www.ers.usda.gov/Briefing/Rurality/RuralUrbCon/).

TABLE 5.6 Data Sources

MEASURE	SOURCE	NOTES
Tobacco leaf sales	Census of Agriculture	Counties with missing data were assumed to have zero tobacco sales; inspection of county urbanization levels and agricultural census data in adjacent years suggests that tobacco leaf sales were missing only in counties with little or no tobacco farming
Tobacco manufacturing earnings	REIS (CA05)	As discussed in appendix text, information from documentary sources was also used in imputing values for counties in which tobacco manufacturing earnings were missing
Tobacco income	Census of Agriculture and REIS	Sum of tobacco leaf sales and tobacco manufacturing earnings
Total earnings	REIS (CA05)	Earnings by place of work
Tobacco dependence ratio	Census of Agriculture and REIS	Tobacco income divided by total earnings
Total number of farms, number and proportion of tobacco farms, total tobacco acreage, mean tobacco acreage per tobacco farm	Census of Agriculture	Mean tobacco acreage per tobacco farm was calculated by dividing the county's tobacco acreage by the number of tobacco farms in the county
Sales of other (nontobacco) agricultural commodities	Census of Agriculture	Total agricultural sales minus tobacco leaf sales
Metropolitan status	USDA ERS Rural-urban influence codes	Metropolitan status and adjacency to metropolitan county, in 1983 and 2003
Population	REIS (CA04)	

TABLE 5.6 (Continued)

MEASURE	SOURCE	NOTES
Per-capita income	REIS (CA04)	Adjusted for inflation
Growth in nonfarm jobs relative to population	REIS (CA04 and CA25)	Coded as 1 for counties in which the 1982–2002 change in number of nonfarm jobs was larger (more positive) than the 1982–2002 change in population
Counties with large increase in long commutes	Decennial Census	Defined as counties in which percentage of workers with a long (more than 45 minutes) commute increased by more than 5 percentage points
New bedroom communities	REIS (population), Decennial Census (long commutes), and Census of Agriculture (farm acreage)	Defined as counties that were nonmetropolitan in 1983 and 2003 and had population growth (1982–2002) above the median, increase in % of long commutes (1980–2000) above the median, and decline in total farm acreage (1982–2002) above the median for all counties in the study sample
Poverty rate	Decennial Census	Percentage of households with income below the poverty line in 1979 and 1999
Change in per-capita transfer income	REIS (CA35)	Percentage change (1982–2002) in inflation-adjusted county-level income from family assistance (primarily AFDC or TANF), SSI, food stamps (SNAP), and unemployment benefits divided by the county population for the corresponding year

See table 5.6 for more information about data sources and variable construction. All sales or income figures are expressed in 2002 dollars.

Problems with missing data arose primarily in the case of earnings from tobacco manufacturing. Data on earnings from tobacco manufacturing are available annually for most years through 1995. This information was suppressed in counties with only a few establishments in this industry; data suppression became more common after 1995. In addition, beginning in 2001, the REIS replaced SIC with NAICS industry codes, which group together tobacco and beverage manufacturing at the two-digit level employed in the REIS; beverage manufacturing had previously been grouped with the manufacture of "food and kindred products." We used a variety of strategies to impute tobacco manufacturing earnings, including interpolation; estimation based on tobacco, beverage, and food earnings before and after the SIC/NAICS transition; and a search of documentary information such as local newspaper accounts of layoffs and plant shutdowns.

To derive the estimates of tobacco dependence in 2025 under the three scenarios, we projected components of the tobacco dependence ratio (tobacco leaf sales, tobacco manufacturing earnings, and earnings by place of work) from 2002 to 2025 and then calculated the ratio using these projected values. The numerator includes income from tobacco leaf sales and tobacco manufacturing. We applied Sumner and Alston's projections of change in total tobacco revenue through 2025 (table 3.4, chapter 3) to county-level tobacco sales receipts in our data. To project tobacco manufacturing earnings, we multiplied county-level tobacco manufacturing earnings in our data by Espinosa and Evans's projected percentage changes in tobacco production employment (table 4.2, chapter 4) and inflated the resulting figures to reflect an annual wage increase of 2.1 percent based on the estimates from chapter 4. The denominator, county-level earnings by place of work, was projected forward to 2025 by assuming a 3.2 percent rate of growth.

NOTE

1. This criterion is admittedly arbitrary, but it is within the range of thresholds used in previous studies (Gale 1999). Setting too high a threshold would result in a measure that is relatively insensitive to change in the tobacco industry because it excluded so many counties. To take an extreme example, if the threshold were set at 0.50, only two counties would be classified as tobacco dependent in any year. Even a more moderate increase in the threshold, to 0.10, would exclude 39.3 percent of counties considered tobacco dependent by the 0.05 standard in 1982, 68.7 percent in 1987, 63.6 percent in 1992, 68.0 percent in 1997, and 79.3 percent in 2002. Moreover, using the 0.10 threshold would exclude some counties generally associated with the tobacco industry, such as Forsyth County (Winston-Salem), North Carolina, in 1997 and 2002, and Richmond,

Virginia, in 1987–2002. Because the aim of the chapter is to address concern about the economic consequences of tobacco control policy, it is important to avoid the perception that we are defining away the problem by using too limited a definition of tobacco dependence. On the other hand, a lower threshold (e.g., 0.01) may appear too inclusive. In addition, because the Census of Agriculture and Census of Manufacturing suppress reporting of income in counties with small numbers of farms or establishments, setting the threshold too low makes the measure more sensitive to missing data; at present, we have imputed values of zero for counties with missing data on tobacco sales and for counties with missing data on tobacco manufacturing (except in instances where documentary evidence indicates a nonzero value).

6

FALLING CIGARETTE CONSUMPTION IN THE UNITED STATES AND THE IMPACT ON TOBACCO RETAILER EMPLOYMENT

KURT M. RIBISL, WILLIAM N. EVANS, AND ELLEN C. FEIGHERY

This chapter addresses the economic implications of markedly reducing cigarette consumption in the United States for the retail establishments that sell tobacco products. Understanding the economic impact on tobacco retailers is important because retailers have often opposed tobacco control measures, such as increased cigarette excise taxes, out of concern that these policies would reduce their business income. Moreover, policymakers want to understand the impact of tobacco control measures because retail establishments selling tobacco employ several million Americans. This chapter reviews the types of establishments where tobacco products are sold, describes employment trends in these establishments, and estimates the impact on retail employment of two policy scenarios that would reduce cigarette consumption. To our knowledge, this is the first national-level analysis of how reducing cigarette consumption would affect retailers in the United States.

WHERE TOBACCO IS SOLD IN THE UNITED STATES

Tobacco products are currently sold in a variety of retail establishments, including convenience stores, gas stations, liquor stores, supermarkets, pharmacies, bowling alleys, doughnut shops, bars, and smoking paraphernalia shops known as "head shops" (Ribisl 2004). Tobacco products are also sold by Internet and mail-order vendors (Ribisl, Kim, and Williams 2001). The exact number of retail and Internet tobacco vendors is unknown because the United States does not have a mandatory licensing system for establishments that sell tobacco products. However, the U.S. Department of Commerce conducts an Economic Census every five years that provides data on the number and types of payroll establishments (i.e., stores with paid employees) selling tobacco products, their employment, and their tobacco product revenues. A caveat: these data include *all* types of tobacco products, including cigars, tobacco, and smokers' accessories as well as cigarettes; we cannot retrieve data solely on cigarette sales or cigarette retailer employment. However, most tobacco products sold in the United States are cigarettes. In 2004 the U.S. Department of Agriculture reported that 92.6 percent of consumer spending on tobacco products was for cigarettes, 3.4 percent for cigars, and the remaining 4 percent for other tobacco products.[1]

In 2002 there were 221,173 payroll establishments that sold tobacco products, accounting for $50.86 billion in annual sales (U.S. Department of Commerce 2006). The Economic Census reports use a business classification system called the North American Industry Classification System, or NAICS (http://www.census.gov/epcd/www/naics.html). According to figures classified using the NAICS categories, in 2002 there were over forty kinds of businesses that sold tobacco products, including auto parts dealers, sporting goods stores, and florists. Most of these, however, derived very little revenue from tobacco products.

Table 6.1 shows retail establishment types with annual tobacco product sales of more than $1 billion in 2002, or more than 2 percent of overall tobacco product sales. Food and beverage stores accounted for more than a quarter of tobacco sales. Within this category, supermarkets had the highest sales, but cigarettes were less than 2 percent of total supermarket sales; in contrast, cigarettes were almost a quarter of convenience store sales. Beer, wine, and liquor stores accounted for $1.2 billion in tobacco sales and were less dependent on tobacco sales. Pharmacies and other health and personal care stores sold $1.5 billion in tobacco products—0.86 percent of revenue for these establishments. Almost half of all tobacco products were purchased from gas stations, with the vast majority of sales in gas stations with convenience stores. General merchandise stores accounted for $7.1 billion in tobacco sales, about 1.60 percent of total revenues in this industry. The last subsector in table 6.1 is miscellaneous store retailers, in which most tobacco sales were from stores that specialize in the sale of tobacco products. Not surprisingly, the most tobacco-dependent category was tobacco stores: these stores sold $5.7 billion in tobacco products in 2002, almost 87 percent of total sales in the industry.

This chapter examines the impact of declining cigarette consumption on retail employment. We selected four key categories of establishments that together

TABLE 6.1 Establishments Selling Over $1 Billion of Tobacco Products in the United States, 2002

NAICS CODE SUBSECTOR	NAICS CODE INDUSTRIES	INDUSTRY DESCRIPTION	NUMBER OF ESTABLISHMENTS SELLING TOBACCO PRODUCTS[a]	SALES OF TOBACCO PRODUCTS ($1,000)	SALES, RECEIPTS, OR REVENUE FOR ALL PRODUCT LINES ($1,000)[b]	PERCENTAGE OF SALES FROM TOBACCO PRODUCTS
445		Food and beverage stores	90,126	$13,370,359	$456,942,288	2.93%
	44511	Supermarkets and other grocery stores (except convenience stores)	51,343	$7,683,683	$395,233,897	1.94%
	44512	Convenience stores	27,871	$4,527,232	$20,379,975	22.21%
	4453	Beer, wine, and liquor stores	13,177	$1,237,603	$28,246,426	4.38%
446		Health and personal care stores (includes pharmacies and drug stores)	17,761	$1,525,046	$177,947,091	0.86%
447		Gasoline stations	94,897	$22,173,329	$249,141,412	8.90%
	44711	Gasoline stations with convenience stores	86,152	$21,153,629	$186,735,177	11.33%
	44719	Other gasoline stores	8,745	$1,019,700	$62,406,235	1.63%

TABLE 6.1 (Continued)

NAICS CODE			NUMBER OF ESTABLISHMENTS SELLING TOBACCO PRODUCTS[a]	SALES OF TOBACCO PRODUCTS ($1,000)	SALES, RECEIPTS, OR REVENUE FOR ALL PRODUCT LINES ($1,000)[b]	PERCENTAGE OF SALES FROM TOBACCO PRODUCTS
SUBSECTOR	INDUSTRIES	INDUSTRY DESCRIPTION				
452		General merchandise stores (e.g., department stores, warehouse clubs)	6,991	$7,107,737	$445,224,985	1.60%
453		Miscellaneous store retailers	8,132	$5,804,021	$90,811,742	6.39%
	453991	Tobacco stores	6,184	$5,674,466	$6,527,871	86.93%

Notes: Tobacco products are sold in over 40 types of establishments in the United States. Table 6.1 includes all establishments selling over $1 billion of tobacco products in 2002 according to the 2002 Economic Census. The total sales, receipts, or revenue for tobacco products was $50,860,948,000 in nominal 2002 dollars.

[a] Tobacco products are defined as NAICS code 20150 "Cigars, cigarettes, etc. & smokers accessories excluding sales from vending machines."

[b] This figure also includes revenue from establishments that do not carry product line 20150 (tobacco products as defined above). For example, there are 86,152 gasoline stations with convenience stores that sell product line 20150, which were a subset of 93,691 gasoline stations with convenience stores (number not listed in table above) that had sales of $186.7 billion for all product lines. The revenue figure in this column is for the 93,691 establishments.

Source: Census of Retail Trade, 2002.

account for approximately $47.4 billion, just over 93 percent, of all tobacco sales. These four categories combine industries with similar patterns of tobacco sales and represent a continuum ranging from high to low dependency on tobacco product sales. The categories are shown in table 6.2, arranged in order of their dependence on tobacco revenue. The first is tobacco stores, which are highly dependent on cigarette sales. The second category, "all convenience stores," includes convenience stores and gasoline stations with convenience stores. This combined category accounts for $25.68 billion, or 50.5 percent of all tobacco product sales in the United States; it is moderately dependent on tobacco, with tobacco sales accounting for 12.4 percent of total revenues. The third industry is beer, wine and liquor stores, in which tobacco sales represented more than 4 percent of total sales in 2002. The fourth category combines the supermarket and general merchandising categories. These two industries had a similar dollar value of cigarette sales in 2002, similar aggregate sales from all products, and hence a very similar fraction of sales from cigarettes—less than 2 percent in both cases.

In addition to these specific categories, we construct a residual category called "other retail industries," which represents all retail minus the four industry categories listed above. This residual category accounted for about 7 percent of tobacco sales in 2002; only 0.18 percent of its total revenues are from tobacco products. The final category we examine is the "combined retail" grouping, which includes all retail establishments in the Economic Census. Across the retail sector as a whole, the $50.8 billion in tobacco sales is 1.7 percent of the $3.1 trillion in sales revenue.

We assess the economic impact of tobacco control policy on the retail sector by looking at the implications of the IOM-based and "high-impact" policy scenarios for retail employment. The impact of declining cigarette sales on employment is not expected to be uniformly negative across these industry categories. Some types of stores may be unaffected whereas others may actually see an increase in employment as consumers shift their expenditures from cigarettes to other products. We expect the largest effect on employment in establishments such as tobacco stores that are relatively highly dependent on tobacco sales.

Our analysis has three main steps. First, as a baseline, we project trends in employment in these six retail categories between 2005 and 2025 in the absence of significant policy change. Second, to understand how potential tobacco policy changes are likely to affect retail employment, we analyze the effect that excise tax increases had on tobacco consumption and retail employment between 1990 and 2004. Third, we combine the baseline employment projections with estimates of the effect of tobacco consumption changes on retail employment to project employment impacts by industry between 2005 and 2025.

TABLE 6.2 Grouping of Retail Establishments for Statistical Analysis, 50 States, 2002

INDUSTRY GROUP	PERCENTAGE OF SALES FROM TOBACCO PRODUCTS	NUMBER OF ESTABLISHMENTS SELLING TOBACCO PRODUCTS[a]	SALES OF TOBACCO PRODUCTS (BILLIONS)	SALES, RECEIPTS, OR REVENUE FOR ALL PRODUCT LINES[b] (BILLIONS)
1. Tobacco stores (45399l)	86.9%	6,184	$5.7	$6.6
2. All convenience stores (44512 and 44711)	12.4%	114,023	$25.7	$207.1
3. Beer, wine, and liquor stores (4453)	4.4%	13,177	$1.2	$28.2
4. Supermarkets and general merchandise (44511 and 452)	1.8%	58,334	$14.8	$840.4
5. All other (retail minus the stores in rows 1–4)	0.18%	29,455	$3.5	$1,972
6. Combined retail sector	1.7%	221,173	$50.8	$3,054

[a] Tobacco products are defined as NAICS code 20150 "Cigars, cigarettes, etc. & smokers accessories excluding sales from vending machines."
[b] This figure also includes revenue from establishments that do not carry product line 20150 (tobacco products as defined above). For example, there are 86,152 gasoline stations with convenience stores (number not listed in table above) that had sales of $186.7 billion for all product lines. The revenue figure in this column is for the 93,691 establishments.
Source: Census of Retail Trade, 2002.

TRENDS IN TOBACCO RETAILER EMPLOYMENT AND CIGARETTE CONSUMPTION

This section of the chapter reviews trends in employment for our six retail categories in order to develop baseline projections of retail employment between 2005 and 2025 under the status quo policy scenario. The employment data in figures 6.1–6.7 come from the Bureau of Labor Statistics (BLS) Current Employment Statistics, which provide annual averages of employees per month by industry. A description of the data can be found at http://www.bls.gov/ces/home .htm#overview. In the graphs, the solid lines are actual BLS employment numbers, and the dashed lines are projections through 2025. In most cases we restrict our attention to 1990 and later because comparable data for retail subsectors are not available prior to 1990. In 2002 the BLS began to use the NAICS occupational classification system; although employment data for 1990 to 2002 were reclassified based on the new system, consistent data series extending back before 1990 cannot be constructed except where SIC and NAICS codes are comparable, as they are for the retail industry as a whole.

Trends for aggregate industry groups show a clearer pattern than trends in more disaggregated industries. Because we exploit these patterns when predicting industry trends, our presentation will move from more to less aggregate levels. Figure 6.1 shows the total industry employment for the retail sector between 1960 and 2002. Notice that employment growth is close to linear over this period. A regression of employment levels on a simple time trend generates an R^2 of 0.98. Over the entire period, employment growth averaged about 2.2 percent per year. Between 1990 and 2006, however, the average annual growth rate in employment was only about 1 percent per year. In this study, we assume this 1 percent growth rate will persist until 2025. This assumed growth rate is identical to the projections of the BLS through 2014 (http://www.bls.gov/opub/mlr/2005/11/art 4full.pdf). Between 2006 and 2025, we project that retail employment would increase from 15.3 to 18.6 million under the status quo scenario.

Figure 6.2 shows trends in supermarket and general merchandise employment. Between 1990 and 2004, this industry category grew steadily in a nearly linear fashion. The distinctions between these two sectors have blurred in recent years as many big box retailers in the general merchandising categories have added grocery stores to their establishments. This led to employment reductions in the supermarket sector and increases in general merchandise, but in the aggregate, as figure 6.2 shows, employment growth has been steady. To predict the growth in this sector, we regressed employment in this sector over the 1990–2004 period on a cubic polynomial in total retail employment; using these coefficients plus the predicted retail employment in figure 6.1, we predict employment through 2025. The initial regression fits well with an R^2 of 0.96, and as the

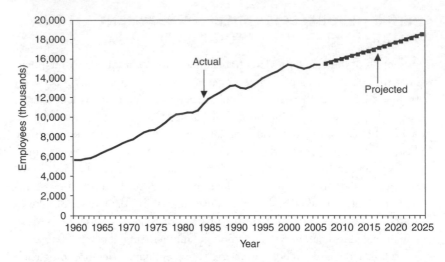

FIGURE 6.1 Actual and Projected Employment: Retail Trade (NAICS 44–45)

Sources: Bureau of Labor and Statistics, Census of Employment and Wages, www.bls.gov/cew/, and authors' calculations.

numbers in figure 6.2 indicate, the model predicts nearly linear growth in employment in this sector through 2025. We expect that employment in this combined sector will grow from 5.2 million in 2004 to 6.1 million workers in 2025, for an average annual growth rate of about 0.8 percent. The BLS predicts that the average annual growth rate in the supermarket sector will be about 0.64 percent per year through 2025 (http://www.bls.gov/oco/cg/cgs024.htm) and about 1 percent per year in general merchandise (http://www.bls.gov/oco/cg/cgs022 .htm), consistent with our estimate of roughly 0.8 percent annual growth in employment for this combined category.

Figure 6.3 shows that after a small dip after 1990, employment in tobacco stores rose steadily until it leveled off starting in 2000 at approximately 27,000 employees. The BLS does not make projections for tobacco store employment, but growth in this sector since 1990 mirrors growth in retail sales overall. Based on data from 1990–2004, a regression of tobacco store employment on total retail sector employment generates an R^2 of about 0.94. Since retail sales are expected to increase by 1 percent per year and tobacco store employment tracks well with retail employment, we project tobacco store employment will grow at an annual rate of about 1 percent per year through 2025, rising from 27,500 workers in 2004 to about 33,900 workers in 2025.

In figure 6.4 we graph actual and projected convenience store employment. Convenience store employment peaked in 1998 and then declined steadily,

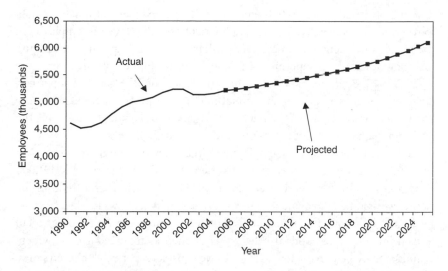

FIGURE 6.2 Actual and Projected Employment: Supermarkets (NAICS 44511) and General Merchandise (NAICS 452)

Sources: Bureau of Labor and Statistics, Census of Employment and Wages, www.bls.gov/cew/, and authors' calculations.

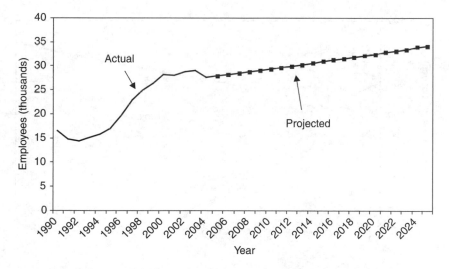

FIGURE 6.3 Actual and Projected Employment: Tobacco Stores (NAICS 453991)

Sources: Bureau of Labor and Statistics, Census of Employment and Wages, www.bls.gov/cew/, and authors' calculations.

leveling off in 2004 at 900,000 employees. The BLS does not make separate projections for convenience store employment growth. However, employment trends in convenience stores are very similar to those in supermarkets. Figure 6.5 shows the ratio of supermarket to convenience store employment over the 1990–2004 period; this ratio is roughly constant. The BLS projects supermarket employment will grow at an annual rate of 0.64 percent per year; because convenience store employment tracks supermarket employment, we assume the same annual rate of increase for convenience store employees.

In figure 6.6 we graph the employment in beer, wine, and liquor stores. Notice that since 1990, employment has varied from 135,000 to roughly 141,000 employees, with little trend in employment. Given the lack of a trend in the series, we assume employment in this sector will persist at this level.

Figure 6.7 shows the actual and predicted employment for all other retail establishments. This residual category is defined as total retail employment minus employment in the four categories we consider separately (tobacco stores, all convenience stores, liquor stores, and general merchandise and supermarkets). To project employment after 2004 in this category, we subtract from the predicted total retail employment series the sum of the predicted values for the four industry groups. The annual growth rate in employment for this residual category is about 1 percent per year.

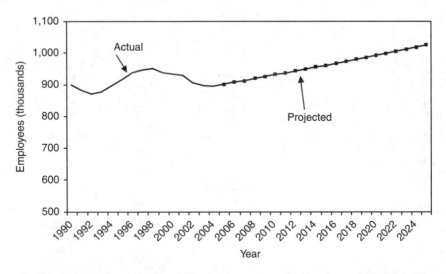

FIGURE 6.4 Actual and Projected Employment: Convenience Stores (NAICS 44512) and Gas Stations with Convenience Stores (NAICS 44711)

Sources: Bureau of Labor and Statistics, Census of Employment and Wages, www.bls.gov/cew/, and authors' calculations.

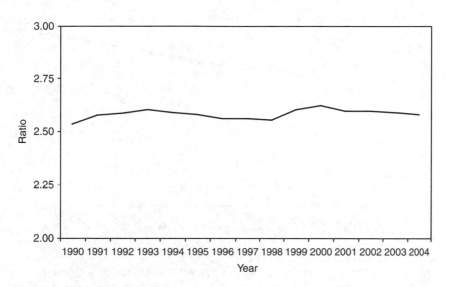

FIGURE 6.5 Ratio of Supermarket to All Convenience Store Employment

Sources: Bureau of Labor and Statistics, Census of Employment and Wages, www.bls.gov/cew/, and authors' calculations.

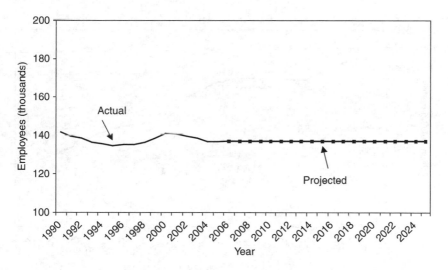

FIGURE 6.6 Actual and Projected Employment: Beer, Wine, and Liquor Stores (NAICS 4453)

Sources: Bureau of Labor and Statistics, Census of Employment and Wages, www.bls.gov/cew/, and authors' calculations.

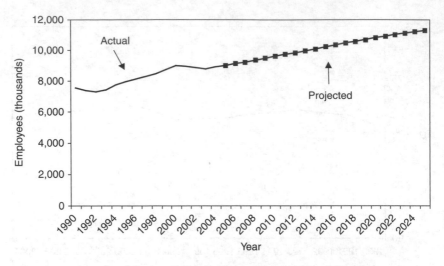

FIGURE 6.7 Actual and Projected Employment: All Other Retail Establishments

Sources: Bureau of Labor and Statistics, Census of Employment and Wages, www.bls.gov/cew/, and authors' calculations.

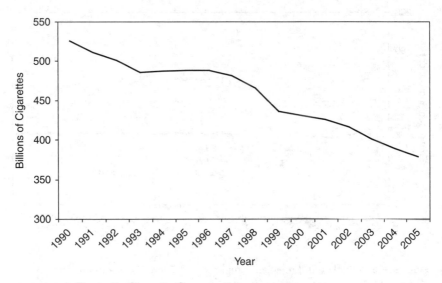

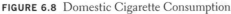

FIGURE 6.8 Domestic Cigarette Consumption

Source: Orzechowski and Walker, "The Tax Burden on Tobacco," various years.

Figure 6.8 displays domestic consumption of cigarettes between 1990 and 2005. Domestic cigarette consumption declined steadily during this period. If tobacco retailer employment were strongly linked to cigarette consumption, figures 6.1–6.4 and 6.6–6.7 would have shown declining employment in each of the establishment types. However, despite a decline in cigarette consumption of 26 percent between 1990 and 2004, none of the four establishment types showed noticeably lower employment figures in 2004 compared to 1990. Employment in the beer, wine, liquor grouping was stagnant, but employment rose for the other three groupings. The rest of this chapter draws on past data to develop more sophisticated multivariate models and employment projections.

RELATIONSHIP BETWEEN CIGARETTE PRICES, TAXES, CONSUMPTION, AND RETAIL EMPLOYMENT

Our ultimate goal is to simulate how retail employment might change under alternative tobacco control scenarios. To do this, we look retrospectively at how employment has been affected in the past by changing cigarette consumption. For some retail sectors we expect that a drop in cigarette consumption would reduce employment. In tobacco stores, 87 percent of sales are for tobacco products; thus, falling cigarette consumption should negatively impact employment in these stores. For other retail sectors the results are less predictable. If consumers purchase fewer cigarettes, they have more money to spend on other goods and services. If consumers shift their consumption to other products purchased at retail establishments, then falling cigarette consumption might actually increase employment at some types of stores.

Estimating the relationship between consumption and retail employment is a difficult task. It is tempting to estimate a model with state-level retail employment as the dependent variable and state-level cigarette consumption as the key covariate to obtain the necessary gradient. However, it is likely such a model would produce biased estimates. A key assumption in ordinary least squares (OLS) regression models is that the dependent variable, retail employment in our case, cannot have a direct "feedback" effect on the independent variable of interest, cigarette consumption. However, it is possible that growth in retail outlets might promote cigarette consumption by making cigarettes more widely available, decreasing the nonmonetary cost of procuring cigarettes, and thereby increasing consumption. Growth in retail outlets might also mean more competition and, hence, lower prices, raising consumption. On the other hand, fewer retail outlets could lead to greater sales volume at remaining stores, prompting greater price discounts from manufacturers, which would decrease price and increase consumption. Few studies have examined empirically the relationship between the number of cigarette retail outlets and cigarette consumption (Burton et al. 2005).

Given these concerns, we need to develop a model that is less susceptible to this type of bias. Here, we seek to isolate the effect of policy-induced changes in consumption on retail employment by examining whether tax-induced changes in consumption also generated changes in retail employment in a variety of sectors.

Cigarettes are taxed at the federal, state, and local levels, and much of the variation in cigarette prices, both across geographic areas and over time, is determined by the size of these excise taxes. Over the last 20 years, there have been frequent and sometimes very large changes in state and federal excise taxes on cigarettes. Between 1990 and 2004, state excise tax rates on cigarettes were changed 104 times. In a few cases, tax rates declined, and in about 30 percent of the cases, taxes increased by less than 10 cents per pack (a nominal amount). In more recent years, however, states have implemented large changes in cigarette tax rates. Econometric evidence has clearly demonstrated that demand falls when tax rates rise (Chaloupka and Warner 1999; Task Force on Community Preventive Services 2005; U.S. Department of Health and Human Services 2000). In this section we exploit the frequent tax changes imposed at the state level and the persistent relationships among cigarette taxes, prices, and consumption to assess the impact of cigarette sales on retail employment. As demonstrated below, we can easily replicate results from prior studies showing that higher taxes reduce cigarette consumption. We then examine whether employment levels in various retail sectors also changed when tax rates were altered. Because the only impact these tax changes should have on retail employment is through changes in cigarette consumption, we can then combine these two parameters to estimate how much retail employment changes when there are policy-induced changes in cigarette consumption.

The data for this section come from a variety of sources. First, annual data on the consumption of cigarettes at the state level from 1990 through 2004 were obtained from the annual publication "The Tax Burden on Tobacco" (Orzechowski and Walker, various years). This publication also lists state and federal excise taxes on cigarettes per year. Next, we obtain annual data on employment in various retail sectors at the state level from the BLS Quarterly Census of Employment and Wages. This program publishes quarterly counts of employment and average weekly earnings reported by employers covering 98 percent of U.S. jobs. The data are available at the county, metropolitan area, state, and national levels by industry.[2] Employment and cigarette consumption are scaled by state population.[3]

Initially, we use state-level data on per-capita cigarette consumption, prices, and excise taxes to estimate models similar to those in past studies of the price elasticity of demand for cigarettes. In these analyses, we use OLS models and regress the real or inflation-adjusted price of cigarettes (measured in cents per pack in 1982 dollars) and the log of per-capita cigarette consumption on the real cigarette excise tax (state + federal, measured in cents per pack). The models also include year and state effects and other covariates. The year effects are included in the model to capture influences on demand for cigarettes that are common to all states but vary over time. These influences include changing concerns about the health effects of smoking or the increase in the retail price of cigarettes brought about by the Master Settlement Agreement, the settlement of the state Medicaid cases against the tobacco companies (Sloan and Trogdon 2004). The state effects include state characteristics that are constant over time within a state but vary across states. For example, Utah has low per-capita consumption because of the high fraction of the population that is Mormon. In contrast, states like North Carolina and Virginia tend to have higher than average per-capita consumption because of their historic ties to the cigarette industry. We also control for cyclic variation in the purchasing power of the population with measures of the state's real per-capita income and the number of jobs in the nonretail sector divided by the number of adults.[4]

In table 6.3 we report the basic results from these preliminary regressions for the first retail category, tobacco stores. These results are presented in detail to illustrate the computations for the basic model. (Table 6.4 summarizes results for all industry types.) The numbers in parentheses are standard errors that reflect the sampling variation inherent in the model. The standard errors are constructed so as to allow for arbitrary correlation in errors within a state over time. The one to three asterisks indicate statistical significance at p values of 0.1, 0.05, and 0.01, respectively. These tables report only the coefficients on real cigarette excise taxes.

In column 1 of table 6.3, the dependent variable is the real price of cigarettes. The results indicate that tax hikes are passed on to consumers nearly penny for penny. A 10 cent tax hike (in real 1982 dollars) is estimated to increase retail prices by 9.4 cents. This parameter is precisely estimated, but we cannot reject the null hypothesis that the coefficient equals 1—in other words, that 100 percent of a tax hike is passed on to consumers in the form of higher prices. The fact that taxes increase retail prices nearly dollar for dollar has been noted by a number of other authors (Evans, Ringel, and Stech 1999; Sullivan 1985; Sumner 1981).

In column 2 the outcome of interest is the log of per-capita purchases of cigarettes. The coefficient on real excise taxes is −0.00692 with a very small standard error. These estimates suggest that a 10 cent increase in the price of cigarettes reduces cigarette consumption by 6.9 percent. The average retail price of cigarettes in our sample is 141 cents (in real 1982 dollars); if a 10 cent tax hike increases prices by 9.4 cents, that tax hike represents roughly a 6.7 percent increase in price. In this sample, then, the elasticity of demand for cigarettes—in other

TABLE 6.3 Estimates of the Relationships Between Cigarette Taxes, Prices, Per-Capita Sales, and Tobacco Store Employment, Continental 48 States, 1990–2004

INDEPENDENT VARIABLE	ESTIMATION METHOD[a]	COEFFICIENT AND (STANDARD ERROR) FOR INDEPENDENT VARIABLE IN MODELS WITH THE FOLLOWING DEPENDENT VARIABLES:				
		REAL PRICE OF CIGARETTES (CENTS/PACK)	LN (PER-CAPITA CIGARETTE SALES)	LN (EMPLOYMENT PER CAPITA)	LN (ESTABLISHMENTS PER CAPITA)	LN (EMPLOYEES PER ESTABLISHMENT)
		1	2	3	4	5
Real tax on cigarettes (cents/pack)	OLS	0.9435*** (0.0681)	−0.00692*** (0.00073)	−0.00948*** (0.00353)	−0.00091*** (0.00291)	0.00044 (0.00224)
ln (per-capita cigarette sales)	2SLS			1.349*** (0.528)	1.411*** (0.448)	−0.0620 (0.3340)

*Statistically significant at $p < 0.10$; **Statistically significant at $p < 0.05$; ***Statistically significant at $p < 0.01$.

[a] OLS, ordinary least squares regression; 2SLS, two-stage least-squares regression. Numbers in parentheses are standard errors, which are calculated to allow for arbitrary correlation in errors within a state over time.

Sources: Orzechowski and Walker, "The Tax Burden on Tobacco," various years; Bureau of Labor Statistics, Census of Employment and Wages.

TABLE 6.4 2SLS Estimates of the Relationships Between Per-Capita Cigarette Sales (Consumption) and Tobacco Retailer Employment, Establishments, and Employment per Establishment, Continental 48 States, 1990–2004

INDUSTRY	SAMPLE TOTALS IN 2004		2SLS COEFFICIENTS ON LN (PER-CAPITA CIGARETTE SALES) IN EQUATIONS WITH THE FOLLOWING DEPENDENT VARIABLES[a]		
	EMPLOYEES (THOUSANDS)	ESTABLISHMENTS[b]	LN (EMPLOYEES PER CAPITA)	LN (ESTABLISHMENTS PER CAPITA)	LN (EMPLOYEES PER ESTABLISHMENT)
Tobacco stores	27	5,203	1.349*** (0.528)	1.411*** (0.448)	−0.0620 (0.3340)
All convenience stores	881	114,683	0.0766 (0.0807)	0.0597 (0.0828)	0.0168 (0.1122)
Beer, wine, and liquor stores	135	25,103	−0.3450** (0.1590)	0.0158 (0.1582)	−0.3608** (0.1729)
General merch./supermarkets	5,123	106,149	0.00036 (0.00076)	0.000076* (0.000045)	−0.1210 (0.1176)
Other retail establishments	8,807	775,727	−0.0296 (0.0317)	0.0321 (0.0452)	−0.0632 (0.0529)
All retail	14,971	1,026,865	0.00246 (0.02554)	0.0485 (0.0447)	−0.0460 (0.0517)

*Statistically significant at $p < 0.10$; **Statistically significant at $p < 0.05$; ***Statistically significant at $p < 0.01$.

[a] 2SLS, two-stage least-squares regression. Numbers in parentheses are standard errors, which are calculated to allow for arbitrary correlation in errors within a state over time.

[b] Establishments data differ from table 6.2 because that table featured establishments selling tobacco, and this table is all establishments, regardless of whether they sold tobacco. Also, this table is 2004 data on 48 continental states rather than 2002 data on all 50 states.

Source: Orzechowski and Walker, "The Tax Burden on Tobacco," various years; Bureau of Labor Statistics, Census of Employment and Wages.

words, the percentage change in consumption for every 1 percent change in price—is roughly −1. This is higher than others have estimated in the past; like our analysis, more recent state-level data on per-capita cigarette sales also show a larger increase in the estimated elasticity of purchases (Goolsbee, Lovenheim, and Slemrod 2010).

Column 3, row 1 shows how a tax increase would affect employment in tobacco stores, using OLS models like those reported in the first two columns. The coefficient on excise taxes is a statistically significant −0.00948, indicating that a 10 cent increase in excise taxes would reduce employment in tobacco stores by 9.5 percent. We use these results to estimate how changing cigarette consumption would affect employment. Recall that the coefficient in column 2 of table 6.3 indicates how changes in cigarette taxes would reduce the demand for cigarettes. The corresponding coefficient in column 3 identifies how tobacco store employment would change if taxes were raised. The ratio of these two coefficients (column 3 divided by column 2) therefore provides an estimate of the impact of changing cigarette consumption on employment in this industry.[5] For the tobacco stores model we estimate a large elasticity of employment given a change in sales. As shown in the second row of column 3, a 10 percent drop in cigarette consumption is estimated to reduce employment in tobacco stores by 13.5 percent. Because cigarette sales represent nearly 87 percent of sales in tobacco stores, a large elasticity was to be expected.

To examine whether employment changes are due to changes in the number of stores or the average number of employees per store, we also present data on the number of establishments per capita (column 4) and the number of employees per establishment (column 5). In the second row, the coefficient for the number of establishments per capita is nearly identical to that for employees per capita, while the coefficient for employees per establishment is small and statistically insignificant. Together, these estimates suggest that virtually all of the job losses in tobacco stores result from a reduction in the number of establishments rather than fewer employees per establishment.

In table 6.4 we report the impact of changes in tobacco consumption (per-capita cigarette sales) on employment, establishments, and employment per establishment for all six industry groups considered in this analysis. The models include state and year effects, the natural log of real per-capita income, and jobs in the nonretail sector divided by the number of adults. In the equation for convenience stores, we also add the log of per capita gallons of gasoline consumed to control for another factor that might affect retail employment in that sector.[6] The first row repeats the results for tobacco stores, discussed above. In row 2 are the estimates for convenience stores. The elasticity of employment with respect to cigarette consumption is a positive 0.08, meaning a 10 percent reduction in cigarette consumption is expected to generate a 0.8 percent reduction in employment in this sector;

this coefficient is not statistically significant. In row 3 we report estimates for beer, wine, and liquor stores, a grouping with modest tobacco dependence. Interestingly, we find that employment in this industry is actually negatively related to cigarette sales, suggesting that some of the money freed up by declining cigarette sales may be spent on alcohol. The coefficient on the log of per-capita cigarette sales is roughly -0.345, meaning that a 10 percent decline in cigarette sales is predicted to boost employment in this sector by 3.45 percent. This result is statistically significant at conventional levels.

In the remaining three rows, the estimated effects are small and not statistically significant; we cannot be certain these effects are nonexistent. For the combined general merchandise/supermarket sector, shown in row 4, the coefficient of 0.00086 suggests that for every 10 percent reduction in cigarette sales, employment in this sector would fall by less than 0.1 percent. In the model for the "other retail" sector, which has very low dependence on tobacco for sales, the coefficient is negative, suggesting that the money freed up by reducing cigarette consumption may be spent on other consumer goods. The effect is small, indicating a 0.3 percent increase in employment for every 10 percent reduction in cigarette sales. The coefficient for all retail establishments indicates a 0.02 percent increase in employment for every 10 percent reduction in cigarette sales. In the aggregate, these results suggest that even large-scale reductions in cigarette sales would have negligible effects on retail sales employment.

The key result from this analysis is that overall retail employment is expected to change little with decreasing consumption of cigarettes, but there are likely to be distributional consequences for the sector. Some store types, such as tobacco stores and convenience stores, would lose sales in an important product line. These lost sales are likely to translate into lower employment in these types of stores, particularly in tobacco stores. However, this money will be spent somewhere else; beer, wine, and liquor stores in particular may see an increase in employment if cigarette sales decline.

In the final two columns of table 6.4 we report estimates of the impact on the number of establishments per capita and employment per establishment. There are three statistically significant results in these two columns. The first is for tobacco stores: as discussed above, the primary driver for any reduction in employment for this store type will be a reduction in the number of stores. For general merchandise/supermarkets, the coefficient for the number of establishments per capita suggests a drop in the number of establishments per capita of less than 1 percent; this coefficient was significant only at the $p < 0.10$ level. Finally, there was a statistically significant coefficient in the employees per establishment equation among liquor stores, indicating that any increase in employment would occur because existing stores added employees, not because of an increase in the number of stores.

PROJECTING EMPLOYMENT OVER TIME
FOR THE TWO POLICY SCENARIOS

This section presents employment projections through 2025 for all six retail categories in the analysis and estimates how employment would be affected by the two policy scenarios—the IOM recommendations (table 6.5) and the "high-impact" scenario (table 6.6). The first three rows in each table show data from the SimSmoke projections under the baseline case and the policy scenario. The key result is the percentage change in cigarette consumption.

Next, we present results for each of the six retail categories. Each block of results includes four rows. The first gives our employment projections for the baseline (status quo) case. These projections were already reported graphically in figures 6.1–6.7. The second and third rows show the expected number of jobs lost and the expected change in employment under the given policy scenario.[7] The final row of results for each industry group shows the lower and upper 95 percent confidence interval estimates, assuming the only source of error is the parameter estimate of the elasticity. Error in these projections may be quite high due to the inherent "noise" in many of the variables used for these projections, such as our baseline projections in employment, the SimSmoke estimates, and the estimated elasticity. We present these for illustrative purposes to indicate the large amount of uncertainty we have about each of these projections. In reality, uncertainty in these other variables will increase considerably the variance in these projections.

The results in tables 6.5 and 6.6 indicate that the primary job loss from a reduction in cigarette demand will come in the two sectors that are most heavily dependent on tobacco. If the IOM tobacco control recommendations had been adopted in 2006, we estimate that 23,000 workers in tobacco shops and 39,300 workers in convenience stores would have lost their jobs by 2025. We project a much smaller reduction in employment in supermarkets and general merchandise stores (2,600). Some of these losses would be made up by growth in employment in stores that sell alcohol (23,700 workers) and in other retail industries. In the bottom four rows of the table, we report results for the entire retail sector. In aggregate, our best estimate is that by 2025, a net total of 22,900 retail workers would have lost their jobs as a result of reduced cigarette sales if the IOM recommendations had been adopted, with most of these in the tobacco store sector. It is important to remember that the retail sector employs over 18.6 million workers, and 22,900 represent a very small fraction of that total. We also want to caution that many of the results in the table are based on models that have statistically insignificant coefficients. The confidence intervals for most of the predictions are very large, and the predicted employment changes in the retail sector range from a decrease of 489,200 jobs to an increase of 443,300 jobs.

TABLE 6.3 Simulated Impact of Falling Demand for Cigarettes on Employment of Workers in the Retail Sector Under the IOM-Based Scenario

VARIABLE	2005	2010	2015	2020	2025
	Cigarette consumption figures				
Baseline domestic cigarette cons. (millions of packs)	19,377	18,910	18,271	17,459	16,770
Δ in domestic consumption (millions of packs)	0	−7,492	−8,022	−8,275	−8,414
% Δ in domestic consumption	0%	−39.6%	−43.9%	−47.4%	−50.2%
	Tobacco store employees				
Baseline employment (thousands)	27.8	29.2	30.7	32.3	33.9
Δ in employment from baseline (thousands)	0	−15.6	−18.2	−20.6	−23.0
% Δ in employment from baseline	0%	−53.4%	−59.2%	−63.9%	−67.7%
Confidence interval, Δ in employment (thousands)	(0, 0)	(−3.6, −27.6)	(−4.2, −32.1)	(−4.8, −36.5)	(−5.3, −40.6)
	All convenience store employees				
Baseline employment (thousands)	899.1	928.3	958.3	989.4	1,021.5
Δ in employment from baseline (thousands)	0	−28.1	−32.2	−33.9	−39.3
% Δ in employment from baseline	0%	−3.0%	−3.4%	−3.6%	−3.8%
Confidence interval, Δ in employment (thousands)	(0, 0)	(30.0, −86.2)	(34.3, −98.7)	(38.2, −110.0)	(41.8, −120.3)
	Beer, wine, and liquor store employees				
Baseline employment (thousands)	136.4	136.4	136.4	136.4	136.4
Δ in employment from baseline (thousands)	0	13.7	20.7	22.3	23.7
% Δ in employment from baseline	0%	13.7%	15.1%	16.4%	17.3%
Confidence interval, Δ in employment (thousands)	(0, 0)	(35.5, 1.8)	(39.4, 2.0)	(42.5, 2.2)	(45.0, 2.3)

TABLE 6.5 *(Continued)*

VARIABLE	2005	2010	2015	2020	2025
	General merchandise and supermarket employees				
Baseline employment (thousands)	5,195.5	5,342.1	5,511.3	5,745.0	6,097.7
Δ in employment from baseline (thousands)	0	–1.8	–2.1	–2.3	–2.6
% Δ in employment from baseline	0%	–0.03%	–0.04%	–0.04%	–0.04%
Confidence interval, Δ in employment (thousands)	(0, 0)	(1.3, –5.0)	(1.5, –5.7)	(1.7, –6.3)	(1.9, –7.2)
	Other retail establishment employees				
Baseline employment (thousands)	8,950.0	9,458.4	10,163.0	10,753.6	11,267.9
Δ in employment from baseline (thousands)	0	111.8	132.1	150.9	167.4
% Δ in employment from baseline	0%	1.2%	1.3%	1.4%	1.5%
Confidence interval, Δ in employment (thousands)	(0, 0)	(346.7, –123.0)	(409.3, –145.2)	(467.5, –165.8)	(518.7, –184.0)
	All retail employees				
Baseline employment (thousands)	15,208.8	15,984.6	16,800.0	17,656.9	18,557.6
Δ in employment from baseline (thousands)	0	–15.6	–18.1	–20.6	–22.9
% Δ in employment from baseline	0%	–0.11%	–0.11%	–0.12%	–0.12%
Confidence interval, Δ in employment (thousands)	(0, 0)	(301.1, –332.3)	(351.1, –387.8)	(398.3, –439.5)	(443.3, –489.2)

Source: Authors' calculations.

TABLE 5.6 Simulated Impact of Falling Demand for Cigarettes on Employment of Workers in the Retail Sector Under the "High-Impact" Scenario

VARIABLE	2005	2010	2015	2020	2025
			Cigarette consumption figures		
Baseline domestic cigarette cons. (millions of packs)	19,377	18,910	18,271	17,459	16,770
Δ in domestic consumption (millions of packs)	0	−14,241	−13,790	−13,337	−12,955
% Δ in domestic consumption	0%	−75.3%	−75.5%	−76.4%	−77.3%
			Tobacco store employees		
Baseline employment (thousands)	27.8	29.2	30.7	32.3	33.9
Δ in employment from baseline (thousands)	0	−29.2	−30.7	−32.3	−33.9
% Δ in employment from baseline	0%	−100%	−100%	−100%	−100%
Confidence interval, Δ in employment (thousands)	(0, 0)	(−6.9, −52.5)	(−7.3, −55.3)	(−7.7, −58.8)	(−8.2, −62.5)
			All convenience store employees		
Baseline employment (thousands)	899.1	928.3	958.3	989.4	1,021.5
Δ in employment from baseline (thousands)	0	−53.5	−55.4	−57.9	−60.4
% Δ in employment from baseline	0%	−5.77%	−5.78%	−5.85%	−5.92%
Confidence interval, Δ in employment (thousands)	(0, 0)	(56.7, −164.0)	(58.9, −169.7)	(61.6, −177.3)	(64.3, −185.2)

TABLE 6.6 *(Continued)*

VARIABLE	2005	2010	2015	2020	2025
			Beer, wine, and liquor store employees		
Baseline employment (thousands)	136.4	136.4	136.4	136.4	136.4
Δ in employment from baseline (thousands)	0	35.5	35.6	36.0	36.4
% Δ in employment from baseline	0.0%	26.0%	26.0%	26.4%	26.7%
Confidence interval, Δ in employment (thousands)	(0, 0)	(67.5, 3.4)	(67.7, 3.5)	(68.5, 3.5)	(69.3, 3.5)
			General merchandise and supermarket employees		
Baseline employment (thousands)	5,195.5	5,342.1	5,511.3	5,745.0	6,097.7
Δ in employment from baseline (thousands)	0	-3.5	-3.6	-3.8	-4.1
% Δ in employment from baseline	0%	-0.06%	-0.06%	-0.07%	-0.07%
Confidence interval, Δ in employment (thousands)	(0, 0)	(2.5, -9.5)	(2.6, -9.8)	(2.8, -10.3)	(3.0, -11.1)
			Other retail establishment employees		
Baseline employment (thousands)	8,950.0	9,458.4	10,163.0	10,753.6	11,267.9
Δ in employment from baseline (thousands)	0	212.9	227.0	243.2	257.7

% Δ in employment from baseline	0%	2.23%	2.23%	2.26%	2.29%
Confidence interval, Δ in employment (thousands)	(0, 0)	(659.5, −233.9)	(703.6, −249.5)	(753.6, −267.2)	(798.6, −283.2)

All retail employees

Baseline employment (thousands)	15,208.8	15,984.6	16,800.0	17,656.9	18,557.6
Δ in employment from baseline (thousands)	0	−29.7	−31.2	−33.2	−35.3
% Δ in employment from baseline	0%	−0.19%	−0.19%	−0.19%	−0.19%
Confidence interval, Δ in employment (thousands)	(0, 0)	(572.9, −632.1)	(633.5, −665.9)	(642.0, −708.4)	(682.4, −753.0)

Source: Authors' calculations.

Table 6.6 presents comparable figures for the "high-impact" tobacco control policy scenario. As the first few rows of table 6.6 indicate, under this policy scenario tobacco consumption would fall by 75 percent almost immediately with a total drop from baseline consumption of 77 percent by 2025. Because the employment/cigarette use elasticity for tobacco shops is almost 1.4, these large changes imply that the tobacco store industry would be eliminated, with a cut of almost 33,900 jobs. The mean expected job loss in convenience stores is estimated to be about 60,000 workers, with another 4,000 jobs lost in supermarkets and general merchandising. In the aggregate, we estimate job loss in the retail sector of 35,300—about the projected size of the tobacco store sector in 2025 under the baseline scenario. Most of the job loss is again concentrated in the tobacco-intensive establishments, and half of the total job loss is compensated for by rising employment in other sectors of the economy.

Our key findings—that there are no major retail employment losses, but there are distributional consequences resulting from lower cigarette consumption—have also been reported by others. Gottlob (2003) estimated the economic impacts on New Hampshire of raising the state cigarette excise tax by one dollar, from $0.52 to $1.52. This study estimated that the dollar price increase would lead to an 11 percent decline in cigarette sales in the state, resulting in an increase of about 184 retail jobs and 857 jobs in all industries "as money not spent on cigarettes is spent on goods and services with a greater multiplier impact on the local economy" (p. 3). A study from Australia (Junor, Collins, and Lapsley 2004) examined the economic impact of a 25 percent reduction in cigarette consumption and concluded that the impact on retail employment would be very minor.

LIMITATIONS OF THE RESEARCH

Some limitations of this research should be noted. Our analysis is based on sales from brick-and-mortar retailers and does not include mail order/Internet vendors. This is not a major limitation because, according to the 2002 Economic Census, the 219 "electronic shopping and mail-order houses" accounted for only $398,450,000, or 0.78 percent of total tobacco product sales. A nationally representative sample of U.S. smokers showed that only 1.3 percent of smokers purchased their cigarettes from the Internet in 2003 (Hyland et al. 2006); although this figure may have increased (Hrywna, Delnevo, and Staniewska 2004), the 2010 passage of the Prevent All Cigarette Trafficking (PACT) law is expected to curb such sales. Thus, it is unlikely that our focus on brick-and-mortar retailers has biased our findings. In fact, some retail outlets also operate online stores. In 2001, 30.7 percent of Internet vendors operated a retail store (Ribisl, Kim, and Williams 2001), although this proportion has dropped over time (Ribisl, Kim, and Williams 2007). In addition, as mentioned earlier, the Economic Census data are based on all tobacco products and not solely cigarettes. This is not a major limitation because about 93 percent of tobacco product sales are for cigarettes. Third, our analysis assumes that the existing distribution of tobacco sales across types of stores would be unaffected by changes in tobacco control policy. This may not be realistic: for instance, an excise tax increase could shift consumption to tobacco store retailers, many of whom offer discount prices.

Because of data availability, our analyses using data from the Economic Census were restricted to tobacco retailers with payroll. The exact number of tobacco retailers with and without payroll is not known precisely, but it has been estimated by others. When the U.S. Food and Drug Administration (FDA) claimed jurisdiction over tobacco products, it estimated the economic impact of the proposed rules on tobacco retailers (U.S. Department of Health and Human Services 1996). The FDA had estimated that there were 280,883 payroll establishments and 127,035 nonpayroll establishments selling tobacco products over the counter. These nonpayroll establishments are likely to be smaller (e.g., family-run corner store) and to have a lower sales volume. The extent to which the inclusion of nonpayroll establishments would alter our findings is unknown, but we see no reason to assume these establishments would be affected differently than payroll establishments. The most likely effect of excluding these businesses is to understate the total job loss due to the tobacco control policy scenarios, but the extent of the understatement depends on the distribution of these nonpayroll establishments across store type, and thus the extent of their dependence on tobacco sales.

Finally, our analysis of economic impact focused on how consumption declines would affect sales of tobacco products, but retailers could also be affected by changes in direct payments from cigarette manufacturers. Approximately two-thirds of stores selling tobacco products receive payments from the tobacco companies. The tobacco industry provides more money to retailers than manufacturers of other consumer products, such as snack foods and soft drinks (Feighery et al. 1999, 2003, 2004). In one study of small retailers in California, the average retailer reported receiving $2,462 annually (1997 dollars) in incentive payments for premium shelf space and price discounts on volume purchases (Feighery et al. 1999). Thus, retailers profit directly by selling tobacco products to smokers and indirectly by displaying and merchandising tobacco products in prime locations in their stores (Bloom 2001). We should point out that the price discounts, or "buydowns," are passed on to the consumer and do not yield direct profit for the retailer, other than the fact that they serve as a stimulus to increase cigarette sales. The retailer lowers the price of cigarettes by a set amount, and the manufacturer rebates the discount amount back to the retailer (Feighery et al. 2003).

These payments have increased substantially over the last several decades, even as cigarette consumption has declined, as other avenues for marketing have been restricted (Bloom 2001; Federal Trade Commission 2007). According to the most recently released report by the Federal Trade Commission (2009), total spending at retail outlets (i.e., point-of-sale, price discounts, promotional allowances-retailers, retail value-added) had declined slightly from $11.13 billion in 2005 to $10.71 billion in 2006; price discounts represented $9.21 billion, or 73.7 percent of expenditures in 2006. Because contracts between retailers and cigarette companies are confidential, there are no standardized longitudinal data sets that can be used to model the increase or decrease in retailer payments. It is unclear whether tobacco companies facing a substantial reduction in consumption would raise payments to retailers in an effort to stimulate demand or lower these payments as the industry is scaled down.

CONCLUSIONS

To our knowledge, this is the first national study of the implications of tobacco control policies for the retail sector. Given the concern frequently expressed about the impact of excise taxes and other tobacco control measures on small retail businesses, this study makes an important contribution.

Over the period from 1990 to 2004, we estimate the relationship between cigarette consumption and retail employment levels and use these estimates to simulate demand for retailer employment through 2025 under two policy scenarios. If the IOM's recommended tobacco control policies had been adopted in 2006, cigarette consumption would be predicted to fall by 50.2 percent by 2025, generating the following percent changes in retail-sector employment: a 67.7 percent drop in tobacco stores, a 3.8 percent drop in convenience stores, a 17.3 percent increase in beer/wine/liquor stores, a 0.04 percent increase in supermarkets/general merchandise, and a 0.12 percent increase in all retail. The change in aggregate retail employment we estimate is essentially equal to the drop in employment in tobacco stores. Although there would be distributional consequences of policies to markedly reduce cigarette consumption in the United States, given the vast size of the retail sector (18.6 million employees) the impact on overall employment for all retailers shows little evidence of serious economic harm.

NOTES

1. http://www.ers.usda.gov/Briefing/Tobacco/Data/table21.pdf.
2. More information about the data is available on the BLS Web page at http://www.bls
.gov/cew/home.htm.

3. These data are available from the U.S. Bureau of the Census, http://www.census.gov/popest/states/.

4. Both of these variables are downloadable from the Bureau of Economic Analysis Web page, http://www.bea.gov/bea/regional/data.htm.

5. In an econometric model, this is equivalent to running a two-stage least-squares (2SLS) model with log employment as the dependent variable (column 3) on log per capita packs of cigarettes and other variables, then using real cigarette taxes as an instrument for log per capita packs of cigarettes. Because this is an exactly identified model, the ratio of the two tax variables exactly produces the 2SLS estimate.

6. Gallons of gasoline purchased at state level are available from the U.S. Department of Transportation, Federal Highway Administration's annual publication *Highway Statistics* (http://www.fhwa.dot.gov/policy/ohpi/hss/index.htm).

7. To calculate the percentage change in employment, we multiplied the estimated percentage change in cigarette consumption from the SimSmoke model by the results from the 2SLS model that estimates the percentage change in employment given a percentage change in consumption. For example, from table 6.5, SimSmoke estimates that cigarette consumption would be 39.6 percent lower in 2010 if the IOM policy recommendations were adopted. In the 2SLS results, for tobacco stores we estimated an employment elasticity with respect to consumption of 1.349, which means a 10 percent drop in consumption would reduce employment by 13.49 percent. To get the percentage change in employment in this scenario, we simply multiply 1.349 by 0.396 to get 0.534 (in other words, a 53.4 percent reduction).

7

NATIONAL ECONOMIC IMPACT OF CLEAN INDOOR AIR REGULATIONS ON THE HOSPITALITY INDUSTRY

ANDREW HYLAND, MARK TRAVERS, AND BRIAN FIX

R egulation of smoking in public places began in the United States more than 35 years ago, in 1973, when Arizona became the first state to pass a statewide smoking control law to restrict smoking in public places (U.S. Department of Health and Human Services 1989). The following year, Connecticut became the first state to restrict smoking in restaurants (U.S. Department of Health and Human Services 1991). As the deleterious health effects of secondhand smoke became more widely known in the 1980s (National Research Council 1986; U.S. Department of Health and Human Services 1986) and early 1990s (U.S. Environmental Protection Agency 1992), nonsmokers' rights organizations began to lobby for laws to protect nonsmokers from secondhand smoke (Centers for Disease Control 1991). State and local governments passed scores of laws that prohibited or significantly limited smoking in all types of public places ranging from government buildings to private worksites. A major advance in smoke-free regulation took place in 1995, when the state of California implemented a law requiring all restaurants to be smoke-free, and New York City made restaurants with more than 35 seats smoke-free. As of April 2010, 17,628 municipalities—and home to about three-quarters of the country's population—were covered by a 100 percent smoke-free state or local provision in workplaces, restaurants, or bars (American Nonsmokers' Rights Foundation 2010). These laws have attracted widespread public support across a range of contexts (e.g., Bernat et al. 2009; Friis and Safer 2005; Rayens et al. 2008).

The expansion of smoke-free legislation may have gained impetus from the 2006 U.S. Surgeon General's report on the health consequences of exposure to tobacco smoke. This report summarized research on the link between second-hand smoke and heart disease, lung cancer, and a variety of other diseases in both adults and children, and concluded that there is no safe level of exposure (U.S. Department of Health and Human Services 2006). More recently, the Institute of Medicine (2009) reviewed the evidence on secondhand smoke and cardiovascular disease and concluded that smoking bans reduce the risk of heart attacks. Secondhand smoke is a particular concern for employees in the hospitality industry. Studies have shown that hospitality workers experience substantial exposure to secondhand smoke and are at heightened risk for lung cancer (Siegel and Skeer 2003). Smoking bans are associated with improvement of air quality in hospitality settings and with a reduction in environmental tobacco smoke exposure and an improvement in workers' respiratory health (Abrams et al. 2007; Bondy et al. 2009; Eisner, Smith, and Blanc 1998; Farrelly et al. 2005b; Lee et al. 2007).

Despite their health benefits, smoke-free regulations often generate considerable debate because of concern that the hospitality industry will be adversely affected (Anonymous 1995). Restaurants, bars, and other hospitality-related businesses are said to face as much as a 30 percent loss in business. Unlike tobacco farming and cigarette manufacturing, which represent small and regionally concentrated sectors, the hospitality industry is a significant share of the national economy: in 2010 the restaurant industry was expected to comprise 4 percent of the U.S. gross domestic product and 9 percent of the U.S. workforce (National Restaurant Association 2010). As the industry grows, so will the number of employment opportunities; restaurant employment is projected to expand by 1.3 million jobs between 2010 and 2020 (National Restaurant Association 2010). If the hospitality industry is indeed hurt by smoke-free legislation, the economic impact could be considerable.

This chapter reviews the existing evidence in order to estimate the net economic impact of a national-level clean indoor air policy on business indicators for the hospitality industry overall and by specific industry subgroup. The chapter includes a review of the existing research in this area. In addition, we report a new empirical analysis that compares hospitality employment trends in U.S. states that have and have not adopted smoke-free regulations. Our conclusion discusses the implications of this evidence for the economic impact of tobacco control policy.

A REVIEW OF PREVIOUS RESEARCH

In 2003 Scollo et al. published a review of 97 studies of the economic impact of smoke-free hospitality regulations. Most of these studies examined smoke-free restaurant policies; only a few examined bars or hotels. Overall, the results of these studies were mixed: some concluded that smoke-free regulations were bad for business, while others concluded they had no effect. A different picture emerged when the authors examined only the most methodologically rigorous studies. There were 21 studies that met the most rigorous study-design criteria: they used objective measurements, had sufficient pre- and postlaw data, and used statistical methods to control for underlying economic trends and other factors that could also have affected business indicators. None of these well-designed studies concluded that smoke-free regulations caused adverse economic outcomes in the hospitality industry.

Although the Scollo et al. paper is the most thorough review available for this topic, it included few studies of nonrestaurant hospitality businesses, and many of the studies it reviewed were conducted before the most recent smoke-free policies had been implemented. No current study quantitatively assesses the potential economic impact of smoke-free regulations across multiple states that have passed smoke-free regulations. To fill these gaps, this chapter updates the Scollo et al. review. As in the previous review, we evaluated the quality of each study's research design as well as its conclusions about the economic impact of smoke-free regulations.

This analysis includes the studies listed in a wide-ranging summary created by the VicHealth Centre for Tobacco Control (http://www.vctc.org.au/tc-res/Hospitalitysummary.pdf). Studies examining the economic outcomes of smoke-free policies in the hospitality industry were identified through electronic databases and Internet searches. Studies included in this analysis were published before July 2005. All of them used quantitative measures of the economic impact of smoke-free policies on the hospitality industry; measures of impact included changes in revenue, employment, number of establishments, bankruptcy figures, patron reports of changes in their habits, and proprietors' estimates of changes in sales and patronage. These studies came from both peer-reviewed and non-peer-reviewed sources. If we have omitted studies published during this time frame, we suspect these omitted studies are likely to have found no effect on economic indicators; because studies reporting a negative impact often generate a lot of attention in the media, they are more likely to have come to our attention.

Two researchers (Brian Fix and Anita Lal from the Cancer Council Victoria, Melbourne, Australia) independently classified study results and study design characteristics. We analyzed all studies together and also conducted separate analyses for four business types: restaurants, bars, hotels, and gaming venues. The outcome of interest was whether the study concluded that smoke-free regulations were associated with a negative economic impact. The economic effect indicated by each study was classified as positive, negative, or null based either on the stated conclusion or, if the outcome was not explicitly stated, the mutual interpretation of the two reviewers. In all, the updated review examined 122 studies of the economic impact of smoke-free air policies on the hospitality industry, including all studies originally considered in the Scollo et al. paper.

As the previous review by Scollo et al. (2003) shows, study conclusions can vary dramatically based on the methodological rigor of the study. Based on previous work, we used four criteria to rate the quality of the study design: (1) the use of objective data such as employment, taxable sales, or licensure statistics, rather than subjective measures such as consumer self-reports of the likelihood of patronizing establishments or proprietor estimates of revenue change; (2) the inclusion of data both before and after implementation of smoke-free air legislation; (3) the use of regression or other statistical methods; and (4) the use of controls for economic trends that could also affect business indicators. Studies that met all four of these criteria were deemed to have a more rigorous study design. In addition, studies published in peer-reviewed journals were more credible because they have undergone review by experts in the relevant field. Studies that met the four quality criteria and/or were published in peer-reviewed journals were considered the most credible. The intent in making these distinctions was not to evaluate the relative importance of each specific criterion but rather to use these criteria together to identify the more rigorous studies.

To supplement these comparisons, we include analyses by two additional indicators. The first is one of our four study-design criteria, the use of objective measures rather than subjective measures. We also sought to identify the funding source for each study by examining its acknowledgements. If no funder was acknowledged, other efforts were made to establish whether study authors had ever received monetary support from the tobacco industry or any group affiliated with the tobacco industry by searching publicly available industry documents at www .tobaccodocuments.org.

We used SPSS 14.0 to analyze data on the association between study conclusions and study quality measures. Chi-square values and odds ratios were used to compare the studies that did or did not report a negative economic impact. No statistical tests were performed for subgroups with fewer than 10 studies.

RESULTS

Of the 122 studies examined in this analysis, 47 percent used objective outcome measures and 24 percent were peer-reviewed. Thirty-one studies (25 percent) met all four of our criteria for methodological quality. Of the 122 studies, 36 (31 percent) were funded directly by the tobacco industry or by a group with ties to the tobacco industry. Five studies did not disclose their funding source. Some studies examined outcomes in more than one type of hospitality location (e.g., restaurants and bars); thus, the sum of studies across all four industry types is greater than 122.

TABLE 7.1 Findings of Higher-Quality Studies

	CONCLUSION OF NEGATIVE IMPACT?		
	YES	NO	*p*-VALUE
Met All Four Study Design Criteria (n = 31)	3.2% (1/31)	96.8% (30/31)	< 0.01
Bars [9, 11, 31, 46, 51, 57, 99, 117]	0.0% (0/8)	100.0% (8/8)	0.04
Restaurants [7, 8, 9, 10, 11, 12, 31, 46, 53, 54, 56, 57, 58, 61, 65, 66, 68, 69, 88, 95, 103, 104, 112, 116, 117, 120]	0.0% (0/26)	100.0% (26/26)	< 0.01
Hotels [52, 57, 99, 112]	0.0% (0/4)	100.0% (4/4)	0.03
Gaming venues [57, 84, 100]	33.3% (1/3)	66.7% (2/3)	N/A
Peer Reviewed (n = 29)	3.4% (1/29)	96.6% (28/29)	< 0.01
Bars [9, 11, 13, 14]	0.0% (0/4)	100.0% (4/4)	0.16
Restaurants [7, 9, 10, 11, 13, 14, 27, 30, 38, 53, 54, 56, 62, 65, 66, 67, 68, 69, 71, 73, 110, 111, 112, 115, 119, 120]	3.8% (1/26)	96.2% (25/26)	< 0.01
Hotels [52, 112]	0.0% (0/2)	100.0% (2/2)	0.18
Gaming venues [13, 55, 84]	0.0% (0/3)	100.0% (3/3)	N/A
Met All Four Study Design Criteria AND Peer Reviewed (n = 15)	0.0% (0/15)	100.0% (15/15)	< 0.01
Bars [9, 11]	0.0% (0/2)	100.0% (2/2)	N/A
Restaurants [7, 9, 10, 11, 53, 54, 56, 62, 66, 69, 71, 112, 120]	0.0% (0/13)	100.0% (13/13)	< 0.01
Hotels [52, 112]	0.0% (0/2)	100.0% (2/2)	N/A
Gaming venues [84]	0.0% (0/1)	100.0% (1/1)	N/A

Source: Reference numbers of studies in each industry segment are from appendix 7.1 and are given in square brackets.

Table 7.1 presents the conclusions of the studies by indicators of study quality. Of the 31 studies that met all four of the methodological criteria, only one reported a negative economic impact of smoke-free policies, whereas the other 30 reported either no impact or a positive impact. Of the 29 peer-reviewed studies, 28 found no economic impact. Fifteen studies met all four methodological criteria and were peer reviewed; none of these concluded that smoke-free regulations were harmful to the hospitality industry overall or for any industry subset.

Table 7.2 examines the correlates of studies that found a negative economic impact of smoke-free regulations. These studies were significantly more likely to

TABLE 7.2 Selected Study Quality Indicators by Study Conclusion of a Negative Impact

	STUDIES FINDING A NEGATIVE OUTCOME	STUDIES NOT FINDING A NEGATIVE OUTCOME	*p*-VALUE
% Using Subjective Outcome Measures Only	77.5% (31/40)	41.5% (34/82)	< 0.01
Bars	75.0% (12/16) [3, 4, 19, 20, 29, 39, 41, 74, 82, 83, 87, 91, 107, 108, 109, 118]	44.1% (15/34) [2, 5, 9, 11, 13, 14, 15, 16, 17, 18, 26, 28, 31, 32, 33, 36, 40, 46, 47, 48, 49, 51, 57, 60, 61, 92, 94, 97, 98, 99, 101, 104, 117, 121]	0.04
Restaurants	80.6% (29/36) [1, 3, 4, 19, 20, 21, 22, 29, 34, 38, 39, 41, 44, 45, 50, 72, 74, 75, 76, 79, 80, 81, 82, 86, 87, 89, 90, 91, 96, 102, 105, 106, 109, 114, 118, 119]	39.4% (26/66) [2, 6, 7, 8, 9, 10, 11, 12, 13, 14, 16, 17, 18, 23, 24, 25, 27, 28, 30, 31, 32, 35, 37, 40, 46, 53, 54, 56, 57, 58, 59, 60, 61, 62, 63, 64, 65, 66, 67, 68, 69, 70, 71, 73, 77, 78, 85, 88, 92, 93, 95, 97, 98, 99, 103, 104, 110, 111, 112, 113, 115, 116, 117, 119, 120, 121]	< 0.01
Hotels	71.4% (5/7) [1, 3, 4, 42, 75, 105, 118]	25.0% (2/8) [2, 16, 24, 40, 52, 57, 99, 112]	0.08
Gaming venues	0.0% (0/2) [100, 118]	66.7% (4/6) [2, 13, 55, 57, 84, 93]	N/A
% Funded by the Tobacco Industry or a Group Supported by the Tobacco Industry	97.2% (35/36)	2.4% (2/82)	< 0.01
Bars	91.7% (11/12) [3, 4, 19, 20, 29, 41, 74, 82, 83, 87, 109, 118]	2.9% (1/34) [2, 5, 9, 11, 13, 14, 15, 16, 17, 18, 26, 28, 31, 32, 33, 36, 40, 46, 47, 48, 49, 51, 57, 60, 61, 92, 94, 97, 98, 99, 101, 104, 117, 121]	< 0.01

TABLE 7.2 *(Continued)*

	STUDIES FINDING A NEGATIVE OUTCOME	STUDIES NOT FINDING A NEGATIVE OUTCOME	p-VALUE
Restaurants	96.9% (32/33) [1, 3, 4, 19, 20, 21, 22, 29, 34, 38, 41, 44, 45, 50, 74, 75, 76, 79, 80, 81, 83, 86, 87, 89, 90, 96, 102, 105, 106, 109, 114, 118, 119] .	3% (2/66) [2, 6, 7, 8, 9, 10, 11, 12, 13, 14, 16, 17, 18, 23, 24, 25, 27, 28, 30, 31, 32, 35, 37, 40, 46, 53, 54, 56, 57, 58, 59, 60, 61, 62, 63, 64, 65, 66, 67, 68, 69, 70, 71, 73, 77, 78, 85, 88, 92, 93, 95, 97, 98, 99, 103, 104, 110, 111, 112, 113, 115, 116, 117, 119, 120, 121]	< 0.01
Hotels	100.0% (7/7) [1, 3, 4, 42, 75, 105, 118]	0.0% (0/8) [2, 16, 24, 40, 52, 57, 99, 112]	< 0.01
Gaming venues	100.0% (2/2) [100, 118]	0.0% (0/6) [2, 13, 55, 57, 84, 93]	N/A
% Not Peer Reviewed	97.5% (39/40)	65.9% (54/82)	< 0.01
Bars	100.0% (16/16) [3, 4, 19, 20, 29, 39, 41, 74, 82, 83, 87, 91, 107, 108, 109, 118]	88.2% (30/34) [2, 5, 9, 11, 13, 14, 15, 16, 17, 18, 26, 28, 31, 32, 33, 36, 40, 46, 47, 48, 49, 51, 57, 60, 61, 92, 94, 97, 98, 99, 101, 104, 117, 121]	0.16
Restaurants	97.2% (35/36) [1, 3, 4, 19, 20, 21, 22, 29, 34, 38, 39, 41, 44, 45, 50, 72, 74, 75, 76, 79, 80, 81, 83, 86, 87, 89, 90, 91, 96, 102, 105, 106, 109, 114, 118, 119]	65.2% (43/66) [2, 4, 7, 8, 9, 10, 11, 12, 13, 14, 16, 17, 18, 23, 24, 25, 27, 28, 30, 31, 32, 35, 37, 40, 46, 53, 54, 56, 57, 58, 59, 60, 61, 62, 63, 64, 65, 66, 67, 68, 69, 70, 71, 73, 77, 78, 85, 88, 92, 94, 95, 97, 98, 99, 103, 104, 110, 111, 112, 113, 115, 116, 117, 119, 120, 121]	< 0.01
Hotels	100.0% (7/7) [1, 3, 4, 42, 75, 105, 118]	75.0% (6/8) [2, 16, 24, 40, 52, 57, 99, 112]	0.18
Gaming venues	100.0% (2/2) [100, 118]	50.0% (3/6) [2, 13, 55, 57, 84, 93]	N/A

Source: Reference numbers of studies in each industry segment are from appendix 7.1 and are given in square brackets.

use subjective measures and to be funded by the tobacco industry or by an agency with ties to the industry, and less likely to be published in a peer-reviewed journal. Subgroup analysis revealed a similar pattern for bars, restaurants, and hotels, although some of these comparisons were not statistically significant.

Like the Scollo et al. study, this updated review shows the importance of taking study quality into account in examining the economic impact of smoke-free laws. Among studies with weaker designs, half reported that smoke-free laws had a negative effect. Among the 31 studies that met all four study design criteria, only one—a study of gaming establishments—concluded that smoke-free laws were detrimental to business. More research is needed on the impact on bars, hotels, and gaming establishments, as there were few well-designed studies of these types of venues; for gaming establishments in particular, there were only a handful of studies, and the results were mixed.

EMPIRICAL ANALYSIS

Although many studies have evaluated the impact of smoke-free regulations in specific locations, few have examined business indicators for the hospitality industry across a large geographic area to estimate the overall net impact of comprehensive smoke-free regulations. Here, we focus on one set of indicators: employment in restaurants and bars. We compare changes in employment for states that have and have not adopted comprehensive smoke-free regulations, using monthly data from 1990 to 2005.

DATA AND MEASURES

The Quarterly Census of Employment and Wages (QCEW) program is a cooperative program involving the Bureau of Labor Statistics (BLS) of the U.S. Department of Labor and the State Employment Security Agencies (SESAs). The QCEW program produces a comprehensive tabulation of employment and wage information for workers covered by state unemployment insurance (UI) laws and federal workers covered by the Unemployment Compensation for Federal Employees (UCFE) program. The QCEW program serves as a near census of monthly employment information as this program includes 99.7 percent of all wage and salary civilian employment. Publicly available files include data on the number of establishments, monthly employment, and quarterly wages by North American Industry Classification System (NAICS) industry, by county, and by ownership sector for the entire United States.

For this study, all available monthly employment data from January 1990 through June 2005 were obtained for all 50 U.S. states, the District of Columbia,

TABLE 7.3 Implementation Dates of Statewide Restaurant and Bar Laws

	SMOKE-FREE RESTAURANT LAW IMPLEMENTATION DATE	DATE *RESTLAW* INDICATOR VARIABLE IS SET TO 1	SMOKE-FREE BAR LAW IMPLEMENTATION DATE	DATE *BARLAW* INDICATOR VARIABLE IS SET TO 1
California	January 1, 1995	January 1995	January 1, 1998	January 1998
Connecticut	October 1, 2003	October 2003	April 1, 2004	April 2004
Delaware	November 27, 2002	December 2002	November 27, 2002	December 2002
Florida	July 1, 2003	July 2003	N/A	N/A
Idaho	July 1, 2004	July 2004	N/A	N/A
Maine	January 1, 2004	January 2004	January 1, 2004	January 2004
Massachusetts	July 5, 2004	July 2004	July 5, 2004	July 2004
New York	July 24, 2003	August 2003	July 24, 2003	August 2003
Rhode Island	March 1, 2005	March 2005	March 31, 2005	April 2005
Utah	January 1, 1995	January 1995	N/A	N/A

Source: American Nonsmokers' Rights Foundation. "Chronological Table of U.S. Population Protected by 100% Smokefree State or Local Laws," http://www.no-smoke.org/pdf/EffectivePopulationList.pdf.

Puerto Rico, and the Virgin Islands for the following NAICS industry classifications: Food Service and Drinking Places subsector (NAICS code 722); Full-Service Restaurants industry group (7221); Limited-Service Restaurants industry group (7222); and Drinking Places industry group (7224). In addition, employment data for the Retail Trade sector (44–45) were also obtained. Data were restricted to private employment only. The BLS withholds publication of UI-covered employment and wage data for any industry level when necessary to protect the identity of employers. As a result, data are missing for certain combinations of month, state, and industry, although the amount of missing data is small.[1]

We created a set of variables indicating the presence of statewide smoke-free restaurant and bar laws using a list of smoke-free laws and implementation dates obtained from www.no-smoke.org. Table 7.3 shows the laws that went into effect between January 1990 and June 2005, the period included in this analysis. The table also shows for which month the indicator variables RESTLAW and BAR-LAW were changed from 0 to 1.

DESCRIPTIVE STATISTICS

Our descriptive analyses compared the level of employment before and after statewide smoke-free regulations were implemented overall and by industry subtype and state. For the nine states that passed statewide smoke-free restaurant laws as well as the six states that passed statewide smoke-free bar laws by July 1, 2004, we calculated annualized rates of employment change for the pre-law and postlaw periods. Prelaw comparisons are made by comparing the average monthly employment level for the 12 months of the baseline data year (January to December 1990) to the average for the 12-month period immediately before the passage of the given smoke-free law for a given state. This figure describes trends in hospitality employment prior to passage of the smoke-free law. Comparisons for postlaw periods are made from the average employment of the 12 months prior to implementation of the law to the period between July 2004 and June 2005. The annualized rate of change between these two periods was then calculated and compared. We also calculated average rates of prelaw and postlaw employment change across these states, weighted by the baseline employment level in each state as well as the fraction of months a given policy was in effect. In other words, larger states and those with laws in effect for longer periods of time contributed greater weight to the summary employment change statistic. In addition, the annualized rate of change in employment was also calculated for all states that did not have a state smoking policy implemented during the study period. No formal statistical tests were performed in this descriptive analysis.

The hospitality sector comprises both full- and limited-service restaurants, which account for about 85 percent of all hospitality employment; only about 5 percent of hospitality employees work in bars or taverns. Employment has increased in the hospitality industry in general, but the trend for the bar and tavern industry subsector has been negative. If smoke-free restaurant regulations were harmful to business, then one would expect to see a decrease in hospitality and restaurant employment, and possibly an increase in bar employment as some patrons switched from dining in restaurants to bars. Smoke-free regulations in bars should have the opposite effect.

Tables 7.4 and 7.5 present employment data before and after implementation of statewide smoke-free restaurant and bar laws by hospitality industry subsector. Compared with states that did not pass a statewide smoke-free law, the states that implemented smoke-free restaurant and bar laws had generally lower employment growth rates across all industry subsectors both before and after smoke-free laws passed. Although there is variability across states in employment trends, the range of observed changes is relatively modest. For example, across the entire hospitality industry (NAICS Code 722), the annualized percentage change in employment across states before a smoke-free law was implemented ranged from 0.8 percent to 6.2 percent, whereas the range after the smoke-free laws was 0.9 percent to 5.1 percent. Full-service restaurants experienced faster employment growth after the passage of smoke-free restaurant laws. Employment growth in limited-service restaurants was approximately the same before and after smoke-free laws, whereas bar employment declined more quickly after such laws were passed. Hospitality and full-service restaurant employment also increased after passage of smoke-free bar laws, but employment indicators for limited-service restaurants and bars were less favorable after smoke-free bar laws were passed.

MULTIVARIATE ANALYSIS

Although tables 7.4 and 7.5 provide a descriptive overview, a more detailed statistical analysis is needed to consider how smoke-free policies may have influenced changes in employment. Changes in the logarithm of monthly employment in each of four industries (722, 7221, 7222, 7224) for each of the 53 states, district, and territories (the 50 U.S. states, the District of Columbia, Puerto Rico, and the U.S. Virgin Islands) were modeled as a linear function of several predictor variables. In addition, we constructed four other outcome measures: the monthly employment in each industry divided by the total monthly retail trade employment (NAICS 44–45) for each state. These outcomes, including retail employment, were multiplied by 100 for scaling purposes. (See appendix 7.2 for more detail on this multivariate analysis.)

TABLE 7.4 Changes in Hospitality Employment by Industry Type and State Before and After Smoke-Free Restaurant Laws Were Implemented, 1990–2005

INDUSTRY CODE	STATE	DATE OF RESTAURANT LAW	JAN.–DEC. 1990 EMPLOYMENT LEVEL	LAW DATE EMPLOYMENT LEVEL	JULY 2004–JUNE 2005 EMPLOYMENT LEVEL	ANNUAL % CHANGE PRE-LAW[a]	ANNUAL % CHANGE POST-LAW[a]	OVERALL WEIGHTED ANNUAL % CHANGE IN STATES WITH SMOKE-FREE LAWS PRE-LAW[b]	POST-LAW[b]	ANNUAL % CHANGE IN STATES WITH NO SMOKE-FREE LAW[c]
722	All States							1.9%	2.5%	2.7%
Overall sector	California	Jan. 1995	766,054	790,751	1,011,927	0.8%	2.4%			
	Connecticut	Oct. 2003	78,321	89,478	92,782	1.0%	2.2%			
	Delaware	Dec. 2002	26,142	26,478	28,740	4.0%	3.2%			
	Florida	July 2003	376,481	494,277	545,822	2.2%	5.1%			
	Idaho	July 2004	25,822	39,528	40,684	3.2%	2.9%			
	Maine	Jan. 2004	33,053	39,421	39,965	1.4%	0.9%			
	Massachusetts	July 2004	170,114	210,082	212,259	1.6%	1.0%			
	New York	Aug. 2003	371,510	437,071	455,240	1.3%	2.1%			
	Utah	Jan. 1995	42,411	53,854	70,453	6.2%	2.6%			
	All States							2.1%	3.1%	3.8%
7221	California	Jan. 1995	363,593	349,934	483,032	–1.0%	3.1%			

TABLE 7.4 (Continued)

INDUSTRY CODE	STATE	DATE OF RESTAURANT LAW	JAN.–DEC. 1990 EMPLOYMENT LEVEL	LAW DATE EMPLOYMENT LEVEL	JULY 2004–JUNE 2005 EMPLOYMENT LEVEL	ANNUAL % CHANGE PRE-LAW[a]	ANNUAL % CHANGE POST-LAW[a]	OVERALL WEIGHTED ANNUAL % CHANGE IN STATES WITH SMOKE-FREE LAWS PRE-LAW[b]	POST-LAW[b]	ANNUAL % CHANGE IN STATES WITH NO SMOKE-FREE LAW[c]
Full-service restaurants	Connecticut	Oct. 2003	35,661	44,626	45,482	1.8%	1.1%			
	Delaware	Dec. 2002	8,499	13,541	14,699	1.2%	4.4%			
	Florida	July 2003	190,751	274,125	299,801	2.9%	4.6%			
	Idaho	July 2004	11,608	18,878	19,109	3.7%	1.2%			
	Maine	Jan. 2004	17,512	22,624	22,697	2.0%	0.2%			
	Massachusetts	July 2004	79,779	106,115	107,013	2.1%	0.8%			
	New York	Aug. 2003	183,039	224,196	231,126	1.6%	1.6%			
	Utah	Jan. 1995	14,150	19,540	30,004	8.4%	4.2%			
	All States							2.5%	2.4%	2.5%
7222	California	Jan. 1995	319,960	369,468	457,303	3.7%	2.1%			
Limited-service restaurants	Connecticut	Oct. 2003	26,454	32,158	34,621	1.5%	4.5%			
	Delaware	Dec. 2002	9,175	10,581	11,813	1.2%	4.4%			
	Florida	July 2003	134,073	179,616	201,124	2.4%	5.8%			
	Idaho	July 2004	11,431	16,746	17,655	2.9%	5.4%			

	State	Date				%a	%b	%c
	Maine	Jan. 2004	12,622	14,178	14,757		0.9%	2.7%
	Massachusetts	July 2004	61,255	75,451	77,077		1.6%	2.2%
	New York	Aug. 2003	110,341	144,200	155,051		2.2%	3.9%
	Utah	Jan. 1995	24,589	29,211	35,390		4.4%	1.8%
	All States					−0.7%	−1.2%	−0.6%
7224 Drinking places	California	Jan. 1995	28,326	26,642	24,055		−1.5%	−1.0%
	Connecticut	Oct. 2003	4,004	2,572	2,506		−3.4%	−1.5%
	Delaware	Dec. 2302	1,188	964	654		−20.4%	−14.0%
	Florida	July 2003	24,646	17,369	17,938		−2.8%	1.6%
	Idaho	July 2004	1,750	2,508	2,523		2.7%	0.6%
	Maine	Jan. 2004	984	932	845		−0.4%	−6.3%
	Massachusetts	July 2004	11,699	8,933	8,251		−2.0%	−7.5%
	New York	Aug. 2003	20,574	18,943	17,581		−0.7%	−3.8%
	Utah	Jan. 1995	1,766	2,494	2,696		9.0%	0.7%

Notes: The baseline employment levels for Delaware for industries 722 and 7224 are for January–December 2001 instead of January–December 1990 because earlier data were unavailable from the Bureau of Labor Statistics.

[a] Annualized percentage change in employment level based on the number of months the policy was in effect.

[b] Post-law annual percentage employment change is weighted by the January–December 1990 average employment level for each state as well as months the smoking policy was in effect.

[c] Annualized percentage change in employment for all states/district/territories without a statewide smoke-free restaurant law (excluded states are California, Connecticut, Delaware, Florida, Idaho, Maine, Massachusetts, New York, Rhode Island, and Utah). In addition, Alabama is excluded from industry 722. New Hampshire, North Dakota, Virginia, and Wyoming are excluded from industry 7224. 722 (n = 42), 7221 (n = 43), 7222 (n = 43), 7224 (n = 39).

Source: U.S. Department of Labor, Bureau of Labor Statistics, Quarterly Census of Employment and Wages.

TABLE 7.5 Changes in Hospitality Employment by Industry Type and State Before and After Smoke-Free Bar Laws Were Implemented, 1990–2005

INDUSTRY CODE	STATE	DATE OF BAR LAW	JAN.–DEC. 1990 EMPLOYMENT LEVEL	LAW DATE EMPLOYMENT LEVEL	JULY 2004–JUNE 2005 EMPLOYMENT LEVEL	ANNUAL % CHANGE PRE-LAW[a]	ANNUAL % CHANGE POST-LAW[a]	OVERALL WEIGHTED ANNUAL % CHANGE IN STATES WITH SMOKE-FREE LAWS PRE-LAW[b]	POST-LAW[b]	ANNUAL % CHANGE IN STATES WITH NO SMOKE-FREE LAW[c]
722	All States							1.5%	2.2%	2.7%
	California	Jan. 1998	766,054	857,303	1,011,927	1.6%	2.2%			
Overall sector	Connecticut	April 2004	78,321	90,517	92,782	1.1%	2.0%			
	Delaware	Dec. 2002	26,142	26,478	28,740	1.4%	3.2%			
	Maine	Jan. 2004	33,053	39,421	39,965	1.4%	0.9%			
	Massachusetts	July 2004	170,114	210,082	212,259	1.6%	1.0%			
	New York	Aug. 2003	371,510	437,071	455,240	1.3%	2.1%			
	All States							1.5%	2.8%	3.8%
7221	California	Jan. 1998	363,593	386,001	483,032	0.9%	3.0%			

Full-service restaurants	Connecticut	April 2004	35,661	44,920	45,482	1.8%	1.0%			
	Delaware	Dec. 2002	8,499	13,541	14,699	4.0%	3.2%			
	Maine	Jan. 2004	17,512	22,624	22,697	2.0%	0.2%			
	Massachusetts	July 2004	79,779	106,115	107,013	2.1%	0.8%			
	New York	Aug. 2003	183,039	224,196	231,126	1.6%	1.6%			
	All States							2.5%	2.0%	2.5%
7222	California	Jan. 1998	319,960	402,432	457,303	3.3%	1.7%			
Limited-service restaurants	Connecticut	April 2004	26,454	32,803	34,621	1.6%	4.4%			
	Delaware	Dec. 2002	9,175	10,581	11,813	1.2%	4.4%			
	Maine	Jan. 2004	12,622	14,178	14,757	0.9%	2.7%			
	Massachusetts	July 2004	61,255	75,451	77,077	1.6%	2.2%			
	New York	Aug. 2003	110,341	144,200	155,051	2.2%	3.9%			
	All States							-1.2%	-2.3%	-0.6%
7224	California	Jan. 1998	28,326	27,030	24,055	-0.7%	-1.5%			

TABLE 7.5 (*Continued*)

INDUSTRY CODE	STATE	DATE OF BAR LAW	JAN.-DEC. 1990 EMPLOYMENT LEVEL	LAW DATE EMPLOYMENT LEVEL	JULY 2004-JUNE 2005 EMPLOYMENT LEVEL	ANNUAL % CHANGE PRE-LAW[a]	ANNUAL % CHANGE POST-LAW[a]	OVERALL WEIGHTED ANNUAL % CHANGE IN STATES WITH SMOKE-FREE LAWS PRE-LAW[b]	POST-LAW[b]	ANNUAL % CHANGE IN STATES WITH NO SMOKE-FREE LAW[c]
Drinking places	Connecticut	April 2004	4,004	2,533	2,506	-3.4%	-0.8%			
	Delaware	Dec. 2002	1,188	964	654	-20.4%	-14.0%			
	Maine	Jan. 2004	984	932	845	-0.4%	-6.3%			
	Massachusetts	July 2004	11,699	8,933	8,251	-2.0%	-7.6%			
	New York	Aug. 2003	20,574	18,943	17,581	-0.7%	-3.8%			

Notes: The baseline employment levels for Delaware for industries 722 and 7224 are for January–December 2001 instead of January–December 1990 because earlier data were unavailable from the Bureau of Labor Statistics.

[a] Annualized percentage change in employment level based on the number of months the policy was in effect.

[b] Post-law annual percentage employment change is weighted by the January–December 1990 average employment level for each state as well as months the smoking policy was in effect.

[c] Annualized percentage change in employment for all states/district/territories without a statewide smokefree restaurant law (excluded states are California, Connecticut, Delaware, Florida, Idaho, Maine, Massachusetts, New York, Rhode Island, and Utah). In addition, Alabama is excluded from industry 722. New Hampshire, North Dakota, Virginia, and Wyoming are excluded from industry 7224. 722 (n = 42), 7221 (n = 43), 7222 (n = 43), 7224 (n = 39).

Source: U.S. Department of Labor, Bureau of Labor Statistics, Quarterly Census of Employment and Wages.

The results of our multivariate model of employment are presented in table 7.6, in which the outcome is the logarithm of employment, and table 7.7, in which the outcome is employment per 100 retail sector employees. The predictors included indicator variables for statewide smoke-free restaurant and bar laws, interactions between smoke-free air laws and the time trend, indicators for states, interactions between states and the time trend, and an indicator for month (to adjust for seasonal variation in hospitality services). The coefficients for the interaction variables $RESTLAW \times YEAR$ and $BARLAW \times YEAR$ measure the change in the slope of the time trend after the implementation of a smoke-free restaurant or bar law, respectively.

Results shown in table 7.6 do not show clear and consistent trends for changes in employment levels after smoke-free regulations were implemented. As coefficients for the $YEAR$ variable show, employment in restaurants has increased over time, while employment in bars and taverns has dropped. Smoke-free restaurant laws appeared to have a significant positive association with restaurant and bar employment ($RESTLAW$ variable), although the interaction term ($REST-LAW \times YEAR$) indicates that the positive effect grew smaller over time. This pattern of findings appeared for each industry segment. Smoke-free bar laws, on the other hand, had a negative association with hospitality employment overall and with employment in limited-service restaurants; for bars and taverns the effect was positive but not statistically significant. As with smoke-free laws in restaurants, the effect of smoke-free laws in bars became smaller over time.

These results do not provide much indication of economic loss following passage of smoke-free laws. In fact, restaurant employment tended to be higher after the passage of laws restricting smoking in restaurants, while bar employment appeared to be unaffected by laws restricting smoking in bars. These estimated effects were small; the largest coefficient for a main effect ($RESTLAW$ or $BARLAW$ variables) of a smoke-free law in any model implied a change of less than 5.9 percent, and the largest effect of any interaction term ($RESTLAW \times YEAR$ or $BARLAW \times YEAR$ variables) implied a change of less than 0.6 percent. These results provide no evidence of large changes in employment following smoke-free regulations.

It is possible, however, that underlying economic trends are obscuring the effect of smoke-free laws. For instance, if the states passing smoke-free laws were also characterized by more robust economic growth, this rise in consumer spending might offset a decline in business related to smoke-free regulations. To adjust for state-level economic trends, we fit models predicting trends in the level of hospitality employment per 100 retail employees. These results are generally similar to the results in table 7.6, although fewer parameter estimates are statistically significant and more point estimates are in the positive direction. These results are consistent with the hypothesis that underlying economic trends may

TABLE 7.6 Results from Linear Regression Models Estimating Log Employment Levels Before and After Statewide Smoke-Free Regulations by Industry Type, 1990–2005

INDUSTRY/PREDICTORS	MODEL R^2 β, UNSTANDARDIZED (SE)	SIGNIFICANCE LEVEL
Food service and drinking places (722)	Model R^2 = 0.999	
RESTLAW	0.125 (0.011)	< 0.001
RESTLAW × YEAR	−0.010 (0.001)	< 0.001
BARLAW	−0.078 (0.023)	0.001
BARLAW × YEAR	0.007 (0.002)	< 0.001
YEAR	0.036 (0.001)	< 0.001
Full-service restaurants (7221)	Model R^2 = 0.998	
RESTLAW	0.136 (0.014)	< 0.001
RESTLAW × YEAR	−0.013 (0.001)	< 0.001
BARLAW	−0.037 (0.031)	0.228
BARLAW × YEAR	0.006 (0.002)	0.009
YEAR	0.056 (0.001)	< 0.001
Limited-service restaurants (7222)	Model R^2 = 0.998	
RESTLAW	0.127 (0.014)	< 0.001
RESTLAW × YEAR	−0.010 (0.001)	< 0.001
BARLAW	−0.093 (0.030)	0.002
BARLAW × YEAR	0.007 (0.002)	0.001
YEAR	0.027 (0.001)	< 0.001
Drinking places (7224)	Model R^2 = 0.995	
RESTLAW	0.112 (0.023)	< 0.001
RESTLAW × YEAR	−0.004 (0.002)	0.049
BARLAW	0.089 (0.050)	0.073
BARLAW × YEAR	−0.014 (0.004)	< 0.001
YEAR	−0.071 (0.001)	< 0.001

Notes: RESTLAW = main effect of statewide smoke-free restaurant law; RESTLAW × YEAR = restaurant law by time (in years) of interaction; BARLAW = main effect of statewide smoke-free bar law; BARLAW × YEAR = bar law by time (in years) of interaction; YEAR = main effect of time (in years). The dependent variables are the natural logarithms of the following NAICS industries: 722, Food Service and Drinking Places; 7221, Full-Service Restaurants; 7222, Limited-Service Restaurants; 7224, Drinking Places. Models are controlled for time (in years), month (not shown), state (not shown), and time-by-state interaction (not shown).
Source: U.S. Department of Labor, Bureau of Labor Statistics, Quarterly Census of Employment and Wages.

TABLE 7.7 Results from Linear Regression Models Estimating Employment per Retail Employment Levels Before and After Statewide Smoke-Free Regulations by Industry Type, 1990–2005

INDUSTRY/PREDICTORS	MODEL R^2 β, UNSTANDARDIZED (SE)	SIGNIFICANCE LEVEL
Food service and drinking places (722)	Model $R^2 = 0.986$	
RESTLAW	1.273 (0.491)	0.010
RESTLAW × YEAR	0.046 (0.045)	0.304
BARLAW	−2.146 (1.072)	0.067
BARLAW × YEAR	0.026 (0.081)	0.750
YEAR	1.073 (0.033)	< 0.001
Full-service restaurants (7221)	Model $R^2 = 0.982$	
RESTLAW	0.414 (0.303)	0.173
RESTLAW × YEAR	−0.004 (0.028)	0.881
BARLAW	0.283 (0.661)	0.668
BARLAW × YEAR	−0.029 (0.050)	0.562
YEAR	0.797 (0.019)	< 0.001
Limited-service restaurants (7222)	Model $R^2 = 0.962$	
RESTLAW	0.759 (0.294)	0.010
RESTLAW × YEAR	0.011 (0.027)	0.685
BARLAW	−1.280 (0.640)	0.046
BARLAW × YEAR	0.020 (0.048)	0.681
YEAR	0.358 (0.018)	< 0.001
Drinking places (7224)	Model $R^2 = 0.986$	
RESTLAW	0.018 (0.067)	0.786
RESTLAW × YEAR	0.014 (0.006)	0.018
BARLAW	0.211 (0.146)	0.149
BARLAW × YEAR	−0.036 (0.011)	0.001
YEAR	−0.106 (0.004)	< 0.001

Notes: RESTLAW = main effect of statewide smoke-free restaurant law; RESTLAW × YEAR = restaurant law by time (in years) of interaction; BARLAW = main effect of statewide smoke-free bar law; BARLAW × YEAR = bar law by time (in years) of interaction; YEAR = main effect of time (in years). The dependent variables are the following NAICS industries, divided by total retail employment (NAICS 44–45), times 100: 722, Food Service and Drinking Places; 7221, Full-Service Restaurants; 7222, Limited-Service Restaurants; 7224, Drinking Places. Models are controlled for time (in years), month (not shown), state (not shown), and time-by-state interaction (not shown).
Source: U.S. Department of Labor, Bureau of Labor Statistics, Quarterly Census of Employment and Wages.

account for the observed variation in employment. Again, the results show in-creasing employment in restaurants and declining employment in bars and tav-erns. For the overall hospitality industry as a whole and for limited service restau-rants, we estimated a small, statistically significant increase in employment following smoke-free restaurant laws, whereas smoke-free laws affecting bars were associated with lower employment in limited service restaurants. Smoke-free laws had no effect on full-service restaurants. A small increasing trend in bar employ-ment per retail employment was observed after smoke-free restaurant laws, but a small decreasing trend was observed after smoke-free bar regulations; these ef-fects were very small, implying differences of fewer than 3.6 bar employees per 10,000 retail employees per year.

We also looked for evidence of short-term effects by examining year-over-year changes in employment and using regression models that included indica-tors for each month after the smoke-free laws, and found little evidence of short-term impacts. For example, the changes in hospitality employment for each of the 12 months after the statewide laws were within 1.4 percentage points of each other; for bars and taverns, these differed by no more than 0.1 percentage points. Multivariate analyses confirmed these descriptive findings. In other words, the rate of employment growth in the months shortly after smoke-free laws took effect was very similar to growth rates over the longer term.

LIMITATIONS

Several caveats about these analyses are important to keep in mind. First, we did not take account of smoke-free policies adopted at the city or county level; for most states the employment data were not available below the state level by indus-try subsector. This omission is most likely to be important in three states, Califor-nia, Massachusetts, and New York, where municipalities have been very active in pursuing smoke-free regulations. These are among the largest states, with smoke-free policies in force for a relatively long period of time. Omitting measures of local smoke-free policies results in some degree of misclassification of states' smoking policies; if smoke-free laws do affect business indicators, the analytic ap-proach used here is likely to underestimate those effects, which are generally in the positive direction for restaurant employment. Attempts to run analyses ex-cluding these three states did not produce robust or consistent results because there were too few postlaw data points available for analysis.

Second, we could not observe trends in industry subsegments. For example, certain types of drinking places, such as small, owner-operated taverns, could be differentially impacted by a smoke-free bar law; the data did not permit us to examine variation in outcomes within the broad categories of full-service res-taurants, limited-service restaurants, and bars. In addition, the employment data do not include self-employed individuals, such as sole proprietors of very small restaurants or bars. Although we have no reason to believe that smoke-free laws would have a differential effect on very small bars or restaurants, the reader should keep this limitation in mind.

Third, employment data may be less responsive to change than other indicators such as taxable sales data. For example, if a smoke-free law was harmful to business, employers may cut costs by reducing employee hours without laying employees off; the employment data would not detect this decline in hours and earnings because part-time and full-time employees are counted equally. Examining other business indicators in conjunction with employment data would be a better way to evaluate the impact of a smoke-free law; however, other indicators are generally not available in comparable formats by industry subgroups across states.

Fourth, with the exception of California's law, smoke-free bar regulations are relatively new; thus, there are relatively few postlaw data points available for analysis. Given this point, as well as the small size of the bar and tavern industry, inferences about this industry subsegment are more limited than for the hospitality industry as a whole or for restaurants. More satisfactory analyses will be available in future years as more data become available.

Fifth, it is important to note that the definition of "smoke-free" differs across states and has changed over time. Smoke-free regulations implemented in the 1980s and early 1990s often had significant loopholes. For example, New York City's 1995 smoke-free law applied only to restaurants with more than 35 seats; thousands of smaller restaurants were exempt from the law. At the time New York City had one of the strongest smoke-free laws in the nation. By today's standards, however, that law is quite weak, as most laws being passed now cover all workplaces, including bars and restaurants, with few exemptions. The results presented in this chapter do not take into account differences in the strength of smoke-free laws.

In sum, this empirical analysis finds little evidence that employment in the hospitality industry has been affected by the passage of statewide smoke-free regulations, whether we consider hospitality employment overall or within major industry categories. The descriptive statistics presented earlier indicate that the absolute rates of employment growth following a smoke-free restaurant or bar law were within 1 percentage point of prelaw growth rate trends. Multivariate statistical analysis confirmed these results, showing no clear trend toward increased or decreased employment levels for all industry subgroups in places that have adopted smoke-free regulations after adjusting for temporal and underlying economic factors. There are numerous factors that influence hospitality business indicators, and although we have controlled for underlying economic trends, there could be other important unmeasured factors that are not included in the models. Nonetheless, the employment data presented here provide an objective measure that is collected in a timely, comprehensive, and uniform manner across all states. Although these data may make it difficult to identify small changes in employment, they offer us a useful tool for assessing the likelihood of large changes and for comparing the consistency of results across different states over time.

TOBACCO CONTROL POLICY AND
THE HOSPITALITY INDUSTRY

The rationale for adopting smoke-free regulations is to improve public health and to protect workers and the public from exposure to a proven carcinogen (California Environmental Protection Agency 2005). Studies show that these regulations are effective in dramatically reducing secondhand smoke exposure (Repace 2004; Travers et al. 2004) and improving employee health (Eisner, Smith, and Blanc 1998). Therefore, it is expected that a comprehensive nationwide secondhand smoke policy would succeed in achieving its main goal of reducing exposure and improving health.

Our charge in this chapter was to assess the likely economic impact of a nationwide clean air policy—one component of the tobacco policy scenarios considered in this volume—on the hospitality industry. Studies of the restaurant industry, and to a lesser extent of bars and hotels, indicate that smoke-free regulations do not cause adverse economic outcomes; to date the evidence on gaming venues is inconclusive. Complementing the literature review, the analysis of employment presented here provides quantitative estimates of the impact of statewide smoke-free laws on hospitality employment. Like those developed by other researchers, these estimates should be interpreted with caution because there are other reasons besides smoke-free regulations that hospitality employment might change, and without an experiment it is difficult to rule out these alternative explanations. However, our results do suggest that any change in employment levels would be modest and that hospitality employment might even benefit from smoke-free laws.

More recent studies, not included in the literature review for this chapter, do not substantially change these conclusions. A recent paper by Cowling and Bond (2005) finds that California's smoke-free law was associated with statistically significant increases in restaurant and bar revenues between 1990 and 2002. A study by Adams and Cotti (2007) used county-level data for 2001–2004 that are similar to the state-level data presented here; they concluded that bar employment decreased by 4.3 percent in smoke-free counties relative to other counties but found no difference in restaurant employment between counties with and without smoke-free laws. Differences in the time period, outcome measures, and analytical approaches used may help account for the slightly different conclusions across studies. It is notable, however, that no study reports the large decreases in employment or revenues that are often feared as a consequence of smoke-free regulations. The evidence remains very limited for establishments other than restaurants and bars. Studies of gaming establishments have found mixed results (Alamar and Glantz 2006a; Garrett and Pakko 2009; Pakko 2006; Pyles and Hahn 2009). More research would be helpful to clarify the impact if any of clean air laws on gaming establishments.

It is worth noting that most existing studies of smoke-free laws examine local-level regulations. In these contexts, smokers can relatively easily cross jurisdictional borders to patronize businesses that suit their smoking preference, making it more likely that we would observe an adverse economic impact of clean air laws, yet this is not what most studies find. Under a comprehensive uniform nationwide policy, there would be no incentive for border crossing; thus, hospitality establishments would be even less likely to lose business than they are under the current, piecemeal approach. A comprehensive policy would also avoid the legal and political impediments that can arise when multijurisdiction communities seek to enact smoke-free laws on a local or regional level (Cork and Forman 2008).

The goal of this chapter was to examine the potential economic impact of smoke-free regulations on the hospitality industry as a whole and on broad subsectors of this industry. Our study is designed to identify changes in business indicators that are quantitatively significant and can be attributed to a smoke-free law. Given the limitations of our data there may be smaller economic effects either industrywide or affecting industry segments or individual business owners that we do not measure. In addition, whereas this chapter is concerned only with the economic impact of smoke-free laws, these laws may have other impacts in areas such as compliance, education, enforcement, behavior, and occupational health. For example, a restaurateur may be required to post signage in order to comply with the law; local smoking cessation and health care services may see an increase in the demand for services as more smokers seek help in quitting; rates of disease related to secondhand smoke may decline, particularly among hospitality workers. This review does not assess the costs or benefits associated with these indirect outcomes.

APPENDIX 7.1: REFERENCES INCLUDED IN LITERATURE REVIEW

1. Advantage Marketing Information. Rhode Islander's attitudes towards smoking in restaurants and hotels: Working paper 1. Wickford, RI: Advantage Marketing Information, 1997.
2. Allen K., Markham V. Public opinions and attitudes towards creating smokefree bars in Western Australia. West Perth, Western Australia: Australian Council on Smoking and Health, 2001.

3. Applied Economics. Economic impact of the City of Mesa smoke-free ordinance: Working paper 1. Scottsdale, AZ: Applied Economics, 1996.
4. Applied Economics. Economic impact of the City of Mesa smoke-free ordinance: Working paper 2. Scottsdale, AZ: Applied Economics, 1996.
5. August K., Brooks L. Support for smoke-free bars grows stronger in California. *Business Wire* (Sacramento: California Department of Health Services), October 16, 2000.
6. Auspoll. Philip Morris Opinion Survey. Philip Morris, January 2000.
7. Bartosch W. J. The economic effect of Boston's restaurant smoking regulation, 1992–2000. Boston: Arnold Worldwide Inc. for the Commonwealth of Massachusetts Department of Public Health Tobacco Control Program, 2002. Available from: http://www.bphc.org/reports/pdfs/report_100.pdf.
8. Bartosch W., Pope G. Preliminary analysis of the economic impact of Brookline's smoking ban. Waltham, MA: Center for Health Economics Research, 1995.
9. Bartosch W., Pope G. The economic effect of smoke-free restaurant policies on restaurant businesses in Massachusetts. *Journal of Public Health Management and Practice* 5(1) (1999): 53–62.
10. Bartosch W. J., Pope G. C. *Analysis of the Adoption of Local Tobacco Control Policies in Massachusetts, Final Report.* Waltham, MA: Center for Health Economics Research, 2000.
11. Bartosch W., Pope G. The effect of smoking restrictions on restaurant business in Massachusetts, 1992–1998. *Tobacco Control* 11 (Supplement II) (2002): ii, 38–42.
12. Bialous S., Glantz S. Tobacco control in Arizona. San Francisco: Institute for Health Policy Studies, University of California, 1997.
13. Biener L., Fitzgerald G. Smoky bars and restaurants: Who avoids them and why? *Journal of Public Health Management and Practice* 5(1) (1999): 74–78.
14. Biener L., Siegel M. Behavior intentions of the public after bans in restaurants and bars. *American Journal of Public Health* 87(12) (1997): 2042–44.
15. Blackley M. Pubs in Scotland "will make a packet." *The Scotsman*, July 11, 2005.
16. Boulder County. Tax receipt data. Boulder, CO, 1996.
17. Bourns B., Malcomson A. Economic impact analysis of the non-smoking bylaw on the hospitality industry in Ottawa. Los Angeles: KPMG, 2001.
18. Bourns B., Malcomson A. Economic impact analysis of the non-smoking bylaw on the hospitality industry in Ottawa. Los Angeles: KPMG, 2002.
19. California State Board of Equalization. Report. Sacramento: California State Board of Equalization, 1998.
20. CCG Consulting Group Limited. The hospitality sector and a Vancouver smoking ban. Vancouver: CCG Consulting Group Limited, 1995.
21. CCG Consulting Group Limited. The food services and hospitality sector and a metro Toronto smoking ban. Vancouver: CCG Consulting Group Limited, 1996.
22. Chamberlain Research Consultants. Smoking issues in Wisconsin. Madison: Chamberlain Research Consultants, 1998.
23. Charlton Research Group. Pacific Dining Car Restaurant and Southern California Business Association Survey. San Francisco: Charlton Research Group, 1994.
24. Collins J. The economic impact of the Fayetteville, Arkansas smoking ban. Fayetteville: Center for Business and Economic Research, University of Arkansas, 2005.
25. The Conference Board of Canada. The economics of smoke-free restaurants. Toronto: Conference Board of Canada, 1996.
26. Connolly G., Carpenter C., Hillel R., Skeer M., Travers M. Evaluation of the Massachusetts smoke-free workplace law. Cambridge, MA: Division of Public Health Practice, Harvard School of Public Health, Tobacco Research Program, 2005.
27. Corsun D., Young C., Enz C. Should NYC's restaurateurs lighten up? Effects of the city's Smoke-Free Air Act. *Cornell Hotel and Restaurant Administration Quarterly* 37(2) (1996): 25–33.

28. Cowan S., Kruckemeyer T., Baker J., Harr T. Impact of smoke-free restaurant ordinance on revenues for Maryville Missouri. Jefferson City: Health Promotion Unit of the Missouri Department of Health and Senior Services, November 2004.
29. Craig Group Inc. West Virginia restaurants and taverns fear smoking bans would hurt business. Columbus, OH: Craig Group Inc., 1998.
30. Cremieux P., Oullette P. Actual and perceived impacts of tobacco regulation on restaurants and firms. Tobacco Control 10 (2001): 33–37.
31. Dai C., Denslow D., Hyland A., Lotfinia B. The economic impact of Florida's smoke-free workplace law. Gainesville, FL: Bureau of Economic and Business Research, 2004.
32. Decima Research. Focus Group Report on Project Visa for Imperial Tobacco. Montreal: Decima Research, 1988.
33. Decima Research. Ottawa residents back smoking ban by two to one. Montreal: Decima Research, 2001.
34. Deloitte & Touche LLP. The impact of non-smoking ordinances on restaurant financial performance. New York: Deloitte & Touche LLP, October 2003.
35. Douglas County Community Health Improvement Project. Douglas County Business Smoking Survey. Lawrence, KS: Douglas County Community Health Improvement Project. June 2001.
36. Dresser J., Boles S., Lichtenstein E., Strycker L. Multiple impacts of a bar smoking prohibition ordinance in Corvallis, Oregon. Eugene, OR: Pacific Research Institute. 1999.
37. Dresser L. Clearing the air: The effect of smokefree ordinances on restaurant revenues in Dane County. Madison: Tobacco-Free Wisconsin Coalition, 1999.
38. Dunham J., Marlow M. Smoking laws and their differential effects on restaurants, bars and taverns. Contemporary Economic Policy 18(3) (2000): 326–33.
39. Economists Advisory Group Limited. The potential economic impact of a smoking ban in restaurants. London: The Restaurant Association, September 1998.
40. Edwards R. New study: 76% of the North East hospitality trade back smoke free areas & over 90% of publicans recommend other pubs try one. Newcastle: University in New Castle upon Tyne, 2000.
41. Enterprise Marketing and Research Services. The effects of recent events on the Tasmanian hotel industry. Tasmania: Enterprise Marketing and Research Services, November 2001.
42. Eppstein Group. Statewide Hospitality Industry Benchmark Poll. N.p.: Eppstein Group, 1997.
43. Eppstein Group. Texas Restaurant Association Poll. N.p.: Eppstein Group, 1998.
44. Fabrizio McLaughlin and Associates Inc. Impact of smoking bans on smokers dining out patterns derived from national survey of adult smokers. Alexandria, VA: Fabrizio McLaughlin and Associates Incorporated, 1995.
45. Fabrizio McLaughlin and Associates Inc. Survey of New York City restaurateurs. Alexandria, VA: Fabrizio McLaughlin and Associates Incorporated, 1996.
46. Ferrence R., Luk R., Gmel G. The economic impact of a smoke-free bylaw on restaurant and bar sales in Ottawa, Canada. Toronto: Ontario Tobacco Research Unit, 2003.
47. Field Research Corporation. A survey of California adults age 21 or older about smoking policies and smoke-free bars. San Francisco: California Department of Health Services, 1997.
48. Field Research Corporation. A survey of California bar patrons about smoking policies and smoke-free bars. San Francisco: California Department of Health Services, 1998.
49. Fletcher J. An analysis of sales tax receipts from restaurants with bars and free standing bars in Chico, California 1995–1997. Sacramento: California Department of Health Services, Tobacco Control Section, 1998.
50. Gambee P. Economic Impacts of Smoking ban in Bellflower, California. Bellflower: California Business and Restaurant Alliance (CBRA), 1991.

51. Glantz S. Effect of smokefree bar law on bar revenues in California. *Tobacco Control* 9(1) (2000): 111–12.
52. Glantz S., Charlesworth A. Tourism and hotel revenues before and after passage of smoke-free restaurant ordinances. *Journal of the American Medical Association* 281(20) (1999): 1911–18.
53. Glantz S., Smith L. The effect of ordinances requiring smoke-free restaurants on restaurant sales. *American Journal of Public Health* 84(7) (1994): 1081–1085.
54. Glantz S., Smith L. The effect of ordinances requiring smoke-free restaurants and bars on revenues: A follow up. *American Journal of Public Health* 87(10) (1997): 1687–93.
55. Glantz S., Wilson-Loots R. No association of smoke-free ordinances with profits from bingo and charitable games in Massachusetts. *Tobacco Control* 12 (2003): 411–13.
56. Goldstein A., Sobel R. Environmental tobacco smoke regulations have not hurt restaurant sales in North Carolina. *North Carolina Medical Journal* 59(5) (1998): 284–87.
57. Hahn E., Mullineaux D., Thompson E., Pyles M., Chizimuzo O. Economic impact of Lexington's smoke-free law: A progess report. Lexington: University of Kentucky, 2005.
58. Hayslett J., Huang P. Impact of clean indoor air ordinances on restaurant revenues in four Texas cities. Austin: Bureau of Disease, Injury and Tobacco Prevention, Texas Department of Health, 2000.
59. Hild C., Larson E., Weiss L., Fligel M., Sandberg K., Smith S. Review of Municipality of Anchorage Chapter 16.65—Prohibition of smoking in public places. Anchorage, AK: Institute for Circumpolar Health Studies, 2001.
60. Hodges I., Maskill C. Assessing the potential impact of restaurant and bar smoking bans on visitors to New Zealand. *Healthsearch* 18 (January 2001).
61. Huang P. Impact of smoking ban on restaurant and bar revenues—El Paso, Texas, 2002. *Morbidity and Mortality Weekly Report* 53(7) (2004): 150–52.
62. Huang P., Tobias S., Kohout S., Harris M., Satterwhite D., Simpson D., et al. Assessment of the impact of a 100% smoke-free ordinance on restaurant sales—West Lake Hills, Texas, 1992–1994. *Morbidity and Mortality Weekly Report* 44(19) (1995): 370–72.
63. Huron County Health Unit. Huron County Health Unit restaurant survey. Clinton, ON: Huron County Health Unit, 1999.
64. Hyland A. Before and after smoke-free regulations in new taxable sales from eating and drinking places in New York State. Buffalo, NY: Roswell Park Cancer Institute, 2002.
65. Hyland A., Cummings K. Consumer response to the New York City Smoke-Free Air Act. *Journal of Public Health Management and Practice* 5(1) (1999): 28–36.
66. Hyland A., Cummings K. Restaurant employment before and after the New York City Smoke-Free Air Act. *Journal of Public Health Management and Practice* 5(1) (1999): 22–27.
67. Hyland A., Cummings K. Restaurateur reports of the economic impact of the New York City Smoke-Free Air Act. *Journal of Public Health Management and Practice* 5(1) (1999): 37–42.
68. Hyland A., Cummings K., Nauenberg E. Analysis of taxable sales receipts: Was New York City's Smoke-Free Air Act bad for business? *Journal of Public Health Management and Practice* 5(1) (1999): 14–21.
69. Hyland A., Puli V., Cummings K. M., Sciandra R. New York's smoke-free regulations: Effects on employment and sales in the hospitality industry. *Cornell Hotel and Restaurant Administration Quarterly* 44(3) (2003): 9–16.
70. Hyland A., Tuk J. Restaurant employment boom in New York City. *Tobacco Control* 10 (2001): 199–200.
71. Hyland A., Vena C., Cummings K., Lubin A. The effect of the Clean Air Act of Erie County, New York on restaurant employment. *Journal of Public Health Management and Practice* 6(6) (2000): 76–85.
72. International Communications Research. Smoking ban. Dublin: Vintners' Federation of Ireland, 2003. Available from: http://www.faac.ca/content/economic%20impact/New%20York%20Survey.pdf .

73. Jones K., Wakefield M., Turnball D. Attitudes and experiences of restaurateurs regarding smoking bans in Adelaide, South Australia. *Tobacco Control* 8(1) (1999): 62–66.
74. KPMG. Proposed smoking ban: Impacts on Hong Kong hospitality businesses. Hong Kong: Hong Kong Catering Industry Association, 2001.
75. KPMG Barents Group LLC. The expected economic impact on Spain of a ban in smoking in restaurants. Washington, DC: KPMG Barents Group LLC, 1997.
76. KPMG Peat Marwick LLP. The impact of California's smoking ban on bars, taverns and night clubs: A survey of owners and managers. Washington, DC: KPMG Peat Marwick LLP, 1998.
77. Lal A., Siahpush M., Scollo M. The economic impact of smoke-free restaurants and cafes in Victoria. *Australia and New Zealand Journal of Public Health* 27(5) (2003): 557–58.
78. Lam T., Chung S., Tam E., Hedley Y. H. A. Public opinion on smoke-free restaurants. Hong Kong: Department of Community Medicine, The University of Hong Kong, 1995.
79. Laventhol & Horwath. Preliminary analysis of the impact of the proposed Los Angeles ban on smoking in restaurants. Los Angeles: Laventhol & Horwath, October 1990.
80. Lilley W., DeFranco L. Massachusetts restaurant smoking ban 23 cities/towns: Impact on restaurant jobs 1993–1995. Westborough, MA, 1996.
81. Lilley W., DeFranco L. Restaurant jobs in New York City, 1993 through first quarter 1996, and the restaurant smoking ban. Washington, DC, 1996.
82. Lilley W., DeFranco L. The impact of smoking restrictions on the bar and tavern industry in California. Washington, DC: InContext Inc., October 26, 1999.
83. Lund M. Smoke-free bars and restaurants in Norway. Oslo: SIRUS Norwegian Institute for Alcohol and Drug Research, 2005.
84. Mandel L. L., Alamar B. C., Glantz S. A. Smoke-free law did not affect revenue from gaming in Delaware. *Tobacco Control* 14(1) (2005): 10–12.
85. Markham V., Tong R. Reactions and attitudes to health (smoking in enclosed places) regulations 1999 Subiaco, Western Australia: Australian Council on Smoking and Health, 2001.
86. Marlow M. The economic effect of smoking laws on bars and taverns. San Luis Obispo: California Polytechnic State University, 1998.
87. Marlow M. An economic analysis of the Maine smoking ban: Evidence from patrons and owners of businesses. San Luis Obispo: California Polytechnic State University, 1999.
88. Maroney N., Sherwood D., Stubblebine W. The impact of tobacco control ordinances on restaurant revenues in California. Claremont, CA: The Claremont Institute for Economic Policy Studies, 1994.
89. Martin Associates. Analysis of passenger expenditure profiles at Phoenix Sky Harbour International Airport in-concession survey. Lancaster, PA: Martin Associates, 1999.
90. Mason-Dixon Market Research. Maryland smoking regulation survey. Washington, DC: Mason-Dixon Market Research, 1996.
91. Masotti L., Creticos P. The effects of a ban on smoking in public places in San Luis Obispo, California. Evanston, IL: Creticos and Associates, 1991.
92. McGhee S., Hedley A., Lam T. Does the government's proposal to create smoke-free catering facilities in restaurants, cafes, bars and karaokes influence the intentions of tourists to visit Hong Kong and to patronise catering venues? Hong Kong: University of Hong Kong, Health Services Research Group, March 2002.
93. Miller C., Kriven S. Community support for smoking bans in bar and gaming venues in South Australia. Adelaide: Tobacco Control Research Evaluation Unit, 2002.
94. Miller C., Kriven S. Smoke-free dining in South Australia: Surveys of community attitudes and practices after 4 and 18 months. Adelaide: Tobacco Control Research Evaluation Unit, 2002.
95. Moseley F., Schmidt K. The economic impact of Minot's smoke-free restaurant ordinance. Minot, ND: Minot State University, 2003.

96. National Restaurant Association. Smoking in restaurants: A consumer attitude survey. Washington DC: National Restaurant Association, 1993.

97. New York City Department of Finance. The state of smoke-free New York City: A one-year review. New York: New York City Department of Finance, New York City Department of Health and Mental Hygiene, New York City Department of Small Business Services, March 2004.

98. New York City Department of Health and Mental Hygiene. Initial effects of New York City smoking ordinance. New York: New York City Department of Health and Mental Hygiene, July 23, 2003.

99. Pacific Analytics Inc. The economic impacts of the proposed amendment to the ETS regulation. Victoria, BC: Pacific Analytics Inc., 2001.

100. Pakko M. Smoke-free law did affect revenue from gaming in Delaware. Working paper. St. Louis: Federal Reserve Bank of St. Louis, May 2005.

101. Parry J., Temperton H., Flanagan T., Gerhardt L. An evaluation of the introduction of "non-smoking" areas on trade and customer satisfaction in 11 public houses in Staffordshire. *Tobacco Control* 10(2) (2001): 199–200.

102. Penn & Schoen Associates. Survey of restaurant owners and managers about NYC smoking regulations. New York: Penn & Schoen Associates, July 1995.

103. Pope G., Bartosch W. Effect of local smokefree restaurant policies on restaurant revenue in Massachusetts. Waltham, MA: Center for Health Economics Research, April 1997.

104. Price J., Dake J., Ruma J., Butler P. Financial stress faced by bars, bowling alleys and restaurants after passage of clean indoor air acts. Toledo, OH: Department of Health, University of Toledo, 2004.

105. Price Waterhouse LLP. Potential effects of a smoking ban in the State of California. Washington, DC: Price Waterhouse LLP, 1993.

106. Price Waterhouse LLP. New York City restaurant survey. Washington, DC: Price Waterhouse LLP, 1995.

107. Pub and Bar Coalition of Ontario. September Pubco survey confirms severe economic impact, job losses in its member bars and pubs. Ottawa, ON: Pub and Bar Coalition of Ontario, 2001.

108. The Publican. Market report 2001: Smoking 2001. *The Publican*, 2001.

109. Roper Starch. National survey of restaurants and bars/taverns: Smoking policy and regulations. http://www.pmoptions.com/images/NationalSurvey.pdf, 1996.

110. Sciacca J. A mandatory smoking ban in restaurants: concerns versus experiences. *Journal of Community Health* 21(2) (1996): 133–50.

111. Sciacca J., Eckram M. Effects of a city ordinance regulating smoking in restaurants and retail stores. *Journal of Community Health* 18(3) (1993): 175–82.

112. Sciacca J., Ratliff M. Prohibiting smoking in restaurants: Effects on restaurant sales. *American Journal of Health Promotion* 12(3) (1998): 176–84.

113. Shapiro T. Butt of the law hits restaurants. *Business Day*, August 15, 2001.

114. Sollars D., Ingram J. Economic impact of the restaurant smoking ban in the city of Boston, Massachusetts. Mongomery, AL, May 5, 1995.

115. Stanwick R., Thomson M., Swerhone P., Stevenson L., Fish D. The response of Winnipeg retail shops and restaurants to a bylaw regulating smoking in public places. *Canadian Journal of Public Health* 79 (1988): 226–230.

116. Styring W. A study of the Fort Wayne (IN) restaurant smoking ban: Has it impacted the restaurant business? Indianapolis: Hudson Institute, 2001.

117. Taylor Consulting Group. The San Luis Obispo smoking ordinance: A study of the economic impacts of San Luis Obispo restaurants and bars. San Luis Obispo, CA, 1993.

118. Thalheimer R. An analysis of the economic effect of the Lexington-Fayette County, Kentucky smoking ban of 2004. Lexington, KY: Thalheimer Research Associates, 2005.

119. Wakefield M., Roberts L., Miller C. Perceptions of the effect of an impending restaurant smoking ban on dining-out experience. *Preventive Medicine* 29 (1999): 53–56.
120. Wakefield M., Siahpush M., Scollo M., Lal A., Hyland A., McCaul K., et al. The effect of a smoke-free law on monthly restaurant retail turnover in South Australia. *Australia and New Zealand Journal of Public Health* 26(4) (2002): 375–82.
121. Yorkshire Ash. Popularity and impact on trade of smoke-free accommodation in the hospitality trade in Yorkshire. Yorkshire: Yorkshire Ash, 2001.

APPENDIX 7.2: MULTIVARIATE MODEL

For the regression analysis, the natural log of employment was used as the outcome variable and the predictors used included indicator variables for statewide smoke-free restaurant laws, statewide smoke-free bar laws, interactions between smoke-free air laws and the time trend, indicators for states, interactions between states and the time trend, and an indicator for month.

$$employment_{it} = \beta_0 + \beta_1 RESTLAW_{it} + \beta_2 BARLAW_{it} + \beta_3 YEAR_j$$
$$+ \beta_4 (RESTLAW \times YEAR)_{ij} + \beta_5 (BARLAW \times YEAR)_{ij}$$
$$+ \Delta State_i + \Gamma (YEAR \times STATE)_{ij} + \Theta MONTH_k + \varepsilon_{it}$$

RESTLAW is an indicator variable equal to 1 when a statewide smoke-free restaurant law is in effect for state i and time t, and equal to 0 otherwise. Similarly, BARLAW is an indicator equal to 1 when a statewide smoke-free bar law is in effect and equal to 0 otherwise. As an example, California has a smoke-free restaurant law that went into effect on January 1, 1995, and a smoke-free bar law that went into effect on January 1, 1998. Therefore, for California, RESTLAW is equal to 0 until January 1995, when it becomes 1, and BARLAW becomes 1 as of January 1998. If a state has no smoke-free bar or restaurant law, then RESTLAW and BARLAW are equal to 0 throughout. RESTLAW and BARLAW measure the main effect of statewide restaurant and bar laws on employment and indicate the immediate impact of the laws on employment.

YEAR, indexed by j, is equal to 1 for the first year (1990) and increments by 1 each year until reaching 16 in the last year (2005). This measures the secular trend in employment. The coefficients for the interaction variables RESTLAW×YEAR and BARLAW×YEAR measure the change in the slope of the time trend after the implementation of a smoke-free restaurant or bar law, respectively.

$\Delta STATE_i$ is a vector of 52 indicator variables accounting for the 53 states, district, and territories. The state indicators control for state-specific factors that affect employment but do not change over time. $\Gamma (YEAR \times STATE)_{ij}$ is a vector of interactions between *YEAR* and *STATE*. These interactions allow each state to have its own secular trend in employment. $\Theta MONTH_k$ is a vector of 11 indicator variables representing month of the year and controls for seasonal changes in employment. ε_{it} is the state-level random disturbance term.

NOTE

1. There were no missing data for retail trade (44–45), full-service restaurants (7221), or limited-service eating places (7222), while food service and drinking places (722) and drinking places (7224) had 4.0 percent and 6.2 percent missing data, respectively. Notable missing data include: no data for drinking places (7224) in the state of Virginia; no data until January 2001 for Alaska, Delaware, Rhode Island, or Wyoming food service and drinking places (722) or drinking places (7224); no data for New Hampshire, Rhode Island, or Wyoming drinking places (7224) for the first and fourth quarters of 2003 and New Hampshire for any of 2005; and no data for North Dakota drinking places for 2005.

8

TOBACCO INDUSTRY PHILANTHROPY AND THE NONPROFIT SECTOR

PATRICK M. ROONEY AND HEIDI K. FREDERICK

Tobacco companies contribute funds to hundreds of nonprofit organizations each year, ranging from local youth service organizations to nonprofits concerned with world hunger and disaster relief. Altria Group, which owns Philip Morris, the largest tobacco manufacturer in the United States, was ranked third among corporate givers by *BusinessWeek* in 2004 (Byrnes 2005), with contributions of $1 billion in cash and in-kind goods over the previous decade,[1] although charitable giving dropped off substantially after 2005.[2] This philanthropic activity may be in jeopardy if tobacco control policies reduce smoking rates significantly.

In this chapter we examined the implications for philanthropy and the nonprofit sector of declines in cigarette consumption under the three policy scenarios laid out in chapter 1. We drew on three kinds of evidence. First, to situate charitable giving in the context of corporate strategy, we reviewed internal documents that the tobacco industry made public under the Master Settlement Agreement. Second, to identify patterns in the industry's philanthropy, we compiled and analyzed a database of tobacco companies' charitable contributions. Third, we developed a series of projections for tobacco company philanthropy through 2025 under the three scenarios used throughout this volume.

PHILANTHROPY AND CORPORATE STRATEGY:
THE CASE OF THE TOBACCO INDUSTRY

Corporate philanthropy, or corporate charitable giving, is generally defined to include only those donations made to nonprofit organizations that qualify for tax deductions. This means gifts must be made to 501(c)(3) organizations or their equivalent, and the company cannot take a tax deduction for any part of the donation for which the company received a direct value. Corporate philanthropy also includes most giving by corporate-sponsored foundations. These foundations typically act as a "pass through": the company donates funds to the foundation each year, and the foundation then makes smaller grants to nonprofits. In addition, many companies, including tobacco companies, will match gifts to charity made by employees. Only the portion of the gift that the company itself gave (i.e., the match) is counted as a company donation. The employees' gifts are counted as part of individual gifts by the IRS and by scholars. However, the company may report their employees' gifts in their company totals when describing the impact of their corporate giving programs.

According to *Giving USA*, the yearbook of philanthropy produced by the Center on Philanthropy at Indiana University (Brown, Chin, and Rooney n.d.), corporate giving, including giving by corporate foundations, is historically the smallest source of total charitable giving in America. In recent years, corporations have accounted for about 5 percent of total donations. Individuals contribute 75 percent, and charitable bequests and foundations, not including corporate foundations, account for the remainder. Corporations, including the tobacco companies, historically have contributed about 1.2 percent of their pretax profits to charity (Indiana University Center on Philanthropy 2005). Philanthropic contributions, however, are not the only source of revenue for nonprofit organizations. In fact, charitable contributions comprise only about 20 percent of all nonprofit revenue (O'Neil 2002).

Corporations contribute to charitable organizations for a variety of reasons, including both altruistic and strategic. According to a recent study of corporate giving programs, nearly 65 percent of companies use business factors when deciding what to give; 23 percent look at community needs; and 23 percent also look internally to the causes their employees support (Steger 2006). Tobacco companies are no exception. They contribute to charity for social and business reasons including supporting the causes important to their employees, and in response to both external and internal factors. In particular, the tobacco industry's philanthropic activities must be placed in the context of the environment in which the industry operates.

Perhaps no other industry operates in as hostile an environment as the tobacco industry. Federal agencies, states' district attorneys' offices, various lobbying groups, and both domestic and international health organizations have sought to regulate and curb the production and sale of tobacco products. This regulatory pressure began to emerge with the accumulation of evidence about the detrimental effects of smoking on health. The Sloan-Kettering Institute released a series of reports in the early 1950s linking the tar from cigarette smoke to cancer in mice (Miles and Cameron 1982). The landmark 1964 Surgeon General's report outlined the serious health risks of cigarette smoking, including a link to lung cancer. This report spurred a series of governmental regulations, research, and hearings. Beginning in 1965, the Federal Trade Commission began to regulate the tobacco industry's advertising, including a ban on advertising to youth. In 1970 Congress passed the Public Health Cigarette Smoking Act banning all cigarette advertising from radio and television. More recently, in 1998, the four largest tobacco companies signed a Master Settlement Agreement, agreeing to pay more than $200 billion through the year 2025. Other recent tobacco control measures have included increases in taxation of cigarettes, a push for more smoke-free environments, and further prohibitions on advertising and promotions.

To understand how the tobacco industry used philanthropy to respond to this challenging environment, we reviewed internal tobacco documents obtained in the Master Settlement Agreement, which are archived at the Legacy Tobacco Document Library, available at www.legacy.library.ucsf.edu. As of early 2006 the Legacy Tobacco Document Library contained more than 7 million documents, including those posted on tobacco industry Web sites as of July 1999; the archive has continued to expand over time. These documents relate to a wide range of topics including advertising, manufacturing, marketing, sales, and scientific research. We searched document titles using search terms related to philanthropy, including "contribution*," "sponsorship*," "community," "minority," "nonprofit*," "contributions committee," "employee matching," and "corporate social responsibility." These search terms were used singularly and in combination with each other and included some variations in the spelling of terms used.

As these documents show, the tobacco industry has responded vigorously to external threats over the last 50 years. Philanthropy and other forms of support for nonprofit organizations have been an integral part of the industry's response. Motivations for corporate giving among tobacco companies are consistent with the operations and objectives of corporate giving more generally in America. The tobacco documents provide examples of several directions and motivations for giving, but the primary motivation revealed in these internal and external documents is the strategic advancement of the interests of the tobacco industry in the face of significant regulatory pressure. The tobacco industry used philanthropy in several specific ways: to support research that might challenge evidence about the health effects of smoking, to gain political access, to expand its markets, to promote a more positive image for the tobacco industry, and to promote loyalty among employees and in the communities where tobacco firms were located (Miles and Cameron 1982).

As early as the 1950s, responding to growing concern about the health effects of smoking, tobacco companies began to sponsor scientific research on that topic. The purpose of this funding was to build a defense by creating a body of literature from prominent scientists and medical institutions. The industry gained valuable lead time, sponsoring research nearly 15 years before the release of the Surgeon General's report on cigarette smoking. The Council for Tobacco Research—USA (formally the Tobacco Industry Research Committee) gave more than $7 million to 230 scientists in more than 100 universities, colleges, hospitals, and medical research centers between 1954 and 1964 (Miles and Cameron 1982). For instance, the tobacco philanthropy database compiled for this chapter contains gifts made by the American Tobacco Company to the Medical College of Virginia totaling $97,500 between 1950 and 1955 for research related to smoking and health.[3] The American Tobacco Company also gave at least $60,000 to the University of Chicago between 1951 and 1953. In 1956 Philip Morris noted that it, too, would expand company grants to include higher education and to support research in "health, scientific, and agricultural fields" (Miles and Cameron 1982, p. 61). These gifts came in addition to the research supported by the tobacco industry through the Council for Tobacco Research—USA. Perhaps more surprising, P. Lorillard Company made $1 million in gifts to the American Medical Association between 1964 and 1968, just after the release of the Surgeon General's report.[4] In fact, as Miles and Cameron (1982) report, cumulative gifts made to the American Medical Association by the largest six tobacco companies totaled $10 million by 1963 and $18 million by 1975.

In addition, evidence suggests the industry used philanthropy to gain political advantage. A variety of documents from the early 1980s to late 1990s suggest corporate giving intended to limit the political/legislative impact of increasing skepticism about tobacco safety. A lengthy memo written in 1982, titled "Developing a Tobacco Industry Strategy," describes how corporate giving can be the "positive" complement to more aggressive and confrontational responses to public criticism of the tobacco industry.[5] The memo specifically identifies areas in which philanthropic investment can improve public perceptions of the industry and build alliances that can be helpful in fending off potentially costly legislation. This document is put forth as a basis for a "unified tobacco institute strategy" and identifies both "defensive" and "positive" strategies for meeting the new challenges and the tobacco companies' changing needs. It is the most lengthy and direct expression of how nonprofit organizations fit into the tobacco industry's political strategy.

The document begins by analyzing the activities of the anti-tobacco groups' coalition that is perceived as the opposition; it also describes direct responses by the Tobacco Institute to those actions. The second half of the report examines more proactive community programs that the Tobacco Institute could use to its advantage. It presents a variety of programs that could be supported in order to "counteract this negative impression and to demonstrate to the public that we are a responsible industry and are capable of looking beyond our own interests." Two such programs, fire safety and teenage smoking prevention, were seen as directly responsive to criticism of tobacco companies, by addressing fires due to smoking and the problem of youth smoking. The remaining programs—health research, job training, handicapped services, parenting education, and health science education—were seen as addressing emerging community needs that would garner positive press. The documents also discuss utilization of community programs to build positive images of the tobacco industry, and implementation of anti-tobacco education programs to improve the tobacco industry's credibility and to prevent potential increases in tobacco restrictions.

Another type of giving related to improving the political environment revolved around gaining access to lawmakers and key decision makers. One example is a $250,000 gift by Philip Morris to the Kennedy Center on the occasion of its twenty-fifth anniversary, discussed in a memo ("N327") in 1995.[6] The donation was encouraged in order to increase the company's "contributions visibility in Washington," potentially important "now that a number of people who are sympathetic to our company and our position on important issues are in the majority in Congress." This pattern of philanthropy was referred to as the "grasstops" strategy, as opposed to "grassroots." Politically strategic giving also included honoraria or donations on behalf of federal and state lawmakers who participated as visiting speakers or guests at tobacco company functions. Such visits gave tobacco companies access to legislators to encourage them to support industry positions on tobacco regulation. Honorarium committees are mentioned in a variety of depositions in the document library.

In addition to this defensive strategy, the industry sought to expand demand for its products. Philanthropy played a role in this effort as the industry sought to broaden its appeal in ethnic minority markets. As previous research has found (Balbach, Gasior, and Barbeau 2003; Yerger and Malone 2002), the industry used donations and sponsorships to complement its marketing in minority communities. For instance, a 1998 document titled "Proactive Public Relations Plan: African-American & Hispanic Market" describes the response to a proposed bill that would impact how the tobacco industry executed business in different states.[7] In it Philip Morris USA outlined potential ways to gain access to minority communities and lobby them for their support in this legislative debate. Included in its recommendations is the pursuit of sponsorship arrangements with influential nonprofit and advocacy groups in minority communities. R. J. Reynolds also sought to use corporate contributions to reach minority groups. In a 1991 speech, then-CEO Jim Johnston noted, "Black and Hispanics traditionally link their trial and purchase of products, and their legislative and editorial support, directly to their understanding and belief that a company cares about their community and issues."[8] This strategy had been pursued over several decades. For instance, a letter from Thomas McCarthy, dated November 23, 1973, discusses the idea of "do good promotions" as marketing; the document discusses donations to a "Black charity" to improve the company's name recognition in New York City.[9] It stated that initial discussions supported the ethnic charity idea and that the group agreed that "the ethnic/charity concept has greater leverage to solve the problems we face in New York" when compared to concerts and other proposed promotions. R. J. Reynolds also created a Regional Initiative Program to target African American and Hispanic markets.[10] The program was designed to identify, create, and implement marketing plans that would reach ethnic consumers.

In addition to seeking to expand markets, the tobacco companies engaged in philanthropy for more general public relations purposes. Philip Morris (now Altria), for instance, has highlighted its donations to hunger, AIDS, and domestic abuse causes. The public relations intent of this philanthropy is evident from the fact that the resources spent on advertising this philanthropy rivals the amount of the donations themselves. ABC News, for instance, reported in February of 2001 that Philip Morris spent $115 million on charity and $150 million on TV ads to publicize its philanthropy.[11] In response to concerns about its reputation, Philip Morris developed a new corporate strategy, known as PM21, "to burnish the company's image by stressing its humanitarian and environmental good works" (Hirschhorn 2004). More generally, like most large corporations the tobacco companies have developed corporate social responsibility (CSR) statements that address the corporation's impact on society; this broad rubric includes charitable donations as well as fair labor standards, ethical trade, human health, and environmental impact. According to the CSR statement for Philip Morris, "Our goal is to be the most responsible, effective, and respected developer, manufacturer, and marketer of consumer products, especially products intended for adults."[12] This statement includes a broad range of activities including "communicate the health effects of our products," "value our employees," and "help reduce youth smoking."[13] Reynolds American, parent company of R. J. Reynolds, also promotes philanthropic involvement.[14] The company's Web site expresses its commitment to community involvement and the prevention of youth smoking. According to the Tobacco Free Initiative of the World Health Organization, almost every major tobacco company invests in a youth prevention smoking program, and many contribute to education in the form of grants, scholarships, and professorships.[15]

Other patterns in tobacco giving also mirror more general trends in corporate philanthropy. The Committee to Encourage Corporate Philanthropy reported, based on its January 2006 Member Survey, that many corporations were targeting charitable giving in an effort to position themselves as socially and community minded. Corporations in general were aligning their philanthropic giving with the company's business strategy, partners, brand, and customer interest (Steger 2006). Among the consequences has been greater attention to publicizing charitable activity. According to the survey, 71 percent of giving departments use public relations as a communication strategy and 35 percent use marketing and direct advertising. Many companies are promoting their philanthropy more energetically, in part because they have received positive press for their good deeds; failure to report the company's philanthropy can lead to a lack of awareness of these efforts and even criticism that the company is not a good corporate citizen.

As tobacco companies have added new lines of business and new markets, they have extended their philanthropy. In parallel with the addition of food and beverage lines such as Kraft and Nabisco, Philip Morris adopted a new focus on hunger issues, beginning a four-year, $100 million campaign called Fight Against Hunger in 1998. In the campaign, $50 million was provided in cash to help organizations such as food banks and $50 million worth of food was donated though America's Second Harvest (Hyatt 1998). In addition, accompanying the expansion to overseas markets has been a greater emphasis on overseas charitable giving as tobacco companies reach out to new communities and constituents. The tobacco philanthropy database, for instance, contains $4 million worth of contributions by Philip Morris made after 2001 to overseas organizations.

The tobacco industry's philanthropic strategy also includes a more traditional rationale for corporate contributions: employee retention/recruitment and satisfaction. Indeed, in an industry facing so many external threats, responding to internal concerns including employee satisfaction may become a more important consideration. Many giving programs include some sort of employee matching gift program and/or volunteer initiative. An employee matching gift program can account for nearly 50 percent of a charitable contributions budget (Steger 2006). This kind of program ties a company's philanthropic activity to the causes its employees support in the locale in which the company operates. It also means a company tends to gives many small donations—usually less than $1,000—to a variety of local organizations. For instance, Altria has an extensive "Dollars for Doers" program, which awards $1,000 to organizations where employees volunteer, as well as the Philip Morris Employee Community Fund for which employees from every level administer, manage, and direct giving to causes in Virginia and North Carolina. This fund, for example, awarded $16 million in 2000; by 2010, renamed as the Altria Companies Employee Community Fund, it had donated more than $23 million to nonprofit organizations in central Virginia.[16] R. J. Reynolds manages employee-directed giving through the R. J. Reynolds Foundation, which supports grantees that serve residents in communities where significant numbers of

Reynolds American Inc. and R. J. Reynolds employees live and/or work.[17] The foundation focuses its giving on public education, local community campaigns including United Way and the Arts Council, and scholarship programs for children of employees or retirees.

To take another example, Brown & Williamson outlined its contributions policy in several documents explaining the focus of its giving as improving the communities in which its employees live.[18] Several memos and documents from the mid-1970s discuss the key role Brown & Williamson played in United Way campaigns in Louisville during that era.[19] These documents suggest that programs involving employees were looked upon favorably and that community-focused giving is a kind of indirect compensation that may aid in employee retention and recruitment. Reynolds American, which has acquired Brown & Williamson, has continued to emphasize giving in locations where its employees live and work.

PATTERNS OF PHILANTHROPY

To understand more specifically how tobacco control policies might affect the industry's philanthropy, we compiled a tobacco philanthropy database containing all gifts made by the tobacco industry that we could identify. The purpose of this tobacco philanthropy database was to document charitable financial contributions made by tobacco companies and their foundations to nonprofit organizations in order to identify patterns and trends in tobacco philanthropy.

Eight companies (before mergers) are represented in the database. Data came from multiple sources including tobacco corporate foundations' IRS filings (51.7 percent), internal tobacco company records (42.2 percent), and other studies (5.9 percent). Every effort was made to eliminate duplication of gifts. The database does not include financial contributions to individual politicians, political candidates, or political parties because these gifts do not have income tax deductibility status with the IRS. On the rare occasion when information was about a gift to a noncharitable organization, the gift was still recorded but categorized as noncharitable and excluded from the analysis. Finally, no information was collected on in-kind or noncash donations that may have been made by tobacco companies. The database also contains little information on tobacco sponsorships provided to nonprofit organizations except for data gathered by Michael Siegel for the years 1995–1999 (Siegel 2000).

The entire database contains a total of 4,865 gifts or sponsorships totaling $161 million and spanning the years 1950 through 2005. However, 78 percent of gifts were made between 1997 and 2005. There were no gifts found for the years 1956–1962, 1970, 1974, and 1991–1993, and the database also has limited information on gifts made in 1950, 1954, 1965, 1967, 1984, and 1994. This is likely a

TABLE 8.1 Descriptive Statistics, All Tobacco Industry Gifts, 1997–2005

Mean gift	$37,265
Median gift	$5,000
Maximum gift	$15,000,000
Minimum gift	$12
Mode	$1,000
25th percentile	$1,001
75th percentile	$25,000
Total amount	$143,954,819
Number of gifts	3,863

Source: Tobacco philanthropy database compiled by the authors (see chapter discussion for data sources).

reflection of missing information rather than lower levels of charitable giving. Given the inconsistency in data from the earlier years, for the purposes of this chapter we will examine only gifts made between 1997 and 2005.

Table 8.1 displays descriptive statistics for the gifts made between 1997 and 2005. Most gifts were small. Half of all gifts in the database were less than $5,000, and a quarter are $1,000 or less. In fact, the modal donation (most often given) is $1,000. The average (mean) is so much higher because it is skewed upward by very large gifts such as a $15 million donation made to Duke University.

The tobacco industry's philanthropic contributions are similar to national estimates of corporate giving (figure 8.1). Health, human services, and community development organizations received the highest percentage of donations from the tobacco industry and from corporations nationally (42.4 and 47.4 percent, respectively). Environmental organizations received the lowest percentage of donations from corporations nationally at 3.1 percent, compared with 8.9 percent of donations from the tobacco industry. In addition, the tobacco industry directed a higher proportion of its donations to arts and culture (15.9 percent vs. 5.7 percent).

PROJECTED CONTRIBUTIONS UNDER TOBACCO CONTROL POLICY SCENARIOS

We used econometric modeling to predict future tobacco giving under the three tobacco control policy scenarios outlined in chapter 2. Data for this exercise

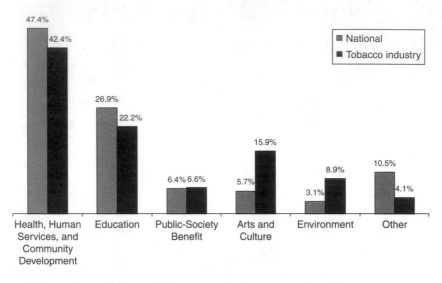

FIGURE 8.1 Giving by Type of Recipient

Source: Tobacco philanthropy database compiled by the authors (see the chapter discussion for data sources). Totals for "Tobacco industry" exceed 100 percent due to rounding.

were taken from IRS records on tobacco/beverage industry income and the tobacco/beverage industry's tax-deductible corporate contributions. Tobacco and beverage manufacturing are currently reported as one industry in the IRS data and cannot be disaggregated. However, inspection of older IRS data, from a period when the two industries were reported separately, indicated that the tobacco industry's philanthropic contributions made up approximately 55 percent of the "tobacco/beverage" industry's contributions.

The three policy scenarios to be examined include the baseline or status quo scenario, which assumes no change in tobacco control policy between 2005 and 2025; the IOM scenario, which incorporates recommendations by the Institute of Medicine and would be expected to lower smoking prevalence to 10.4 percent by 2025; and the "high-impact scenario," a more vigorous set of measures that could reduce smoking prevalence to 5.7 percent by 2025. Tax-deducted contributions by the tobacco/beverage industry in 2002, the latest year for which IRS data were available at the time we conducted this analysis, totaled $347 million.

To project tobacco industry contributions between 2005 and 2025, we employed a model developed for national estimates of corporate giving for *Giving USA*. This model is based on the historical relationship between changes in tax-deductible corporate contributions and changes in gross domestic product (and lagged gross domestic product), corporate pretax profits (and lagged pretax profits), lagged corporate giving, and changes in the top corporate tax rate (and lagged corporate tax rate). All dollar amounts are inflation-adjusted. We ran a series of regressions for each year to determine estimated total itemized tax-deductible contributions for the tobacco/beverage industry through 2025.

Results using this modeling strategy predict that tobacco philanthropy would decline under all scenarios, falling to zero between 2018 and 2023 (see figure 8.2). Some decline in philanthropic contributions might be expected in any event, given the projected decline in smoking prevalence and cigarette consumption under all three scenarios. These specific projections may, however, be overly pessimistic. The models rely on the historical relationship between the industry's net income and contributions, among other factors, and on the predicted decline in the industry's net income over the next two decades. If the industry in fact increases net income, perhaps through further diversification of product lines, increasing the price of cigarettes (at a faster rate than the projected decline in demand), or expanding in overseas markets, contributions are likely to increase rather than decrease. In addition, the industry's historic use of philanthropy as a means of public relations and marketing may suggest the industry will spend a disproportionate share on philanthropy despite declining profits as a means to try to influence public opinion and policy. That is, tobacco companies may give a higher share than they have historically if the industry experiences serious attacks and declines in demand as a method of trying to counter public attitudes and

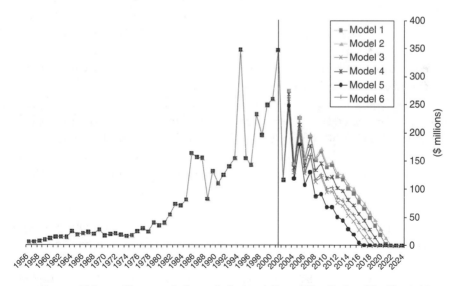

FIGURE 8.2 Tobacco/Beverage Industry Inflation-Adjusted Tax-Deductible Charitable Giving, 1956–2025

Source: Authors' calculations based on the *Giving USA* model (see the chapter text and appendix 8.1).

public policy. This type of phenomenon is not implausible given the industry's vigorous defense and offense, as shown by its past practices. Such factors are, however, beyond the scope of these models.

TOBACCO PHILANTHROPY AND NONPROFIT ORGANIZATIONS

The future of tobacco philanthropy depends most critically on corporate income. If further tobacco control policies decrease the industry's income, the industry's philanthropic contributions are also likely to decrease. As discussed above, there are a number of contingencies that might affect tobacco companies' philanthropic decisions, and it is difficult to project future levels of giving. However, the tobacco industry's philanthropy is not likely to have a significant impact on the nonprofit sector. Because of the small size of most contributions, as well as the minor role that the tobacco industry plays in corporate giving and the relatively small role corporate giving plays as a percentage of total giving from all sources, even a substantial decline in tobacco giving is unlikely to have an appreciable effect on the nonprofit sector overall and most if not all nonprofits specifically. Overall, the tobacco industry's corporate philanthropy represents only about 3.2 percent of all corporate contributions in the United States and only 0.15 percent of total philanthropy. Furthermore, philanthropic contributions are only approximately 20 percent of all revenue generated for the nonprofit sector (O'Neil 2002), so tobacco contributions represent only 0.03 percent of total revenue for the nonprofit sector.

Based on the discussion above, we anticipate two additional developments in tobacco philanthropy. First, as the tobacco industry expands operations internationally, the tobacco industry is increasingly likely to make corporate contributions overseas to create a positive working environment in new countries. Based on the industry's history in the United States, these gifts are likely to be designed to improve the regulatory environment and to create goodwill in the communities in which the companies are recruiting employees and/or marketing to sell their products.

Second, mergers and acquisitions are also known to impact nonprofit organizations, particularly when there is a change in the headquarter city (Rooney, Tempel, and Small 2005). Although Altria has decentralized its corporate contributions and given its subsidiaries, which include Philip Morris USA and Philip Morris International, a larger percentage with which to contribute to charity, 48 percent of contributions from the Altria Group are controlled by local managers of Altria facilities worldwide (Wilhelm 2005). The impact of this decentralization, which began in 2003–2004, has been a decline in Altria grants to the arts and to domestic-violence-prevention organizations, particularly in New York. In addition, Philip Morris USA has increased giving to organizations serving youth, colleges and universities, and charities located near cigarette-manufacturing plants in Richmond, Virginia and Charlotte, North Carolina. This trend will likely continue into the near future, but as Altria facilities change locations and perhaps relocate overseas, so too will donations to local community groups where facilities are located.

CONCLUSION

Tobacco companies have been active participants in corporate philanthropy. Their patterns of giving are in most respects very similar to those of other major corporations, although the documentary evidence suggests that at least some of their philanthropic activity represents an effort to counter the challenging political and regulatory environment the industry has faced over the last half century. Even in the absence of significant change in tobacco control policies, levels of giving would be expected to decline over the next two decades if we assume that corporate income declines along with smoking prevalence (see chapter 2). More vigorous tobacco control policies are likely to accelerate this decline in philanthropy.

However, the nonprofit sector is not likely to be dramatically impacted by these trends. As discussed above, tobacco philanthropy represents only 0.03 percent of the total revenue of nonprofit organizations in the United States. Even if the tobacco industry ended its philanthropic activities, only a few organizations would be impacted significantly, and even then only in the short run (Rooney, Tempel, and Small 2005), whereas the overall effect would be minimal. Those organizations historically receiving funding by the industry would of course be impacted more deeply, as would localities where tobacco manufacturing has been concentrated. In addition, because most gifts were only $5,000 or less, even those receiving gifts historically are unlikely to experience a significant adverse effect.

APPENDIX 8.1: PROJECTING TOBACCO/BEVERAGE GIVING

Predicted tobacco/beverage giving was estimated using an econometric model developed for national estimation of corporate giving for *Giving USA* (Brown, Chin, and Rooney n.d.). A priori use of the *Giving USA* model appears to be appropriate because the tobacco industry's contributions as a percentage of net income are correlated with those of all industries as a percentage of net income (Pearson correlation = 0.440, p-value = 0.002), suggesting the tobacco industry's philanthropic giving is similar to that of U.S. corporations in general. Further,

TABLE 8.2 Assumed Annual Rates of Decline in Tobacco Industry Income by Scenario

	ANNUAL RATE OF DECLINE OF TOBACCO INDUSTRY INCOME	
	2003–2010	2011–2025
Status quo, high: model 1	−0.007	−0.008
Status quo, low: model 2	−0.003	−0.004
IOM, high: model 3	−0.054	−0.018
IOM, low: model 4	−0.027	−0.009
High-impact, high: model 5	−0.096	−0.012
High-impact, low: model 6	−0.048	−0.006

our descriptive analysis indicates that net income is an important driver of the industry's contributions. Changes in giving and changes in corporate income for the tobacco and beverage industries tend to be associated (the Pearson correlation is 0.380, $p = 0.009$). Exceptions may be due to idiosyncratic factors, such as the timing of gift awards (beginning of one year versus the end of another year) and/or unexpected changes in corporate earnings.

The model is:

$$\text{Tobacco Giving}_t = \text{Constant} + \beta_1 \text{Tobacco Industry Income}_t$$
$$+ \beta_2 \text{Tobacco Industry Income}_{t-1} + \beta_3 \text{GDP}_t + \beta_4 \text{GDP}_{t-1}$$
$$+ \beta_5 \text{Tobacco Giving}_{t-1} + \beta_6 \Delta \text{Top Corporate Tax Rate}_t$$
$$+ \beta_7 \Delta \text{Top Corporate Tax Rate}_{t-1} + \varepsilon.$$

Our projections of tobacco/beverage industry income between 2003 and 2025 are based on assumptions made about the impact of three tobacco control policy scenarios. We tested the robustness or stability of our estimates by including two possible income implications for each tobacco control scenario. The first is a modest decline in income, and the second assumes a more dramatic decline in income. The annual rates of decline in tobacco industry income assumed for the three scenarios are shown in table 8.2. We found that the results were relatively insensitive to choice of parameters.

NOTES

1. Altria.com, www.altria.com/responsibility/4_9_contributionscommunities.asp, last accessed April 28, 2006.
2. http://www.accessphilanthropy.com/funderinnews.php?funderID=393.
3. The American Tobacco Company, IRS Forms 990-PF, 1950–1951 and 1953–1955.
4. Blasingame, F. J. L., American Medical Association. P. Lorillard Company, February 12, 1964. Bates No.: 85871453/1454 and T0022590. Legacy Tobacco Document Library, available at www.legacy.library.ucsf.edu.
5. Tobacco Institute, "The development of tobacco industry strategy," 1982. Tobacco Institute. Bates No.: 03673753/3762, 20249566531/6698, 5039081001/8142. Legacy Tobacco Document Library, available at www.legacy.library.ucsf.edu.
6. Bring, Murry, "N327," May 25, 1995. Philip Morris USA. Bates No.: 2045756743. Legacy Tobacco Document Library, available at www.legacy.library.ucsf.edu.
7. "Proactive public relations plan: African-American & Hispanic Market," April 27, 1998. Philip Morris USA. Bates No.: 207183355/59. Legacy Tobacco Document Library, available at www.legacy.library.ucsf.edu.
8. R. J. Reynolds, "Minority affairs presentation to Jim Johnston." March 22, 1991. R. J. Reynolds Tobacco Company. Bates No.: 507701655-1665. Minnesota Tobacco Document Depository, available at www.legacy.library.ucsf.edu.
9. McCarthy, Thomas, "1974 (740000) New York Promotion—Ethnic/Charity Concept," RJ Reynolds Tobacco Company. Bates No.: 500780149. Legacy Tobacco Document Library, available at www.legacy.library.ucsf.edu.
10. R. J. Reynolds, "Summary of MIP/RIP Proposal," 1994. R. J. Reynolds Tobacco Company. Bates No.: 512722664/2667. Legacy Tobacco Document Library, available at www.legacy.library.ucsf.edu.
11. "Corporate Goodwill or Tainted Money?" ABC News, February 8, 2001.
12. Philip Morris USA's mission statement as printed on www.philipmorrisusa.com and accessed April 25, 2006, now reads, "products to adults who use them." The word "choose" was omitted in what became the final statement.
13. Philip Morris USA's mission statement as printed on www.philipmorrisusa.com and accessed April 25, 2006, now also includes "Providing Cessation Information" as a means to achieving their CSR mission.
14. R. J. Reynolds Tobacco Company, http://www.rjrt.com/values/respCore.aspx, last accessed April 29, 2006.
15. Tobacco Free Initiative, World Health Organization. "Tobacco industry and corporate responsibility . . . an inherent contradiction," February 2003. World Health Organization, available at http://www.who.int/tobacco, last accessed April 29, 2006.
16. http://www.altria.com/en/cms/Responsibility/Contributing_to_Communities/Employee_Community_Fund/default.aspx.
17. R. J. Reynolds Foundation Guidelines for Giving, www.rjrt.com/values/communityGuidelines.aspx, last accessed April 25, 2006.
18. Brown & Williamson, 1981. Bates No.: 517002849. Legacy Tobacco Document Library, available at www.legacy.library.ucsf.edu.
19. Brown & Williamson, "Draft Remarks C. I. McCarthy 1977 United Way Kickoff," 1977. Brown & Williamson. Bates No.: 690144128 and 670303332. Legacy Tobacco Document Library, available at www.legacy.library.ucsf.edu.

9

TOBACCO CONTROL POLICIES: THE EFFECT ON STATE AND LOCAL TAXES

HOWARD CHERNICK

Cigarettes are an inviting target for taxation. From the point of view of the revenue collector, they have the twin virtues of being harmful for consumers yet with demand sufficiently insensitive to price to yield large amounts of revenue. As the links between health and smoking, particularly the harmful effects of secondhand smoke, have become more firmly established, the justification for cigarette taxation as a "sin" tax has become stronger. At the same time, the long-term decline in smoking prevalence has reduced the size of the cigarette tax base. The decline means that the marginal revenue productivity of the cigarette tax—the additional revenue that comes from a given increase in the tax rate—has probably fallen. On the other hand, the reduction in the number of smokers and the increased concern about the broader health effects of smoking have made it easier to raise cigarette taxes. McGowan and Mahon (2005) cite recent state polls showing widespread support for increasing tobacco taxes, even among smokers.

In raising their cigarette tax rates, states must evaluate the trade-offs among the additional revenue from higher tax rates, the health benefits from reduced smoking prevalence, and the potential loss in taxable sales through tax avoidance through cross-border shopping, purchases via the Internet, or smuggling. Tax avoidance nullifies the health benefits from reduced smoking while depriving the state of tax revenues. Large differences in tax rates across states encourage illegal smuggling of cigarettes and raise the costs of enforcing excise taxes.

This chapter examines the role of cigarette taxation as a revenue source for state and local governments. Its major goal is to simulate what would happen to state tax revenues under the policy scenarios employed throughout this volume. Both the Institute of Medicine (IOM) and high-impact scenarios include a $2 increase in tobacco excise taxes, and both are projected to reduce cigarette consumption rapidly between 2005 and 2025. The fiscal consequences for the states obviously depend on whether the tax rate increase is imposed at the federal or state level; this chapter considers both alternatives.

The first section of this chapter describes trends in state and local cigarette taxation between 1972 and 2004 and the changing importance of tobacco taxes in state budgets over time. In the second section I estimate the relationship between cigarette tax rates and taxable sales; this analysis is the first step in developing projections of tax revenues under the three policy scenarios. The third section uses these estimated relationships, along with simulation results from chapter 2, to forecast changes in state tax revenues under the common policy scenarios.

CIGARETTE TAXES IN STATE REVENUE SYSTEMS

Although excise taxes have been levied on tobacco at the federal level at least since 1865, the first state tax was not imposed until 1921. By 1961, all states imposed their own cigarette taxes. Federal tax collections exceeded state taxation for more than 100 years, but since 1969 state taxes have been higher than federal levies. In 2006 states collected $13.75 billion while the federal excise tax yielded $7.5 billion. Total state and local tax revenues from cigarettes, including the sales tax on cigarettes, equaled $18.2 billion. In 2006 the federal rate of 39 cents per pack was half of the weighted average state cigarette tax rate of 78.5 cents per pack and a little more than a third of the total state and local rate, including general sales taxes collected for cigarettes (all figures in this paragraph drawn from "The Tax Burden on Tobacco" [Orzechowski and Walker 2006]).

There are three components of the taxation of cigarettes and other tobacco products. All 50 states impose a separate excise tax on cigarettes, set in cents per pack. In addition to the excise tax, 48 states now include cigarettes in the sales tax base. Moreover, in most states, the basis for cigarette taxation under the sales tax is the retail price of cigarettes inclusive of the excise tax. With state sales taxes clustered around 5 percent, the inclusion of the excise tax in the sales tax base means that a given increase in the excise tax rate leverages at least an additional 5 percent increase in the tax rate through the sales tax. Although the cigarette tax is primarily a state-level tax, about 500 local jurisdictions in eight states also levied cigarette excise taxes in 2006. This chapter sets its focus on state taxes.

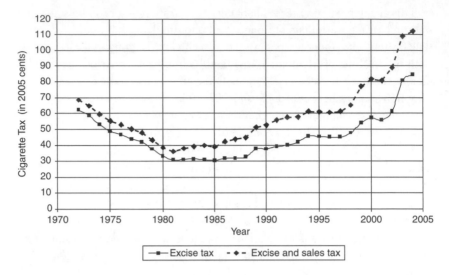

FIGURE 9.1 State and Local Cigarette Tax

Source: Orzechowski and Walker, "The Tax Burden on Tobacco," vol. 39, 2004.

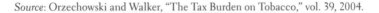

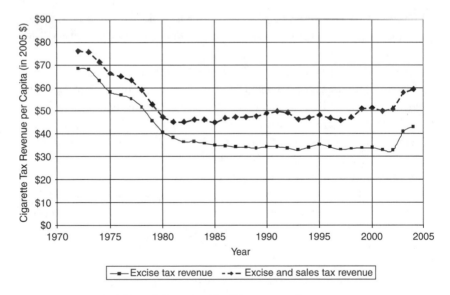

FIGURE 9.2 State and Local Cigarette Tax Revenue per Capita

Sources: Orzechowski and Walker, "The Tax Burden on Tobacco," vol. 39, 2004; U.S. Census Bureau, *Annual Survey of State and Local Government Finances*, http://www.census.gov/govs/estimate/; and U.S. Census Bureau, *Census of Governments*, http://www.census.gov/govs/cog/.

Figure 9.1 displays the mean state cigarette tax rates between 1972 and 2004, showing both the excise tax alone and the excise plus sales tax rate. Tax rates are expressed in terms of cents per pack and are adjusted to 2005 price levels. Average rates declined by about 50 percent between 1972 and 1985 and then increased slowly between 1985 and 1995. In 1997 they began a rapid rate of increase, reaching 85 cents per pack for the excise tax alone and $1.12 for the sales tax inclusive rate—double the rate in 1997. Between 2004 and 2010, 36 states and the District of Columbia raised their excise tax rates, with an average increase of 91.5 cents per pack. The average state excise tax rate in February 2010 was 134.6 cents per pack (figures calculated from Tax Foundation, http://www .taxfoundation.org/taxdata/show/245.html).

Figure 9.2 shows per-capita revenue from state and local tobacco taxes. As the graph shows, per-capita revenues were flat between 1980 and 2001 and only began to increase after 2001. The drop in revenue from 1972 to 1980 reflects both the decline in real (i.e., inflation-adjusted) tax rates and reductions in smoking prevalence. Between about 1980 and 2000, modest increases in tax rates were largely offset by falling smoking rates. Since 2001, however, the rapidly increasing tax rate has outpaced declines in smoking, leading to a marked jump in per-capita tobacco tax revenues. Excise tax revenues from cigarettes have not been this high since the late 1970s.

Figure 9.3 shows state cigarette tax revenues as a share of state tax revenues for the nation as a whole and for the five highest and five lowest states as of 2004. Between 1976 and 2002 cigarette taxes fell from almost 5 percent of state taxes to a little more than 2 percent. In 2002 that share began to rise, reaching 2.7 percent in 2004—the highest since 1986. In high-tax states tobacco taxes were above 7 percent of revenue in 1976, fell rapidly to 4 percent by 1985, declined more slowly between 1985 and 2000, then rose more than a percentage point since 2000, comprising more than 4.5 percent of revenues by 2004. In low-tax states the cigarette tax share fell to about 1 percent of state taxes by the early 1980s and has remained at about that level since.

As shown in figure 9.4, there is considerable variation across states in tobacco taxation. Over time, the highest- and lowest-tax states have become more regionally concentrated. The tobacco-growing states have historically had among the lowest cigarette tax rates in the country: in 1972, the five states with the lowest tax rates (starting with the lowest) were North Carolina, Virginia, Colorado, Kentucky, and Indiana; Kentucky, North Carolina, and Virginia were still among the lowest five in 2004. The five highest-tax states have become more concentrated in the Northeast. In 1972, the five states with the highest cigarette tax rates were Connecticut, New Jersey, Texas, Pennsylvania, and Minnesota; in 2004, the five highest were New Jersey, New York, Rhode Island, Massachusetts, and Connecticut. As figure 9.4 shows, the low-tax states kept their real tax rates practically unchanged for more than three decades. In contrast, the high-tax

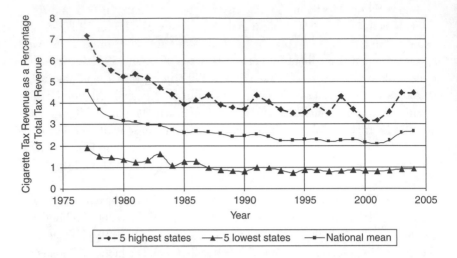

FIGURE 9.3 State Cigarette Excise and Sales Tax Revenue as a Percentage of Total State Tax Revenue: Averages of the Five Highest and Five Lowest States Plus National Mean

Source: Orzechowski and Walker, "The Tax Burden on Tobacco," vol. 39, 2004.

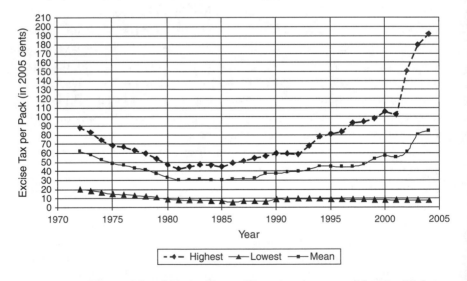

FIGURE 9.4 State and Local Excise Tax on Cigarettes: Averages of the Five Highest and Five Lowest States Plus National Mean

Source: Orzechowski and Walker, "The Tax Burden on Tobacco," vol. 39, 2004.

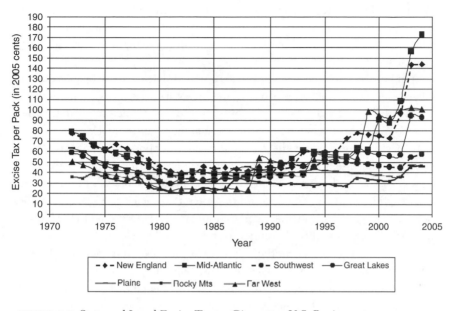

FIGURE 9.5 State and Local Excise Tax on Cigarettes: U.S. Regions

Source: Orzechowski and Walker, "The Tax Burden on Tobacco," vol. 39, 2004.

states converged toward the average until about 1980, but since then the gap between low- and high-tax states has widened, particularly after 2000. The interstate difference in tax rates is a measure of the incentive to smuggle cigarettes from low- to high-tax states, and these figures suggest that by 2004 this incentive was stronger than it had been at any time in the previous 35 years.

Figure 9.5 shows average tax rates over time by seven census regions. Interregional variation in rates was relatively stable until about 1997 and then began to grow sharply. The increase in tax rates since 1997 is concentrated in the Mid-Atlantic region, the New England states, and the Far West. Whereas tax rates have diverged sharply, variation in revenue levels and revenue shares is more muted. Since 2004 substantial excise tax increases have been imposed by states in all regions of the country, suggesting that the excise tax increase in the Northeast is diffusing throughout the country.

EXCISE TAXES AND THE DEMAND FOR CIGARETTES

Many studies have estimated the effect of cigarette taxation on the demand for cigarettes. Consensus estimates are that a 10 percent increase in the retail price of a pack of cigarettes will lead to a decline in demand of about 4.5 percent (Chaloupka and Warner 1999). Some more recent estimates suggest a somewhat higher elasticity of about 0.6 for legal sales (Gruber and Köszegi 2001; Yurekli and Zhang 2000).

A number of studies have found that evasion of state cigarette taxes is quantitatively significant and has grown with the recent increase in cigarette tax rates. Coats (1995) regressed taxable sales on both the pretax price of cigarettes and state tax rates and concluded that 80 percent of the tax effect on taxable sales is a result of cross-border sales rather than falling consumption: in other words, faced with a tax increase, most people seek out lower-tax alternatives rather than cut back on smoking. Likewise, Stehr (2005) compared taxable sales estimates to consumption estimates; he estimated that after a tax increase, 85 percent of the decline in tax-paid cigarette sales comes from tax avoidance rather than changes in consumption. Goolsbee, Lovenheim, and Slemrod (2010) argue that the ability to purchase cigarettes over the Internet has provided an increasingly important means for evading state cigarette taxes. From an informal survey in Ann Arbor, Michigan, Goolsbee and his colleagues concluded that about 90 percent of the tax savings from Internet purchases were passed forward to the consumer, providing a strong financial incentive for smokers to switch to the Internet. They reported that the elasticity of taxable sales has doubled since 1990, while the elasticity of consumption has not changed or may even have decreased. This research implies that the additional revenue states can gain by increasing their cigarette tax rates is severely circumscribed by the ability of smokers to evade higher taxes.

Despite the evidence of sharp increases in avoidance when a state raises its cigarette tax rate, Stehr (2005) found that tax avoidance accounted for less than 10 percent of cigarette sales. Similarly, Thursby and Thursby (2000) reported that smuggling made up less than 7 percent of sales. Because there seems to be a strong behavioral response to changes in the relative prices of alternative sources of cigarettes, the limited share of out-of-state purchases suggests, and the data confirm, that the average tax differential between adjacent states is relatively small. This can be explained by the fact that neighboring states have a strong incentive to mimic each other in setting cigarette tax rates. For example, Rork (2003) finds that a 10 cent per pack increase in the tax rate in neighboring states leads to a 4 to 6 cent increase in own-state tax rates.

METHODOLOGY AND DATA

Following the strategy used by other researchers for estimating the revenue effect of cigarette taxation (Goolsbee, Lovenheim, and Slemrod 2010; Gruber, Sen, and Stabile 2003), I regressed taxable sales on the retail price of cigarettes and the average retail price in neighboring states. The model is estimated for a panel of 48 continental states and includes state-level income and demographic characteristics. The retail price measure includes cigarette excise taxes as well as all applicable sales taxes. All specifications include state fixed effects to account for unobservable differences across states and year effects to account for the secular decline in smoking (Harris 1994). For the subset of years where data on tobacco control policies are available, I perform a separate analysis including various indices of these policies.

In addition to the price variables, the estimating equation included per-capita personal income and several demographic covariates: percent college graduate, percent foreign born, percent African American, percent Hispanic, percent less than 18 years of age, and percent 65 years of age or older. Because smoking rates differ across social and demographic groups, smoking prevalence and hence the potential revenue from cigarette taxation may vary across states according to the social and demographic composition of their populations. The regression analysis shows that several of these state demographic characteristics are significantly related to taxable cigarette sales, although the direction of effect is frequently inconsistent over the two time periods.

A number of studies of the demand for cigarettes have included a measure of the incentive for interstate cigarette smuggling. For example, Becker, Grossman, and Murphy (1994) use the difference between a state's own cigarette tax rate and the rate in the lowest-tax tobacco-producing states, weighted by the distance between the state and the low-taxed states. I do not include a separate term for smuggling in this specification. Because distance is constant, and the low-tax states kept their tax rates approximately constant in real terms over the sample period, own-state tax rate is likely to fully reflect state-specific changes in the incentive to smuggle. National changes in the resources devoted to enforcement of anti-smuggling laws will be reflected in the year effects, and persistent differences across states (related, for example, to differences in religious composition) will be reflected in the state fixed effects.

The model was estimated using data on cigarette tax rates and revenues for the 48 continental U.S. states between 1980 and 2004. (Hawaii and Alaska are excluded because the neighbor effects are less relevant for these states.) Tax rates are measured for the state and its localities and are separated into an excise tax rate and a sales tax rate on cigarettes. Revenues are for the state fiscal year. For years in which the cigarette tax changed during the fiscal year, the tax rate is the weighted average of the tax rates before and after the change, with the weights equal to the percentage of months in the year under each of the two tax regimes. The most comprehensive tax rate is the combined state-local excise plus sales tax rate. All values are expressed in 2005 dollars. (Variable definitions and data sources are presented in table 9.6, found in appendix 9.1.)

As discussed in the literature review, the evidence suggests that taxable sales of cigarettes have become more responsive to increases in price in recent years, relative to cigarette consumption itself. Goolsbee, Lovenheim, and Slemrod (2010) argue that the explanation lies in the increasing ability to purchase cigarettes tax-free on the Internet, whether from Native American tribes or from abroad. The sharp increase in cigarette taxes and in tax differentials in recent years has increased the financial incentive for smokers to seek out cheaper alternatives, just as it has increased the incentive for illegal smuggling of cigarettes.

To address this possible change in the relationship between tax rates and tax revenues, I divided the sample into two periods, 1980–1994 and 1995–2004. This division was based on the discussion by Goolsbee and colleagues (2010) of the timing of diffusion of Internet use and the fact that the pace of excise tax increases accelerated substantially in the late 1990s and early 2000s. (A Chow test rejected at the 1 percent level of significance the hypothesis of equality of coefficients for the two periods. A within-sample prediction exercise comparing predicted to actual values for the 1995–2000 period, using the estimated coefficients from the initial period, also showed substantial overprediction of taxable sales in the second period.) Because the increase in tax rates was particularly rapid from 2000 to 2004, I also estimated a separate regression for that period alone.

The basic regression results are shown in table 9.1. All variables are in log form. The estimated elasticity for taxable sales is −0.84 for the 1980–1994 period. For 1995–2004 the elasticity is −1.54, almost double that for the earlier period. As shown in column 3, a separate regression for 2000–2004 yields an elasticity of −1.37, close to the elasticity for the entire second period. In the period from 1995 to 2004, neighbor price had a significant effect on taxable sales, with the magnitude of the effect almost four times as high as the effect in 1980–1994. In other words, the higher the retail cigarette prices in neighboring states, the more cigarettes are sold in the state in question. Thus, the estimates suggest an increase both in the sensitivity of sales to the price of cigarettes and in cross-border shopping.

The near doubling in the price elasticity of taxable sales suggests that since 1995, the cigarette tax has become less productive as a revenue source for state governments. To test this proposition directly, in columns 4, 5, and 6 of table 9.1, the dependent variable is the log of per-capita cigarette tax revenue. The sample is again divided into two periods, together with a separate regression for 2000–2004. The results show a decline in the revenue elasticity of the cigarette tax between 1980–1994 and 1995–2004, from 0.83 to 0.73. In other words, a 10 percent increase in the tax rate yielded an 8.3 percent increase in per-capita revenues in 1980–1994 and only a 7.3 percent increase in the later period. The effect of neighboring state tax rates also increased in magnitude in the second

TABLE 9.1 Regression of Taxable Packs Sold and Cigarette Tax Revenue on Cigarette Tax Rate

DEPENDENT VARIABLE	TAXABLE PACKS SOLD			CIGARETTE TAX REVENUE		
Sample years	1980–1994	1995–2004	2000–2004	1980–1994	1995–2004	2000–2004
Retail price[a]	−0.84 (.13)**	−1.54 (.18)**	−1.37 (.34)**			
Neighbor retail price	0.15 (.09)	0.57 (.28)*	0.43 (.36)			
Tax rate				0.83 (.02)**	0.73 (.03)**	0.74 (.06)
Neighbor tax rate				0.03 (.03)	0.12 (.07)	0.12 (.07)
R^2	0.96	0.97	0.97	0.96	0.98	0.99
Number of observations	720	480	192	720	480	240

Notes: Taxable Packs Sold and Cigarette Tax Revenue are per capita. All variables are in logarithmic form. All analyses include state-level per-capita income and demographic composition measures.

Instrumented by state and local cigarette tax rate, including sales tax on cigarettes. First-stage equation, estimated separately for each period: Retail Price = 0.18*Cig Tax Rate + State/Year Dummy Variables.

Significance levels: *$p < 0.05$; **$p < 0.01$.

Source: Author's calculations (see appendix 9.1 for data sources).

period but was not statistically significant. The results using only the period 2000–2004 are not significantly different from those for 1995–2004.

The decline in the elasticity of cigarette tax revenues in the 1995–2004 period, as compared with 1980–1994, is consistent with the increased elasticity of taxable sales in this period. It suggests that states are deriving proportionally less revenue from tax increases than they did in the past. Despite the reduced revenue elasticity of the cigarette tax, however, on average an increase in the cigarette tax still yields a substantial revenue increase for states. As discussed in appendix 9.1, the apparent contradiction between the sharp increase in the elasticity of sales on the one hand, and the relatively modest decline in the revenue elasticity on the other, results from the fact that, despite recent increases in tax rates, cigarette taxes still made up only about 21 percent of the retail price in the 1995–2004 period. Evaluated at the mean 2004 state tax rate of $1.00 per pack, a 10 percent increase in cigarette taxation would have increased state cigarette tax revenues by about 8 percent.

The estimated revenue elasticity is a mean value for the sample. To test whether high-tax states are at or close to the limits of their ability to raise additional revenue from the cigarette tax, I reestimated the regression in table 9.1 using only those observations with tax rates at least one standard deviation above the mean for the years 1995–2004. The estimated price elasticity of taxable packs sold was −1.44, not significantly different from the elasticity for the entire sample over that period. The revenue elasticity for the high-tax states was 0.65, compared with 0.73 for the entire sample. The lower revenue elasticity for high-tax states reflects the fact that cigarette taxes are a higher share of the retail price in high- than in low-tax states. Consequently, the elasticity of retail price with respect to the tax rate in high-tax states is 0.28 as opposed to 0.19 for the entire sample. The predicted revenue elasticity for the high-tax states is 0.6, again close to the estimated elasticity of revenues with respect to the tax. The lower revenue elasticity is incorporated into the simulations of the revenue effects.

Tobacco control policies other than excise taxes may influence taxable sales, and if states implement these regulations and policies at the same time they raise excise taxes, the nontax policies could be responsible for some of the decline in sales that we are attributing to tax increases. Alternatively, other tobacco control policies could make tax increases more effective. To examine whether either of these is true, I introduced three different indices of state-level tobacco control policy, all drawn from the ImpacTeen project at the University of Illinois at Chicago (http://www.impacteen.org/). For this analysis the sample is restricted to 1991–2001, the years for which the policy measures were available. The measures include (1) the Alciati index of youth access to smoking, (2) another measure of youth access policies, the Possession-Use-Purchase (PUP) index, which ranges from 0 (least restrictive) to 3 (most restrictive), and (3) the smoke-free (SF) index, which ranges from 0 (least restrictive) to 5 (most restrictive) and measures the extent and strength of smoke-free rules for various types of buildings and activities.

The first column of table 9.2 excludes all policy indexes. Columns 2–4 enter separately the Alciati, PUP, and SF indexes. The last column includes an interaction between retail price and the SF index to test whether price increases have a greater effect on taxable consumption when stricter smoking restrictions are in place. Cigarette sales were lower in states with more restrictive smoke-free laws, but the two youth access measures had no effect on taxable sales. In an analysis (not shown) excluding the year effects, each policy index had a negative effect on sales; because policy indexes tended to increase over the years, it is difficult to distinguish their effects from other year-by-year changes. More important for our purposes, the retail price coefficient is unaffected by the inclusion of anti-smoking policy indexes, suggesting that the effects of cigarette tax rates are not confounded with other tobacco control policy changes.

TABLE 9.2 Taxable Packs Sold: Effect of Tobacco Control Policies, 1991–2001

INDEPENDENT VARIABLE	NO INDEX	ALCIATI	POSSESSION-USE-PURCHASE	SMOKE-FREE	SMOKE-FREE INTERACTED
Retail price[a]	−1.27	−1.28	−1.31	−1.29	−1.26
	(.20)**	(.20)**	(.20)**	(.19)**	(.21)**
Neighbor retail price	0.17	0.31	0.30	0.28	0.28
	(.12)	(.17)	(.17)	(.16)	(.16)
Alciati index		0.001			
		(.001)			
PUP index			0.006		
			(.007)		
SF index				−0.003	0.006
				(.001)**	(.015)
SF index × retail price					−0.002
					(.003)
Observations	528	528	528	528	528
R^2	0.95	0.96	0.96	0.96	0.96

Notes: All cigarette revenues and packs are per capita. All variables are in logarithmic form.
[a] Instrumented by state and local cigarette tax rate, including sales tax on cigarettes. First-stage equation, estimated separately for each period: Retail Price = 0.18*Cig Tax Rate + State/Year Dummy Variables. Significance levels: *$p < 0.05$; **$p < 0.01$.
Source: Author's calculations (see appendix 9.1 for data sources).

CIGARETTE TAXATION IN THE BROADER CONTEXT OF STATE FINANCES

As discussed earlier, over the last several decades cigarette taxation has played only a small role in state government finances. Since the late 1990s, however, its importance has grown, as more states have turned to cigarette tax increases to address fiscal stress in state budgets. In this context, a drop in smoking prevalence could present a greater problem for state budgets now than in the past.

Table 9.3 summarizes recent changes in the role of cigarette taxation in state finance, showing mean and maximum state cigarette tax rates (column 1), cigarette taxes as a share of total state taxes (column 2), the correlation between the cigarette tax rate and the cigarette tax share (column 3), and that between the cigarette tax share and the level of state taxes (column 4). The years are 1996, 2000, and 2004. The first column shows little change from 1996 to 2000 but a sharp increase in average cigarette tax rates between 2000 and 2004. During this

TABLE 9.3 State Cigarette Taxes and Total State Taxes

	STATE CIGARETTE TAX RATE[a] (MAXIMUM) (IN CENTS)	AVERAGE CIGARETTE TAX SHARE[b] (MAXIMUM)	CORRELATION BETWEEN CIGARETTE TAX RATE AND CIGARETTE TAX SHARE	CORRELATION BETWEEN CIGARETTE TAX SHARE AND PER-CAPITA STATE TAXES
1996	51.1 (125)	2.2 % (5.4%)	0.58	−0.25
2000	62.1 (147)	2.1 % (5.4%)	0.51	−0.15
2004	95.1 (250)	2.7 % (5.6%)	0.64	0.12

[a] Includes sales tax on cigarettes.
[b] Cigarette taxes as a share of total state taxes.
Source: Author's calculations (see appendix 9.1 for data sources).

period, cigarette taxes increased more rapidly than other state taxes, with an increase in the cigarette tax share from 2.1 percent to 2.7 percent. The correlation between the cigarette tax rate and the cigarette tax share increased significantly between 2000 and 2004. This increase reflects the fact that a number of states raised cigarette taxes to offset the sharp downturn in state revenues between 2001 and 2003. This fiscal response differed from previous recessions, in which states tended to raise other taxes. Column 4 shows a change in the relationship between the cigarette tax share and the level of state taxes. Before 2000, states more reliant on cigarette taxes tended to have lower overall state tax rates, but since that time states with high cigarette tax shares also had higher overall tax rates.

As table 9.3 shows, although cigarette taxes increased in the early 2000s, in 2004 cigarette revenues still provided less than 3 percent of state tax revenues; when we consider intergovernmental aid and nontax revenues, cigarette taxes provided only 1 percent of total state revenue. Even if smoking were completely eradicated, on average states would have to raise tax revenues by less than 3 percent to offset the loss from cigarette taxes. States with relatively high cigarette tax shares (defined here as at least one standard deviation above the mean) would have to raise other taxes by at least 4 percent to offset the loss in cigarette taxes. Rhode Island, the highest tax state in 2004, would have to increase other taxes by about 6 percent to offset the total loss from cigarette taxation.

SALES TAX OFFSETS TO LOSSES IN CIGARETTE TAX REVENUES

If cigarette consumption fell, the loss in tobacco tax revenues could potentially be offset by increased revenues from other taxes as smokers shift their spending from cigarettes to other taxable goods and services. If cigarettes and alcohol are substitutes for each other, for instance, alcohol tax revenues could rise. In addition to yielding tax revenues, this spending could stimulate the state economy. Because cigarettes are produced in and exported from a few tobacco-growing states, a shift in demand from cigarettes to other goods and services is likely to benefit businesses in nontobacco states. However, because tax rates are much higher for cigarettes than for other consumer goods, any offset is likely to be only partial. In 2006, state cigarette excise taxes averaged 22 percent of the retail price of cigarettes (Orzechowski and Walker 2006, table 13A). The median state sales tax rate was about 5 percent, and states typically exempted a substantial portion of consumption from the general sales tax (Chernick and Reschovsky 1990). Busch et al. (2005) find evidence that as cigarette prices rise, households spend more on food, which is often taxed at a lower rate or exempt from sales tax. Although the tax rate on retail sales understates somewhat the total burden of the sales tax (Ring 1999), and despite offsetting spending on other goods and services, at current tax rates reductions in smoking are still likely to reduce state revenues. (This conclusion is supported by a regression analysis, available from the author upon request, which finds no evidence that lower revenues from cigarette taxation are offset by higher revenues from alcohol or general sales taxes.)

TAX REVENUE PROJECTIONS UNDER THREE POLICY SCENARIOS

In this section I combine the SimSmoke estimates from chapter 2 with the estimated price elasticities from the previous section to simulate the effect of tobacco control policies on state cigarette tax revenues under three alternative scenarios: the status quo, IOM, and high-impact scenarios. As in previous chapters, the status quo scenario assumes no change in tobacco control policy between 2006 and 2025; excise tax rates are assumed to be adjusted for inflation. The IOM scenario includes a moderate package of tobacco control measures, including a $2 increase in the excise tax. The high-impact scenario retains the $2 tax increase but assumes that a stronger set of policies leads to a steeper reduction in smoking rates. Details of the estimation procedures are in appendix 9.1.

For both the IOM and high-impact scenarios, I calculated two sets of estimates: one assumed that the states imposed the tax increase, and the other assumed that the federal government imposed (and retained) the tax increase. The revenue impact for states depends on which level of government raises the tax. The $2.00 per pack increase in taxes leads to a reduction in the tax base for both levels of government. If the rate increase is at the federal level, then the states would lose money because their tax base would decline while tax rates remained the same. If states impose the tax increase, they receive a higher tax rate on a dwindling tax base; whether revenue rises or falls depends on the size of the tax increase relative to the size of the reduction in consumption.

Table 9.4 presents the mean values for per-capita revenues from tobacco excise taxes for all states. Each panel presents values for five scenarios. The first row displays results for the status quo scenario. The second and third rows show results for the IOM and high-impact scenarios assuming that the tax is imposed by the federal government. The fourth and fifth rows project what would happen if the $2 increase in tobacco tax rates was imposed by the states or (alternatively) was collected by the federal government and passed through to the states.

Among all states, per-capita revenues from cigarette taxes are projected to decline from $65 in 2005 to $46 in 2025 under the status quo, reflecting the expected decline in smoking rates because of demographic change and the long-

TABLE 9.4 Mean Per-Capita Tobacco Tax Revenues and Percentage Decline in Total Per-Capita State Tax Revenues Under Alternative Policy Scenarios, All States, 2005–2025

	2005	2010	2015	2020	2025
Per-capita revenues from tobacco					
Status quo	$65	$59	$55	$50	$46
IOM ($2 goes to federal government)	65	35	30	26	22
High-impact ($2 goes to federal government)	65	15	14	12	11
IOM ($2 goes to states)	65	115	98	84	74
High-impact ($2 goes to states)	65	46	43	38	34
Percentage decline in total per-capita state tax revenue[a]					
Status quo		0.2	0.5	0.7	0.9
IOM ($2 goes to federal government)		1.4	1.6	1.8	2
High-impact ($2 goes to federal government)		2.3	2.4	2.4	2.5
IOM ($2 goes to states)		−2.5	−1.7	−1	−0.5
High-impact ($2 goes to states)		0.8	1	1.2	1.4

[a] Positive values indicate a decline in per-capita revenue; negative values indicate an increase in per-capita revenue.
Source: Author's calculations (see appendix 9.1 for data sources).

term effects of previously enacted policy changes. Under the IOM scenario, state revenues from cigarette taxation would decline from $65 to $35 per capita in 2010 and to $22 per capita in 2025 with a federal tax increase. Under the high-impact scenario, the decline in smoking would be much more rapid, with per-capita cigarette tax revenues falling to $15 by 2010. However, if the states imposed the tax increase, the IOM scenario would initially result in a sharp increase in per-capita revenues; although revenues would decline over time as smoking rates fell, the value in 2025 is still substantially higher than under the status quo. Under the high-impact scenario, if the states imposed the tax increase, revenues would fall relative to the status quo scenario, but not as steeply as they would if the federal government imposed the tax.

To understand the fiscal impact of these revenue changes, it is useful to put them in the context of states' total tax revenue streams. The lower panel of table 9.4 shows the percentage decline in per-capita state tax revenues under the five scenarios. These figures assume that inflation-adjusted per-capita tax revenues remain constant; these estimates, although crude, let us compare the magnitude of the fiscal impact across scenarios and across states with different tax regimes. The top panel shows the average across all states. Overall, the changes in per-capita state tax revenue are small. Across all states, under the status quo scenario, total per-capita state tax revenue is projected to decline by 0.9 percent between 2005 and 2025 with no change in tobacco control policy. Under the worst-case scenario for the states—the high-impact scenario with tax increases levied by the federal government—per-capita revenue is projected to decline by 2.5 percent.

Table 9.5 presents these values for the five states with the highest tax rates and the five with the lowest tax rates. The five states with the highest tax rates (Connecticut, Michigan, New Jersey, New York, and Rhode Island) had higher initial values for per-capita revenues, but the projected trends are similar. Again, the states would experience a steeper decline in per-capita revenue if the federal government imposed the tax increase but would see an increase in revenue under the IOM scenario if the state imposed the tax. In the five states with the lowest tax rates (Kentucky, Mississippi, Missouri, North Carolina, and South Carolina), the projected trends were similar. Strikingly, under the IOM or high-impact tax increase, if the states imposed the tax increase these low-tax states would have had the same per-capita tobacco tax revenue as the average across the nation; their higher initial smoking rates would compensate for tax rates that remain relatively low.

Table 9.5 also presents the percentage change in all state tax revenues per capita. The impact is greater for the high-tax states because tobacco taxes currently make up a larger share of their revenue stream. For the five states with the highest tax rates, per-capita tax revenues could decline by as much as 3.5 percent under the high-impact scenario with the tax increase imposed by the federal government. Among states with the lowest tax rates, the negative impact is

TABLE 9.5 Mean Per-Capita Tobacco Tax Revenues and Percentage Decline in Total Per-Capita State Tax Revenues Under Alternative Policy Scenarios, States with Highest Tax Rates and States with Lowest Tax Rates, 2005–2025

	2005	2010	2015	2020	2025
Five states with highest tax rates					
Per-capita revenues from tobacco					
Status quo	$113	$104	$96	$96	$88
IOM ($2 goes to federal government)	113	52	45	45	39
High-impact ($2 goes to federal government)	113	31	28	28	25
IOM ($2 goes to states)	113	137	117	117	101
High-impact ($2 goes to states)	113	56	51	51	45
Percentage decline in total per-capita state tax revenue[a]					
Status quo		0.3	0.7	1	1.3
IOM ($2 goes to federal government)		2.4	2.7	2.9	3.1
High-impact ($2 goes to federal government)		3.1	3.2	3.3	3.5
IOM ($2 goes to states)		−0.9	−0.2	0.5	1
High-impact ($2 goes to states)		2.2	2.4	2.6	2.8
Five states with lowest tax rates					
Per-capita revenues from tobacco					
Status quo	$33	$31	$28	$26	$24
IOM ($2 goes to federal government)	33	20	18	15	13
High-impact ($2 goes to federal government)	33	7	6	6	5
IOM ($2 goes to states)	33	118	101	87	76
High-impact ($2 goes to states)	33	48	44	39	35
Percentage decline in total per-capita state tax revenue[a]					
Status quo		0.1	0.3	0.4	0.5
IOM ($2 goes to federal government)		0.7	0.8	1	1.1
High-impact ($2 goes to federal government)		1.3	1.4	1.5	1.5
IOM ($2 goes to states)		−4.5	−3.6	−2.8	−2.3
High-impact ($2 goes to states)		−0.8	−0.6	−0.3	−0.07

[a] Positive values indicate a decline in per-capita revenue; negative values indicate an increase in per-capita revenue.
Source: Author's calculations (see appendix 9.1 for data sources).

far less: a drop of 0.5 percent under the status quo compared with 1.5 percent under the high-impact scenario (with a federal tax increase).

CONCLUSION

In 2004 cigarette taxes made up an average of 2.7 percent of state tax revenues. Due primarily to a decline in smoking prevalence, cigarette taxes declined steadily in importance from 1975 to 2000. However, cigarette taxes began to rebound in 2001, propelled by large tax increases in a small number of states, mainly in the Northeast. In the five highest-cigarette-tax states these taxes comprised more than 4.5 percent of tax revenues, compared with less than 1 percent in the low-tax states. As a share of total state revenues, including grants and fees, the cigarette tax share is less than half as large.

These numbers suggest that despite the recent increase in tax rates, even a dramatic decline in smoking prevalence would have only a minor effect on overall state revenue systems. The simulations developed for this volume indicate that under the two scenarios that involve a sharp increase of $2.00 in the federal tax rate on cigarettes—the IOM and high-impact scenarios—state cigarette tax revenues would decline by almost half. As a share of total state tax revenues, this would represent a 1.4 percent decline. The impact varies substantially by state because of wide differences in actual tax rates and in consumption and sales patterns. High-tax or high-consumption states would lose more than 2 percent of tax revenues, while low-tax or low-consumption states would lose less than 1 percent of tax revenues. However, a small number of relatively high-tax states would face a considerable fiscal challenge in replacing the lost revenue.

As state tax systems are now structured, the loss in cigarette tax revenues associated with a decline in smoking prevalence is unlikely to be substantially offset by an increase in revenues from taxes on general sales or alcohol. Because cigarettes are among the most highly taxed commodities, changes in consumption patterns away from cigarettes would in general cause states to lose tax revenues.

It is important to note that these simulations do not take into account the recent increase in federal excise tax rates for cigarettes. The analyses developed here suggest that the federal tax increase will reduce state excise tax revenues by reducing smoking prevalence. However, because the federal tax increase is only about a third the size of the $2 rate increase modeled in this chapter, the impact on state revenues will have a much more modest effect than the policy scenarios discussed here.

Several caveats are appropriate to keep in mind. First, although the SimSmoke model discussed in chapter 2 provides national-level projections of smoking prevalence and consumption, it does not (yet) provide state-level projections. As discussed in appendix 9.1, the state-level estimates developed here are valid as long as the ratio between taxable sales and consumption is constant over time and across place, but substantial changes in tax rates or Internet sales could affect the validity of this assumption. Second, in projecting the future impact of various policy scenarios on the loss in tax revenue as a share of total state tax revenues, state tax revenues are assumed to remain constant in real terms. This approach undoubtedly overstates the fiscal impact of any decline in smoking because state revenues are likely to grow in real terms over time. Third, the simulated increase in state revenue from tax increases under the various scenarios is based on estimates from prior years of the revenue–tax rate relationship. If tax avoidance behavior were to become even more important in the future as cigarette tax rates grow, then the revenue effects of an increase in state taxes would be overestimated.

APPENDIX 9.1

The basic equation for estimating effects of cigarette taxes on taxable sales is:

$$\text{Ln}(\text{Packspc}_{st}) = a_1 \, \text{ln}(\text{retail price}_{st}) + a_2 \, \text{ln}(\text{neigh retail price}_{st})$$
$$+ \, a_3 \, (\text{Smoking Suppression Index}_{st})$$
$$+ a_4 \, (Y_{st}) \, a_5 \, (\text{Demographics}_{st}) + a_s + a_t + \text{error}_{st}$$

The retail price is assumed to be equal to the wholesale price $P_{\text{wholesale}}$ plus the cigarette tax rate t. The tax rate, measured in cents per package of 20 cigarettes, is given by $t = t_{\text{cig}} + D_{it} \cong t_{\text{sales}} \, (P_{\text{wholesale}} + t_{\text{cig}})$, where t_{cig} is the sum of the state/local excise tax rate, D_{it} is a dummy variable equal to 1 in those states where cigarettes are included in the sales tax base, and t_{sales} is the general sales tax rate. To take into account possible price discrimination by cigarette producers (Keeler et al. 1996), retail price is instrumented by the combined state and local cigarette tax rate. To take account of unmeasured state effects on the retail price, the first-stage estimating equation also includes state and year effects.

Neighbor retail price is the weighted average of the retail price in a state's geographic neighbors. The weight for each neighbor state is the state's population living in counties that border the state in question as a proportion of the total border population for all of that state's neighbors.

The relationship between the effects on cigarette demand and on tax revenue is mediated by the share of cigarette taxes in the retail price of cigarettes. The revenue elasticity with respect to the tax rate is given by

$$\varepsilon_{\text{rev},t} = 1 - \varepsilon_{Q,P} \bullet \varepsilon_{P,t}$$

where $\varepsilon_{Q,P}$ is the (absolute value of the) elasticity of taxable sales with respect to the retail price, and $\varepsilon_{P,t}$ is the elasticity of the retail price with respect to the tax rate. If $\varepsilon_{P,t}$ were equal to 1, that is, if a 1 percent increase in cigarette tax rates were associated with a 1 percent increase in the retail price, then the revenue elasticity would be exactly equal to 1 minus the taxable sales elasticity, and an elasticity of sales greater than −1 would imply a decrease in revenues when tax rates increase. However, if $\varepsilon_{P,t}$ is less than 1, then the revenue elasticity could still be positive, even with an elasticity of demand greater than 1.

A linear specification of the relationship between the tax rate and the retail price (available upon request) indicates that the cigarette tax is fully passed forward to consumers via price increases. However, in the log-log specifications, the elasticity of the retail price with respect to the tax rate is well below 1. The elasticity ranges from 0.4 if there are no other covariates in the equation to 0.19 if fixed state and year effects are included. The fact that the inclusion of state and year effects lowers the estimated elasticity of the retail price with respect to the tax by a half indicates the importance of factors other than tax rates in causing variation over time and across states. As discussed by Keeler et al. (1996), some of this variation may reflect price discrimination on the part of cigarette manufacturers.

PROJECTING THE EFFECTS OF THE TOBACCO CONTROL SCENARIOS

The IOM and high-impact scenarios both include a $2 per pack increase in the cigarette tax. The $2 tax increase represents a 265 percent increase in the combined state/local rate of taxation of cigarettes. To estimate the effect of this increase on cigarette tax revenues, I use the packs-sold model discussed above to predict the state-specific change in taxable sales and tax revenues resulting from this tax increase. I then use the national consumption estimates from SimSmoke under the IOM and high-impact scenarios and make each individual state's reduction in revenue proportionate to that state's reduction in taxable sales, as compared to the average reduction in taxable sales.

Predicted cigarette revenues are equal to predicted packs sold multiplied by the 2005 state/local cigarette tax rate, inclusive of the sales tax. I use the years 1995–2004 for prediction. Predicted packs for 2005 are obtained using 2005 tax rates to generate retail prices and 2004 values for the other covariates in the model. All values are in per-capita terms.

PREDICTED PACKS SOLD Estimates of packs sold are based on SimSmoke projections of the national decline in per-capita cigarette consumption. At this point SimSmoke does not provide state-by-state projections of prevalence or consumption; therefore, I assume that the scenario-driven consumption trends in each state will mirror national trends and that the ratio of taxable sales to cigarette consumption is constant across states and over time. This assumption is likely to be reasonably accurate if tax rates do not change, as in the status quo scenario. However, if tax rates rise significantly, as in the IOM and high-impact scenarios, then taxable sales are likely to decrease by more than the drop in consumption, and the difference between the two margins of response may differ across states. As discussed earlier, at least 10 percent of cigarette consumption represents purchases from other states, Indian reservations, or smuggled cigarettes. The estimates presented here do not adjust for interstate variation in the difference between taxable sales and consumption.

PROJECTIONS OF REAL PER-CAPITA TAX REVENUES A model projecting future state taxes is beyond the scope of this chapter. Instead, I assume that real per-capita state tax revenues will remain constant throughout the simulation period. This assumption is obviously an underestimate of future state taxes, as taxes tend to rise over time with increases in income and in the relative prices of state and local purchases. Between 1995 and 2004, the average growth rate in per-capita state taxes was 1.3 percent. Hence, our approach will err on the side of overstating the fiscal impact of declining cigarette tax revenues.

DATA SOURCES

Variable definitions and data sources are shown in table 9.6.

COMPONENTS OF VARIABLES

- State population: taken from U.S. Department of Commerce, Bureau of Economic Analysis, Regional Economic Accounts, *State Annual Estimates*, various years, available at http://www.bea.gov/regional/spi/.
- SHR (revenue suffix for share of state and local total tax revenue): U.S. Census Bureau, *Annual Survey of State and Local Government Finances and Census of Governments*, available at http://www.census.gov/govs/estimate/. Interpolated local data for 2001 and extrapolated local data for 2003 and 2004.
- BORD (suffix and weight for border county populations): Border county indicators furnished by Terra McKinnish,, Department of Economics, University of Colorado at Boulder, http://www.bea.gov/regional/reis/, 1969–2003. Data for 2004 were extrapolated from the previous five years. County populations taken from U.S. Department of Commerce, Bureau of Economic Analysis, Regional Economic Accounts, *State Annual Estimates*, various years.

TABLE 9.6 Variable Definitions, Data Description, and Data Sources in 2005 Dollars, 1995–2004

VARIABLE NAME	VARIABLE DEFINITION	MEAN (STANDARD DEVIATION)	RANGE: MIN, MAX
PACKSPC	Taxable cigarette packs consumed per capita	103.11 (29.96)	32.70, 241.29
STLCRETAILSLS	Total retail price for a pack of cigarettes plus total sales tax, which includes state and local cigarette excise and sales tax, in cents	250.38 (85.91)	114.6, 610.4
NBRSTLCRETAILSLS	Average of total retail price and sales taxes of neighboring states, using border county population as weights, in cents	252.34 (84.95)	124.1, 564.5
STLCCIGREVSHR	Net cigarette excise tax revenue as a share of total state tax revenue	0.021 (0.015)	0.001, 0.337
STLCCIGSLSREV	Net state and local cigarette excise and related sales tax revenue per capita	50.258 (22.51) 47.715 (26.24)	12.24, 550.22 0, 735.52
STLCSLSREV	Total state and local sales tax revenue per capita	773.72 (1,331)	0, 20,108
STLCALCREV	State and local alcohol tax revenue per capita	25.286 (16.43)	2.544, 114.28
STLCCIGTAX	Combined state and local cigarette excise tax rate per pack, in cents	41.793 (23.39)	0, 215.74
STLCCIGSLSTAX	Combined state and local cigarette excise tax rate and sales tax per pack, in cents	52.032 (28.9)	9.969, 251.44
STLCSLSTAX	Combined state and local sales tax per pack, in cents	11.0 (8.77)	0, 49.106
STSLSTAXRT	State sales tax rate (%)	3.808 (1.9)	0, 8.6
NBRSTLCCIGTAX	Average of neighboring states' state and local cigarette excise tax, using border county population as weights, in cents	43.24 (20.86)	8.716, 191.91

TABLE 9.6 (*Continued*)

VARIABLE NAME	VARIABLE DEFINITION	MEAN (STANDARD DEVIATION)	RANGE: MIN, MAX
PCTBORD	Percentage of state's population residing in border counties	44.35 (25)	6.713, 100
NBRPCTBORD	Ratio of sum of neighboring states' border county populations divided by own state population	3.629 (5.636)	0.085, 41.543
PCINC	State personal income per capita	23,206 (7,092)	7,478, 48,179
PCTYOUNG	Percentage of state population under 18 years of age	27.992 (3.55)	21.19, 40.04
PCTOLD	Percentage of state population 65 years of age and over	11.847 (2)	6.3, 18.55
PCTBLK	Percentage of state population black	9.918 (9.49)	0.17, 76.18
PCTHSP	Percentage of state population Hispanic	6.062 (8.13)	0.44, 43.68
PCTFOR	Percentage of state population foreign born	4.954 (4.43)	0.4, 26.78
PCTCOLL	Percentage of state population who are college graduates	18.771 (5.92)	6.62, 36.7

VARIABLES

- PACKSPC: Orzechowski and Walker, "The Tax Burden on Tobacco," vol. 39 (Arlington, VA: Orzechowski and Walker, 2004), table 11.
- (STLC)(RETAILSLS), NBR(STLC)(RETAILSLS): Orzechowski and Walker, "The Tax Burden on Tobacco," vol. 39, tables 13, 15.
- (STLC)(CIGSLS)REV, . . . SHR: Orzechowski and Walker, "The Tax Burden on Tobacco," vol. 39, tables 9, 15, 17. Local sales tax revenue from cigarettes was interpolated using sales tax revenue from cigarettes, and aggregate state and local sales tax, and state (see stlcslstaxrev).
- (STLC)(CIGSLS)TAX, NBR(STLC)(CIGSLS)TAX: Orzechowski and Walker, "The Tax Burden on Tobacco," vol. 39, tables 7, 10, 15, 17. An average local excise tax per pack was computed by dividing the aggregate local cigarette revenues by the total tax-paid cigarettes sold in a state. All neighbor states' averages are weighted by county population (see . . . BORD).

- PCTBORD, NBRPCTBORD: see data source for . . . BORD above.
- (STLC)SLSREV, . . . SHR: U.S. Census Bureau, *Annual Survey of State and Local Government Finances*, http://www.census.gov/govs/estimate/, and *Census of Governments*, http://www.census.gov/govs/cog/. Interpolated local data for 2001, and extrapolated local data for 2003 and 2004.
- STSLSTAXRT: Orzechowski and Walker, "The Tax Burden on Tobacco," vol. 39, table 15.
- (STLC)ALCREV, . . . SHR: U.S. Census Bureau, *Annual Survey of State and Local Government Finances* and *Census of Governments*. Interpolated local data for 2001, and extrapolated local data for 2003 and 2004.
- PCINC: Bureau of Economic Analysis, 1980–2004.
- PCTYOUNG, PCTOLD, PCTBLK, PCTHSP, PCTFOR, PCTCOLL: *Statistical Abstracts*, U.S. Census Bureau, 1980–2004, available at http://www.census.gov/compendia/statab/.

PART 2

HEALTH AND LONGEVITY

10

ESTIMATING THE IMPACT OF TOBACCO CONTROL POLICIES ON FUTURE MORTALITY PATTERNS IN THE UNITED STATES

BENJAMIN J. APELBERG AND JONATHAN M. SAMET

Smoking, a significant cause of acute and chronic diseases, is a leading contributor to the burden of avoidable premature death and morbidity in the United States, accounting for approximately 443,000 deaths and 5.1 million years of potential life lost annually (Centers for Disease Control and Prevention 2008). Tobacco control measures could reduce that burden of disease, but the question is: how much, and how fast? Many smoking-caused illnesses have a long latency period; consequently, there is little immediate difference in mortality risk of young smokers and nonsmokers, but after decades of smoking, smokers have far greater risks for morbidity and mortality than never smokers. Moreover, when smokers quit, mortality risks decline slowly after maintained cessation, and for some diseases they never decline to those of never smokers. Consequently, the full benefits of successful tobacco control measures for mortality are only realized decades after their implementation.

To understand the magnitude and timing of this impact, we estimate smoking-attributable mortality for the United States under alternative tobacco control policy scenarios. We examine three scenarios discussed in earlier chapters: the status quo scenario, which holds constant the tobacco control policies in place in 2005, as well as the Institute of Medicine (IOM) and high-impact scenarios. In addition, we consider the implications of a "100 percent cessation" scenario in which all smokers stopped smoking in 2006. Obviously such an abrupt and universal halt to smoking is not a realistic prospect, but it usefully sets an upper bound around the health impacts that tobacco control policy could yield.

We calculate the burden of smoking-attributable mortality for all causes of death and for the major diseases caused by smoking under each of these tobacco control policy scenarios. Our analysis focuses on lung cancer, other smoking-related cancers, and cardiovascular disease. These diseases, along with chronic obstructive pulmonary disease (COPD), make up a substantial burden of premature death due to smoking (Centers for Disease Control and Prevention 2008). Smoking is the predominant cause for some diseases, while others are multifactorial in origin. Most cases of lung cancer, the leading cause of cancer death in men and women in the United States, are attributable to cigarette smoking. Cardiovascular disease, on the other hand, has numerous causes, and the fraction of disease attributable to smoking is lower. However, because cardiovascular disease is the leading cause of death in the United States, reducing a smaller fraction of the mortality burden by reducing smoking would have significant public health benefits. Smoking is also a cause of a number of nonspecific diseases that do not fit into the disease categories listed above. To capture avoided mortality from these diseases, we also include total mortality from all causes.

METHODS

In general, the disease burden is calculated using the population attributable risk (PAR), which is based on two factors: the exposure prevalence, the proportion of people exposed to a given condition, and the additional risk of disease associated with it. For lung cancer, for instance, current and former smokers have about 15 times the mortality risk of never smokers, and the exposure prevalence in adults is approximately 40 percent. The resulting PAR is 85 percent—in other words, smoking accounts for 85 percent of lung cancer cases. Coronary heart disease, on the other hand, has multiple causes, and the proportion of cases attributable to smoking is much lower than for lung cancer. Assuming that current and former smokers have twice the risk of developing coronary heart disease, the PAR is about 29 percent. The PAR statistic is the basis for the Centers for Disease Control's widely used Smoking-Attributable Mortality, Morbidity, and Economic Costs (SAMMEC) model (U.S. Department of Health and Human Services 2004a).[1]

Like the SAMMEC model, our approach is based in the concept of attributable risk and uses prevalence rates over time and the associated relative risks for

MEASURING DISEASE BURDEN: POPULATION ATTRIBUTABLE RISK

The epidemiological measure of disease burden is usually called the population attributable risk (PAR); it is also sometimes called the etiologic fraction, attributable
proportion, or incidence density fraction. Interestingly, the conceptual basis for this
measure was developed initially for the specific example of smoking and lung cancer
(Levin 1953). The calculation of PAR requires knowledge only of the prevalence of
exposure to cigarette smoking (or another risk factor) and the associated relative risk
for disease or death. It can be expressed as:

$$PAR = \frac{(RR-1) \cdot p}{1 + (RR-1) \cdot p}$$

where RR is the relative risk associated with the exposure and p is the exposure
prevalence. The RR is calculated as the incidence of disease (or death) in the exposed group divided by the incidence of disease (or death) in the unexposed. In this
formula, the expression $(RR-1) \cdot p$ represents the additional disease due to the exposure, and the quantity $1 + (RR-1) \cdot p$ represents the total.

As this formula shows, excess mortality depends on both RR and p. An uncommon exposure, even if it carries a high relative risk, contributes only a small proportion of the disease cases in a population. On the other hand, a very prevalent exposure, even if associated with a relatively modest relative risk, can contribute
substantially to the burden of disease. In estimating the PAR, there is an implicit
comparison to an alternative scenario of exposure, in which the value of p is different. This alternative is often referred to as the counterfactual. For tobacco smoking,
the typical counterfactual is that p has the value of zero; that is, no one has ever
smoked. Other counterfactuals are sometimes of interest, particularly for exposures
that could never be reasonably eliminated. For indoor radon, for example, concentrations cannot be reduced to outdoor, background concentrations; some lung cancer cases will always be attributable to radon.

all causes and the major causes of death associated with smoking, other than
COPD. We apply estimates of mortality risk by smoking status and cause to
model the mortality burden between 2006 and 2025. Figure 10.1 provides the
general framework for estimating the mortality burden, which draws on estimates of RR and p, as in the attributable risk formula.

For our simulation we divided the U.S. population into categories or strata
defined by sex, age, and smoking status including, for former smokers, the number of years since cessation. The total population by age and sex is based on
Census Bureau projections. The smoking prevalence rates at the start of the
simulation are based on 2004 National Health Interview Survey data; changes in
prevalence under alternative policy scenarios are based on the SimSmoke projections discussed in chapter 2.

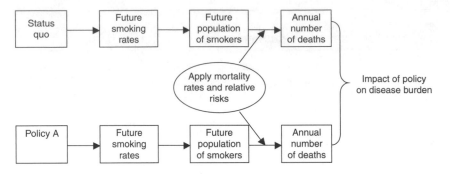

FIGURE 10.1 Framework for Estimating Smoking-Attributable Mortality

The total number of people within each of these strata change as smokers age or stop smoking. For example, figures 10.2 and 10.3 show how two hypothetical smokers would be classified across the years of these projections. In figure 10.2 the smoker continues to smoke as he or she ages. The smoker contributes time as a current smoker from ages 40 to 44 in calendar years 2006–2010, then from ages 45 to 49 in calendar years 2011–2016, and so on. In contrast, figure 10.3 shows a smoker who stops smoking at age 45. In calendar years 2006–2010 this person is counted as a current smoker aged 40 to 44 (upper left table). After permanently quitting at age 45 the person moves into the stratum for former smokers who are 45–49 years of age and who stopped smoking 0–4 years ago. Between 2011 and 2025, as this former smoker ages, he or she moves into strata of greater age and greater time since quitting. As in the SimSmoke model, after individuals have quit, they do not relapse and become current smokers again.

Each stratum has a mortality risk associated with it (table 10.1). As shown, mortality risk drops for a smoker who successfully quits, relative to the smoker who continues smoking. The estimated number of deaths by year for each stratum is the product of the number of persons in that stratum and its mortality rate. For instance, if there were 10 million male current smokers aged 40–44 in 2010, and they had an estimated lung cancer mortality rate of 18 per 100,000, we would expect 1,800 deaths from lung cancer in 2010 among male smokers of those ages (10 million persons × 18 per 100,000). After the number of deaths among current smokers, former smokers, and never smokers per year, by age and gender categories, are generated, these estimates are summed to project the total number of deaths per year. The difference between the projected annual number of deaths for each scenario and the status quo scenario is the number of premature deaths avoided as a result of a particular tobacco control policy. This provides a useful metric for determining the effect of tobacco control policies on future disease burden.

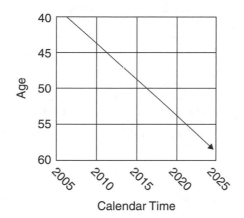

FIGURE 10.2 Tracking a Hypothetical Current Smoker Through the Model

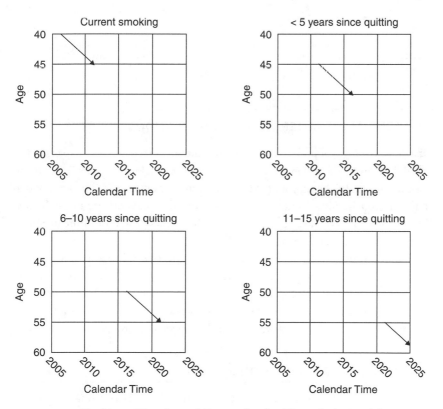

FIGURE 10.3 Tracking a Hypothetical Former Smoker Through the Model

TABLE 10.1 Lung Cancer Mortality Rates and Follow-Up Years Contributed for a Hypothetical Current Smoker and Former Smoker Who Quits at Age 45

AGE GROUP	FOLLOW-UP YEARS CONTRIBUTED	MORTALITY RATE (PER 100,000)[a]	
		CURRENT SMOKER	FORMER SMOKER
40–44	5	18	18
45–49	5	49	30
50–54	5	115	45
55–59	5	230	65
60–64	5	399	90
65–69	5	601	121
70–74	5	788	159
75–79	5	904	202
80–84	5	911	253

[a] Mortality rates are modeled estimates for males, as described in the "Methods" section.
Source: Authors' calculations.

CURRENT AND FORMER SMOKER POPULATIONS

The methodology for projecting prevalence rates of current and ex-smokers in the United States was described in chapter 2. Because smoking has only a small impact on mortality among young adults, we limit our analysis to the U.S. population between 40 and 84 years of age. Estimates of population size in the United States between 2005 and 2025 were obtained from the U.S. Census Bureau, which projects these estimates forward from the 2000 U.S. Census based on predicted immigration, emigration, and birth and death rates (Hollmann, Mulder, and Kaller 2000). Population projections for the United States were available from the Census Bureau by age and gender. These projections are applied to future smoking rates from chapter 2 of this volume to estimate the number of current smokers, ex-smokers, and never smokers under the tobacco control policy scenarios.

SMOKING AND MORTALITY RISK

We used data from the Cancer Prevention Study II (CPS II) to estimate the added risk of mortality caused by smoking. The CPS II is the largest cohort study of smoking and mortality in the United States and is the only data set large enough to provide reliable estimates of smoking-caused mortality by age group, sex, and smoking status. In CPS II, smoking status was assessed at baseline, and study participants were followed up over time for vital status. The 1 million participants in CPS II included over 480,000 never smokers (Garfinkel 1985). We based mortality rates on follow-up results from 1984 to 1991, excluding individuals with cancer, heart disease, or stroke at enrollment. The first two years of follow-up were also excluded to provide a lag period between the measurement of smoking status and identification of mortality outcomes, reducing the likelihood of selection bias, and to reduce the effect of having a disease on smoking status (i.e., reverse causation). People often stop smoking when they become ill, inflating the apparent disease risk of former smokers; excluding the first two years of follow-up reduces this problem. Although follow-up continued after 1991, we did not include these later results because smoking status was not updated after enrollment; over time the risk of misclassification of smoking status would increase.

We calculated mortality rates for never smokers, current smokers, and former smokers by five-year age group and gender for death from all causes, lung cancer, other smoking-related cancers, and cardiovascular disease. Mortality rates for former smokers were also available by age at cessation in 10-year age groupings. We generated relative risks for current and former smokers, respectively, by dividing their respective mortality rates by the mortality rate for never smokers. These relative risks represent the increased chance of dying at a particular age for current and former smokers relative to individuals who never smoked. Mortality rates were pooled across gender before the calculation of relative risks, which are applied to both males and females.

In CPS II, women have a lower relative risk of smoking-related mortality than men. Much of this difference is likely a result of differences in smoking patterns between men and women during the decades leading up to the study (U.S. Department of Health and Human Services 1997). In the current analysis, we model future mortality using projected smoking prevalence in the United States without stratifying on smoking amount. Smoking patterns between men and women are more similar now than in the past, and recent evidence suggests that, after controlling for smoking amount and duration, similar relative risks are observed across gender (Bain et al. 2004; Gandini et al. 2008; Jemal et al. 2003; Kreuzer et al. 2000; Marang-van de Mheen et al. 2001; Nilsson, Carstensen, and Pershagen 2001; Nordlund, Carstensen, and Pershagen 1999; Vollset, Tverdal, and Gjessing 2006). As a result, we apply a pooled relative risk from CPS II.

Even with a study population of more than a million participants, when mortality rates are stratified by age, gender, smoking status, and cause of death, some strata have small sample sizes. The precision of estimated mortality rates and relative risks varies based on the sample size and number of deaths observed in each stratum. To smooth out fluctuations in these estimates, we modeled relative risk

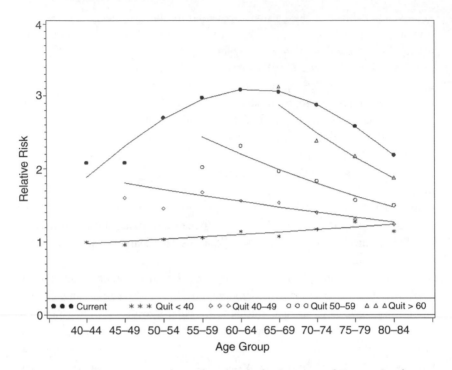

FIGURE 10.4 All-Cause Mortality Relative Risks for Current and Former Smokers

Note: Never smokers in a given age group are the reference group. Points represent observed relative risks, and lines are predicted relative risks. Predictions based on weighted linear regression of log(RR) on age. Age was included as a linear term for former smoker relative risk and a quadratic term for current smoker relative risk. Legend reflects age at cessation.
Source: Cancer Prevention Study II, 1984–1991.

as a function of age for current smokers and time since quitting for former smokers (see appendix 10.1).

Figure 10.4 shows the observed and predicted relative risks of all-cause mortality by age group for current smokers and former smokers. Current smokers have two to three times the mortality risk of never smokers. A smoker's relative risk for all-cause mortality has an inverse-U shape in relation to age, peaking between ages 60 and 69, followed by a decline in the relative risk with older ages. This decline may represent a selection process by which smokers who have survived to older ages are less susceptible to the harmful effects of tobacco and, thus, have a lower excess risk. The relative risk of mortality for former smokers compared with never smokers declines as time since cessation increases. The magnitude of this decline depends partly on the age at cessation. Smokers who quit when they are young gain the most in terms of reduced mortality risk. However, even smokers who quit after age 60 can reduce their relative risk significantly.

A similar pattern is observed in the relationship between lung cancer mortality risk and age among current and former smokers (not shown here). The major difference is the magnitude of the relative risk, which at some ages is almost 25 times that of a never smoker. By contrast, the relative risks for cardiovascular disease are similar to those for all-cause mortality, ranging from about 2 to 6 depending on age. The lower relative risks reflect the fact that there are many other risk factors for cardiovascular disease. The decline in relative risk for cardiovascular disease also occurs at an earlier age; this probably reflects the accumulation of other risk factors such as obesity, diabetes, and hypertension that affect never smokers as well.

It is important to note that the CPS II sample is likely to be healthier than the entire U.S. population. CPS II participants overrepresent individuals in more advantaged sociodemographic and racial categories; 93 percent of the CPS II study population was white, 83 percent were married, and 30 percent were college graduates (Thun et al. 2000). In addition, individuals who volunteer to participate in health studies, such as CPS II, tend to be healthier than the general population (Lindsted et al. 1996). Not surprisingly, crude mortality rates for the CPS II population between 1984 and 1991 were lower than the overall U.S. rates in 1988; disparities in mortality were higher for the older age groups. In fact, CPS II mortality rates were lower in 1984–1991 than the national average in 2002 despite advances in disease prevention and treatment over the last 20 years as well as a significant decline in smoking prevalence. To adjust for this difference in mortality rates, we calibrated our model so that the number of deaths predicted in 2002 equaled the number of deaths reported that year in the United States. We performed this calibration by scaling up the never-smoker mortality rates from CPS-II. This approach assumes that the relative risks of smoking in CPS II are representative of the United States as a whole, even though the absolute risk of death differed.

RESULTS

Our analysis predicts the number of deaths attributed to smoking under each tobacco control policy scenario. It is important to keep in mind that the U.S. adult population is projected to grow by 24 percent between 2002 and 2025, with the largest increases among individuals between the ages of 55 and 84—an age group with high mortality rates. In other words, the number of deaths occurring in the United States will increase in any event. The question we address is how tobacco control policies could shape this increase.

We examine the impacts on future mortality from three different tobacco control policies: (1) the status quo, (2) the IOM best-case recommendations, and (3) the high-impact tobacco control scenario. We also provide an upper-bound estimate of deaths that could be avoided through smoking cessation by model-ing the impact of the complete elimination of smoking in 2006. More detailed descriptions of these policies and their impacts on future smoking rates can be found in chapter 2.

ALL-CAUSE MORTALITY

As figure 10.5 shows, annual all-cause mortality—the total number of deaths—will rise under all scenarios, but the rate of that predicted increase depends on tobacco control policy. Under the status quo scenario, the projected number of deaths from all causes will increase from 1.6 million per year to 2.4 million per year between 2006 and 2025. Under the 100 percent cessation scenario the number would increase by less, to more than 2.1 million. Projected mortality increases for the other two scenarios fall between these two extremes.

Table 10.2 shows the cumulative number of premature deaths avoided, by gen-der, over the 20-year period under the different tobacco control scenarios. The 100

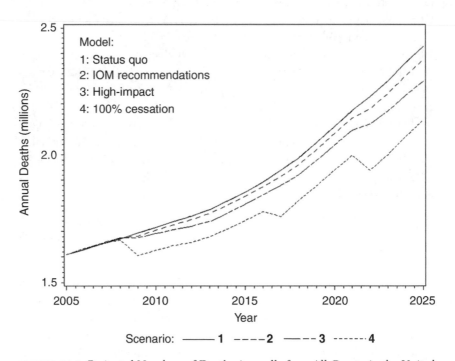

FIGURE 10.5 Projected Numbers of Deaths Annually from All Causes in the United States by Year and Control Scenario: Full Population (Never, Current, and Former Smokers)

Source: Authors' calculations.

TABLE 10.2 Cumulative Number of Premature Deaths Avoided from 2006 to 2025 and Percentage Reduction by Cause of Death and Scenario

SCENARIO	ALL-CAUSE		LUNG CANCER		OTHER SMOKING-RELATED CANCERS		CARDIOVASCULAR DISEASE	
	AVOIDED DEATHS	PERCENTAGE REDUCTION[a]	AVOIDED DEATHS	PERCENTAGE REDUCTION[a]	AVOIDED DEATHS	PERCENTAGE REDUCTION[a]	AVOIDED DEATHS	PERCENTAGE REDUCTION[a]
IOM recommendation								
Male	280,000	1%	110,000	5%	25,000	2%	90,000	2%
Female	175,000	1%	73,000	5%	12,000	2%	49,000	1%
Total	450,000	1%	190,000	5%	37,000	2%	130,000	1%
High-impact								
Male	700,000	3%	290,000	14%	64,000	5%	210,000	4%
Female	430,000	3%	180,000	13%	31,000	4%	120,000	3%
Total	1,100,000	3%	460,000	13%	100,000	5%	330,000	3%
100% cessation								
Male	1,800,000	8%	640,000	31%	150,000	12%	480,000	8%
Female	1,100,000	7%	400,000	29%	74,000	9%	270,000	7%
Total	2,800,000	7%	1,000,000	29%	220,000	11%	750,000	8%

[a] Percentage reduction is based on the total number of cause-specific deaths under the status quo.
Source: Authors' calculations.

percent cessation scenario sets an upper bound on the number of avoided deaths over the next 20 years. If all smoking had ceased in 2006, we estimate that 2.8 million premature deaths from all causes would be avoided over the next 20 years, or about 7 percent of all deaths over that time. Under the high-impact scenario, over 1 million premature deaths, or about 3 percent of all deaths, would be averted. A more realistic scenario might be the achievement of the IOM recommendations, under which we project close to half a million premature deaths avoided.

LUNG CANCER

Lung cancer is currently the leading cause of cancer death for men and women in the United States. In 2002 there were close to 170,000 deaths due to lung cancer in the United States, of which approximately 140,000 occurred among individuals aged 40–84 (authors' calculations from http://wonder.cdc.gov/cmf-icd10.html). Roughly 85 percent of lung cancer cases are attributable to tobacco smoke, suggesting that about 144,000 lung cancer deaths could have been avoided in 2002 if there had been no cigarette smokers in the U.S. population (Centers for Disease Control and Prevention 2005a).

Figure 10.6 shows the projected trend in overall lung cancer mortality (never, current, and former smokers combined) in the United States under the different tobacco policy scenarios. Under most scenarios, the number of lung cancer deaths continues to rise due to population growth and the long-term effects of smoking even among former smokers. The 100 percent cessation scenario, however, would lead to a decline in total lung cancer deaths within the 20-year time frame. The zigzag pattern is an artifact of this scenario, in which all current smokers quit simultaneously and therefore change cessation risk categories at exactly the same time.

As table 10.2 shows, with complete cessation we estimate approximately 1 million lung cancer deaths avoided—close to 30 percent of all lung cancer deaths projected to occur over the next 20 years. Under the high-impact and IOM scenarios, we estimate approximately 460,000 (13 percent of projected deaths) and 190,000 (5 percent) avoided lung cancer deaths, respectively. Tobacco control has a much larger impact on lung cancer deaths than on all-cause mortality because smoking is the key determinant of lung cancer and only one of many determinants of total mortality risk.

OTHER SMOKING-RELATED CANCERS

Smoking causes cancer at many sites in the body besides the lung. In the most recent version of the Surgeon General's report on smoking, the following cancer types, other than trachea, lung, and bronchus, have been identified as being causally related to cigarette smoking: lip, oral cavity, and pharynx; esophagus;

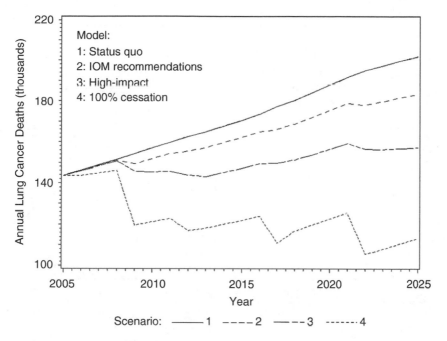

FIGURE 10.6 Projected Numbers of Deaths Annually from Other Lung Cancer in the United States by Year and Control Scenario: Full Population (Never, Current, and Former Smokers)

Source: Authors' calculations.

stomach; pancreas; larynx; cervix; kidney; bladder; and acute myeloid leukemia (U.S. Department of Health and Human Services 2004a). In the United States in 2002 there were 102,976 deaths due to these cancers, of which about 86,000 occurred among individuals between the ages of 40 and 84 (authors' calculations from http://wonder.cdc.gov/cmf-icd10.html).

Figure 10.7 shows the projected trend in mortality from other smoking-related cancers (never, current, and former smokers combined). An overall increase in smoking-related cancers is observed in all scenarios. Under the status quo scenario the annual number of deaths from these causes is projected to rise from about 87,000 in 2006 to 123,000 in 2025. Table 10.2 shows the projected cumulative number of avoided cancer deaths, by gender, for each of the tobacco control scenarios. Under complete cessation we estimate over 200,000 deaths avoided from other smoking-related cancers, representing a decline of 11 percent from the status quo. Under the high-impact and IOM recommendation scenarios, we project 100,000 and 37,000 avoided cancer deaths, respectively. Thus, although lung cancer is the greatest contributor to smoking-related

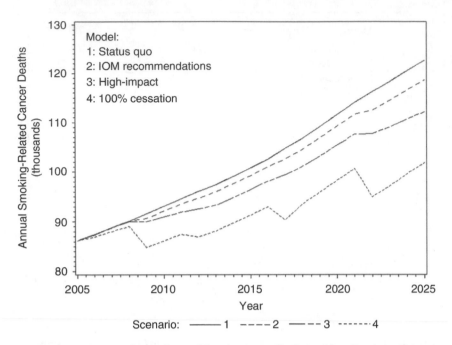

FIGURE 10.7 Projected Numbers of Deaths Annually from other Smoking-Related Cancers in the United States by Year and Control Scenario: Full Population (Never, Current, and Former Smokers)

Source: Authors' calculations.

cancer mortality, a significant number of other cancer deaths could also be avoided over the next 20 years under effective tobacco control policies.

CARDIOVASCULAR DISEASE MORTALITY

Although deaths from cardiovascular disease have been declining over the past several decades, it remains the leading cause of death among adults in the United States (U.S. Department of Health and Human Services 2004a). In 2002 there were over 650,000 deaths due to coronary heart disease (ICD-10: I20–I25) and stroke (ICD-10: I60–I69). Of these deaths over 400,000 occurred among individuals between the ages of 40 and 84 (authors' calculations from http://wonder.cdc.gov/cmf-icd10.html). Although cardiovascular disease has many risk factors, cigarette smoking is an important modifiable risk factor for dying from heart disease and stroke.

Figure 10.8 shows the projected annual number of deaths from cardiovascular disease under different tobacco control policies. These trends assume that cardiovascular disease mortality rates remain constant into the future, an as-

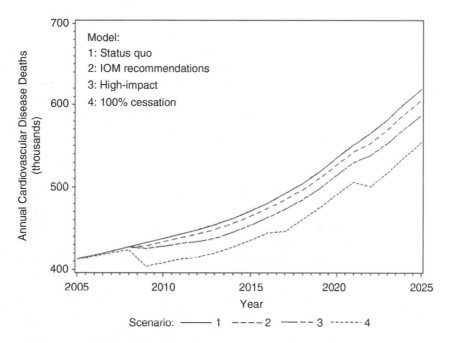

FIGURE 10.8 Projected Numbers of Deaths Annually from Cardiovascular Disease in the United States by Year and Control Scenario: Full Population (Never, Current, and Former Smokers)

Source: Authors' calculations.

sumption we discuss below. The rising trend in the number of deaths under all scenarios, similar to what was observed for other causes of death, reflects the growth and aging of the U.S. population. The cumulative number of avoided cardiovascular deaths by 2025 is shown in table 10.2. If all smoking had ceased in 2006, we project that approximately 750,000 cardiovascular deaths could have been avoided, about 8 percent of the total cardiovascular disease deaths expected between 2006 and 2025. Under the high-impact scenario about 330,000 cardiovascular disease deaths (3 percent) would be avoided, and under the IOM scenario about 130,000 cardiovascular disease deaths (1 percent) would be avoided.

The smaller percentage reductions in cardiovascular disease mortality due to tobacco control policies reflect the multifactorial nature of cardiovascular disease. However, because the incidence of cardiovascular disease in the United States is so high, even minor relative reductions can have large public health impacts on an absolute scale. Complete cessation of smoking in 2006 could have averted about 1 million lung cancer deaths and about 750,000 deaths from cardiovascular disease between 2006 and 2025.

CIGARETTE SMOKING AND LIFE EXPECTANCY

It is clear that a significant number of premature deaths could be avoided by reductions in smoking prevalence. Another way to quantify the effect of a reduction in smoking rates is to consider how much the lives of persons who do not die prematurely would be prolonged by quitting or never starting to smoke. A useful metric for this comparison is the years of potential life lost (or gained) (YPLL) due to tobacco use. Indeed, YPLL can more accurately reflect the public health benefit of an intervention by accounting not only for the number of lives saved but also the extent to which death is delayed.

Several studies have examined the impact of prolonged cigarette smoking on life expectancy. These estimates have been generated using large prospective cohort studies of the health impacts of smoking. The CDC used data from the CPS II to estimate the number of annual deaths attributable to smoking and the years of potential life lost due to this premature mortality. The CDC estimates that between 2000 and 2004, approximately 433,000 deaths per year were attributable to cigarette smoking, corresponding to approximately 5.1 million YPLL, an average of 11.8 years per death (Centers for Disease Control and Prevention 2008). Taylor et al. (2002) used follow-up data from CPS II to estimate the difference in life expectancy by smoking behavior after adjusting for potential confounders. They estimate that lifelong never smokers could expect to gain between 7.4 and 10.5 years of life relative to current smokers, depending on gender. The authors also showed that most of this difference in life expectancy could be gained back by current smokers if they quit smoking by age 35. Quitting smoking even as late as age 65 was associated with a gain in life expectancy relative to continuing smokers (1.4–2.0 years for males and 2.7–3.7 years for females) (Taylor et al. 2002).

Doll et al. (2004) examined the relationship between lifelong smoking and longevity using 50 years of follow-up from the British Doctors Study. This study, begun in 1951, was the first prospective study to examine the relationship between smoking and mortality after the findings of several case-control studies had shown that smoking adversely affected human health. Because of the long follow-up time, the authors could examine survival across the lifespan for study participants based on smoking status. The authors report that lifelong smokers lived, on average, 10 years less than lifelong never smokers. As the CPS II showed, significant gains in life expectancy could be achieved through smoking cessation across the lifespan. Smokers quitting by age 30 had almost the same life expectancy as never smokers. Even those quitting at age 60 gained an average of about three years of life relative to those who continued to smoke.

These findings describe the importance of cessation for reducing premature mortality and the extent to which life years can be gained by cessation. The extent to which future tobacco control policies will result in life years gained across the U.S. population depends predominantly on the age and time since quitting. Under the conservative assumption that only three years of life were gained per premature death averted in our analysis, equivalent to quitting smoking late in life, 1.35 million years of life would be gained under the IOM scenario and 3.3 million years of life under the high-impact scenario. These figures would be much higher if the mean age at cessation were lower and if we continued the simulation for longer than 20 years.

LIMITATIONS AND ASSUMPTIONS

Given the limitations of our data, there were some issues we were unable to address. The most important of these is how the health impacts of tobacco control policy would differ by population categories such as gender or race and ethnicity. Although we did provide separate mortality estimates for males and females, our analysis assumed equal susceptibility in males and females and used a pooled relative risk from CPS II across gender. We predicted more premature deaths avoided among males than females in the U.S. population, primarily because males have a higher baseline risk of mortality. Recent findings have stimulated debate about gender susceptibility to the effects of smoking. When men and women have the same smoking patterns, several cohort studies report either no gender difference or slightly higher risk of smoking-caused illness among males (Bain et al. 2004; Jemal et al. 2003; Kreuzer et al. 2000; Marang-van de Mheen et al. 2001; Nilsson, Carstensen, and Pershagen 2001; Nordlund, Carstensen, and Pershagen 1999). Case-control studies, however, suggest that women are more susceptible than men (Henschke and Miettinen 2004; Khuder 2001; Risch and Miller 2004; Risch et al. 1993, 1994; Zang and Wynder 1996). As we gain better evidence about whether the health impacts of smoking differ by gender, the health implications of tobacco control policy for men and women can be projected more accurately.

We did not specifically examine the distribution of health benefits by racial or ethnic categories. Smoking patterns differ by race and ethnicity; according to national estimates, age-adjusted adult smoking prevalence is highest among American Indian/Alaskan Natives, followed by whites and African Americans, and lowest among Asians. Although smoking prevalence is similar among whites and African Americans, white daily smokers tend to smoke more cigarettes per day, and whites and American Indian/Alaskan Natives begin to smoke at earlier ages (Adams and Schoenborn 2006). The effect of tobacco control policies on group-specific mortality is dependent on two parameters about which our current knowledge is inadequate. The first is race and ethnic differences in the relationship of smoking to mortality. Smoking frequency and age at initiation are key predictors of smoking-related risk, so we might expect whites and American Indian/Alaskan Natives to have the greatest smoking-related excess risk. There is some evidence, however, that the burden of smoking-caused disease, such as lung cancer, is higher among African Americans, which could be due to differences in cigarette types consumed (e.g., menthol use), smoking topography, and/or metabolism (Abidoye, Ferguson, and Salgia 2007; Alberg, Brock, and Samet 2005). The second parameter is race and ethnic differences in response to tobacco control policy. As Balbach and colleagues discuss in chapter 16, the evidence base on this question is very limited.

Any attempt to predict future mortality patterns necessarily involves some uncertainty and requires the analyst to make some assumptions. Some uncertainties can be quantified, while others require a more qualitative assessment. Table 10.3 provides an overview of key assumptions made in this analysis, and the discussion that follows provides more detail.

One set of assumptions concerns the U.S. population size and composition over the period between 2002 and 2025. We used the same population estimates for all three scenarios, when in fact the future population structure would be affected by different tobacco control policies. Because smoking cessation increases longevity, policies that reduce smoking prevalence would result in a larger U.S. population over time. Failure to account for this increase overestimates the number of premature deaths saved relative to the status quo. Sensitivity analyses show that adjusting for population size reduces the estimates of avoided deaths by less than 10 percent.

More significant sources of uncertainty come from the use of the CPS II data to estimate mortality rates. Even with a large number of cases, the sample selection process always introduces some uncertainty. To limit the impact of imprecise estimates of mortality rates and relative risks, we fitted a smooth function to these estimates using weighted regression and then used these smoothed estimates to predict future mortality. We also conducted sensitivity analyses using upper and lower confidence bounds of the smoking relative risks in the estimation of avoided deaths. We found a narrow range in our estimates of avoided deaths when using these bounds, suggesting that statistical uncertainty from the estimation of relative risks was not an important source of uncertainty in our model.

Another caveat concerns the use of the CPS II, a sample of individuals recruited in 1982, to predict mortality risk between 2006 and 2025. Clearly, the past two decades have seen a number of changes in chronic disease risk and treatment protocols that could affect projected mortality, and other changes will undoubtedly occur over the next two decades. The direction and extent of any resulting bias are unclear, however. We assumed that mortality rates among never smokers remain constant into the future; however, these mortality rates could be affected by improvements in detection and treatment of other diseases and changes in

TABLE 10.3 Key Assumptions and Related Uncertainties

Population Projections

- Population growth follows current U.S. Census Bureau projections for all scenarios.

- Projected populations are constant within 5-year age groups.

- Projected smoking rates are constant within 10-year age groups.

Baseline Mortality Rates

- Mortality rates are constant within 5-year age groups.

- No temporal trends in baseline mortality rates among never smokers.

- Trend in mortality rates by age among never smokers is best described by an exponential function.

- Women who are never smokers have lower mortality rates than men (based on CPS II).

- CPS II population is healthier than general U.S. population. Mortality rates from CPS II can be scaled to predict current general population rates (assuming no significant changes in ICD codings).

Smoking Mortality Risk

- Statistical uncertainty from using a random sample from CPS II.

- Men and women are equally susceptible to the effects of active smoking.

- Smoking relative risks derived from CPS II (1984–1991) are applicable to the current U.S. general population and into the future (2006–2025).

- Typical smoking patterns among smokers in CPS II are comparable to future smoking patterns in the U.S. for both genders.

- Log(relative risks) after cessation are best described by a declining linear trend.

- Former smokers defined by time since quitting groups (e.g., ≤ 2 years, 3–5 years, 6–10 years, etc.) are equally distributed among the years in that group.

exposure to secondhand smoke and in other risk factors. Such factors should have little impact on mortality from diseases such as lung cancer, which has very few non-smoking-related risk factors and no effective screening modalities (Manser et al. 2004), and has shown little change in survival rates over time (National Cancer Institute 2005b). However, changes in risk factor prevalence may be especially important for diseases with many causes, such as cardiovascular disease.

As we discussed earlier, the CPS II population is considerably healthier than the general population. To accurately characterize future mortality patterns, we scaled the never smoker mortality rates so that our predicted estimates would match 2002 U.S. mortality rates. This scaling approach assumes that the relative risk of mortality associated with smoking derived from the relatively healthy CPS II population can be generalized to the full U.S. population and used as the basis for smoking-attributable mortality estimates. Given the extensive body of evidence relating smoking to increased mortality in many different settings, it is unlikely that the relative risk estimates observed for CPS II would be dramatically different among the broader U.S. population. However, when we study mortality risk, factors such as health care access and utilization may play a role in the magnitude of the associations observed.

Last, some questions arise from our use of the CPS II sample to estimate mortality rates and relative risks for current and former smokers, irrespective of smoking quantity and duration. The study population followed in CPS II between 1984 and 1991 comprises current and former smokers who began smoking as early as the 1940s and 1950s. By contrast, the population projected in our model would have begun smoking in the 1960s and 1970s. The pattern of smoking in the United States changed over this time: the average age at initiation rose, and the average number of cigarettes consumed per day dropped (U.S. Department of Health and Human Services 1997). These factors are likely to influence the magnitude of the effect of smoking on mortality risk; so are other changes, such as the constituents of cigarettes and the depth of smoke inhalation. Absent offsetting trends, these changes are likely to mean that the relative risk of mortality for smokers and former smokers is overstated.

We used relative risk estimates from CPS II that were unadjusted for potential confounders, aside from age group. Estimates like these are subject to the criticism that smokers may be less healthy than nonsmokers in other health behaviors, such as diet, physical activity, or risk taking. However, research has shown that adjusting for these other factors makes surprisingly little difference to the estimated risk of mortality associated with smoking (Malarcher et al. 2000; Thun, Apicella, and Henley 2000; Vollset, Tverdal, and Gjessing 2006). For instance, Thun, Apicella, and Henley (2000) compared hazard ratios for smoking and cause-specific mortality age-adjusted models in CPS II using multivariate models that adjusted for potential confounders such as socioeconomic status, dietary patterns, body mass index, and occupational exposures. Full adjustment resulted in a less than 10 percent decrease in hazard ratios for lung cancer and ischemic heart disease among current smokers. Among female former smokers multivariate adjustment resulted in increased hazard ratios for lung cancer, ischemic heart disease, and several other causes of death. Overall, the use of multivariate adjusted relative risks resulted in a 1 percent decline in the estimate of smoking-attributable deaths (Thun, Apicella, and Henley 2000). Malarcher et al. (2000) also examined the robustness of smoking-attributable mortality estimates to multivariate adjustment of CPS II relative risks. The authors found that smoking-attributable estimates for four major diseases combined (lung cancer, chronic obstructive pulmonary disease, coronary heart disease, and cerebrovascular disease) remained equal among men and increased among women after multivariate adjustment (Malarcher et al. 2000). These findings suggest that the smoking relative risk and attributable fraction estimates from CPS II are fairly robust to multivariate adjustment after controlling for age.

Finally, this analysis focuses only on the reduction in premature mortality due to effective policies aimed at reducing smoking prevalence. Quitting smoking has been associated with a modest average weight gain (5–10 pounds) (Filozof, Fernandez Pinilla, and Fernandez-Cruz 2004; Rigotti 2002; U.S. Department of Health and Human Services 1990). However, for some, the weight gain may be considerably greater (O'Hara et al. 1998; Swan and Carmelli 1995; U.S. Department of Health and Human Services 1990), which could reduce the likelihood of a quitter remaining abstinent and/or reduce some of the benefits of cessation because of the additional risk of obesity. We did not examine the impact of postcessation weight gain; however, any adverse effects associated with weight gain are more than balanced by the substantial harms caused by smoking and the health benefits of cessation (U.S. Department of Health and Human Services 1990). Nonetheless, the effectiveness of tobacco control strategies could benefit from the promotion of other healthy behaviors such as increased physical activity.

CONCLUSIONS

The 2004 Surgeon General's report has causally linked cigarette smoking to disease in almost every organ of the human body (U.S. Department of Health and Human Services 2004a). It is estimated that more than half of persistent smokers will be killed by their habit and that smokers lose, on average, 10 years of life compared with lifetime nonsmokers (Doll et al. 2004). Although smoking prevalence has declined in the United States, there are still approximately 46 million current smokers 18 years of age and older (Centers for Disease Control and Prevention 2009a), and smoking remains the leading preventable cause of death (Danaei et al. 2009). Effective tobacco control policies could have a substantial impact on health.

To understand the magnitude and timing of these impacts, we examined the potential reduction in premature mortality in the United States over the 20-year period from 2006 to 2025 that could be achieved through various future tobacco control policies. We estimate that the IOM recommendations would result in nontrivial reductions in premature mortality in the United States over this 20-year period. Under this scenario close to 500,000 premature deaths could be avoided, with a substantial portion due to lung cancer and cardiovascular disease.

Under a more aggressive tobacco control scenario, the number of premature deaths avoided could rise to 1 million over this 20-year period. If cigarette smoking were completely eliminated today, we predict that close to 3 million premature deaths could be avoided over the same time frame. Even under this scenario, some smoking-related disease burden would still exist after 20 years, specifically for cancer deaths, because the reduction in risk after cessation declines relatively slowly for cancer.

Of the premature deaths avoided by reducing or eliminating smoking, we project that almost 40 percent would be due to lung cancer and approximately 8 percent would be due to other cancers. Thus, close to half of premature deaths avoided would be from cancer. Another 30 percent of premature deaths avoided would be due to declining cardiovascular disease risk. In addition to the decrease in mortality, reduction in smoking would lead to a significant decline in illness and an improvement in quality of life—benefits not captured by our analysis.

The near-term impact of the policy scenarios we considered is modest: within 20 years, the IOM scenario would reduce deaths from all causes by 1 percent, the high-impact scenario by 3 percent, and the 100 percent cessation scenario by 7 percent. Because the high-impact scenario places most of its emphasis on preventing youth initiation, its near-term impact is relatively limited; tobacco-related illness has a long latency period (Weiss 1997); thus, the reduction in smoking would have little impact on mortality among adults in their 20s and 30s. In our simulation, we modeled excess risk only among 40- to 84-year-olds because, prior to age 40, mortality rates are so low that there is expected to be little excess risk due to smoking. However, policies focused on preventing youth initiation are expected to have much larger benefits over the longer term. A larger near-term reduction in mortality would come primarily from more aggressive promotion of cessation among adult smokers, as mortality risk can decline substantially after cessation (see figure 10.4). Both of these approaches are key components of comprehensive policies to reduce the burden of the tobacco epidemic.

In this chapter we have focused on the impact of smoking on premature mortality. However, smoking causes numerous adverse health effects that may or may not end in death. In addition to cancer and cardiovascular disease, smoking is a cause of respiratory diseases such as COPD, pneumonia, and decreased lung function; adverse reproductive outcomes such as fetal death, reduced fertility, low birthweight, and preterm birth; and a host of other adverse effects including increased risk of cataracts, hip fractures, and poor surgical outcomes. In general, smokers have poorer health and miss more days of work than comparable nonsmokers (U.S. Department of Health and Human Services 2004a). If we include the gain in healthy and productive life through avoidance of smoking, the public health impact of effective tobacco control policies would be significantly greater than reported here.

APPENDIX 10.1

MODELING RELATIVE RISKS

We modeled the relative risks using weighted linear regression (Carroll and Carroll 1988), where the analytical weights were equal to the inverse of the variance of the relative risk, and relative risks were log-transformed prior to modeling. Separate regressions were run for current smokers and former smokers by age at cessation. For current smokers, log relative risks were modeled using a quadratic function of age because the relative risks increased with age but dropped at the oldest ages. For former smokers the decline in log relative risk with age was modeled using linear functions. Using these models we predicted relative risks for each five-year age category and 10-year age at cessation category. In the simulation model, we include a lag period immediately after cessation during which no risk reduction is observed immediately. Because CVD risk declines faster than cancer risk after cessation, we use a two-year lag period for CVD and a three-year lag period for cancer and all-cause mortality.

MODELING MORTALITY RATES AMONG NEVER SMOKERS

Previous research shows that the relationship between rates of cancer mortality and age is well described by an exponential model (Armitage and Doll 1957; Doll 1971; Fisher 1958; Nordling 1952). Empirically, we have found this to be true for other causes as well. Thus, we modeled mortality rates as a function of age among never smokers, using the following general formula:

$$Rate = \beta \cdot age^k \tag{A.1}$$

where *age* is the midpoint of each five-year age group (from 40–44 to 80–84). Because some CPS II rates were based on small numbers, we conducted weighted regressions, using the number of deaths in each age group as the analytical weight. We varied the value of the unknown parameter, k, from 3 to 10 and chose the best-fitting model using the adjusted R^2. Separate regressions were run for males and females for each cause of death.

NOTE

1. This model is used to estimate the burden of smoking-attributable disease at the national and state levels. It incorporates national age- and sex-specific estimates of p and relative risk estimates from the American Cancer Society's Cancer Prevention Study (CPS) II, a nationwide, prospective cohort study begun in 1982, comprising 1.2 million U.S. adults ages 30 and older (Garfinkel 1985; Stellman and Garfinkel 1986; Thun and Heath 1997; Thun et al. 1995, 2000).

11

ASSESSING THE EFFECTS OF TOBACCO POLICY CHANGES ON SMOKING-RELATED HEALTH EXPENDITURES

DOUGLAS E. LEVY AND JOSEPH P. NEWHOUSE

D ecreases in population smoking will lead to improvements in the population's health, as Apelberg and Samet discuss in the previous chapter. One consequence of changes in smoking-related disease rates will be changes in health care expenditures. Based on our estimates, smoking accounts for about 5 percent of all personal health expenditures, or $79 billion in 2004. We use the SimSmoke projections of smoking rates through 2025 under each of the three principal policy scenarios to determine the effects of decreased smoking rates on American health care spending. To generate an upper bound on possible savings, we also consider a "100 percent cessation" scenario in which all smoking ceases in 2006.

Our chapter has three aims. First, we review previous studies that estimate the effect of smoking on personal health expenditures. Second, we quantify the effect of the tobacco control policy scenarios laid out in the SimSmoke model on health expenditures through 2025. We estimate health expenditures attributable to smoking in three populations: noninstitutionalized adults, newborn infants, and nursing home residents. Within each population we distinguish effects on up to five sources of financing. We include two publicly funded programs—Medicare, the federally funded program for the elderly and disabled, and Medicaid, the program for those with low income, which is funded through a combination of state and federal dollars. We also consider care paid for by private purchasers (specifically private third-party payers, such as employer-sponsored insurance), expenses paid out of pocket by consumers, and expenditures covered by other payers. Third, we discuss the implications of our estimates for tobacco control policy, focusing on the causal links among changes in tobacco policy, changes in smoking, and changes in health expenditures, and note the limitations involved in our projections of the effects of tobacco control policies on future spending.

ESTIMATES OF TOBACCO'S IMPACT ON HEALTH CARE SPENDING: PREVIOUS RESEARCH

There has been extensive research on the relationship between smoking and health care expenditures; for detailed reviews, see Warner, Hodgson, and Carroll (1999) and Max (2001). Analysts have used a wide range of strategies, each with a different interpretation and policy application. We begin by discussing some of the key issues in this kind of analysis.

First, it is important to distinguish between two approaches: those based on incidence and prevalence. The incidence approach compares the health expenditures of smokers and never smokers over their entire life spans. This strategy is used to determine the cost smokers impose on society (Hodgson 1992; Lippiatt 1990; Manning et al. 1989; Oster, Colditz, and Kelly 1984; Sloan et al. 2004; Viscusi 1995). Some of these studies focus solely on medical expenditures, with some concluding that smokers have higher lifetime costs (Hodgson 1992; Oster, Colditz, and Kelly 1984) and others that nonsmokers have higher lifetime costs because they live longer (Lippiatt 1990). Others balance smokers' medical costs with other social costs that might be higher or lower because of smokers' reduced life spans. Manning et al. (1989) and Sloan et al. (2004) both found that smokers have higher overall lifetime costs for health care than nonsmokers do, but Manning et al. suggest that at usual discount rates, smokers' excess costs are adequately offset by cigarette excise taxes. Viscusi (1995) performed a similar analysis and concluded that smokers do not impose any additional costs on society.

The prevalence approach, by contrast, compares the health care costs of current, former, and never smokers, using this comparison to determine the percentage of health care costs attributable to smoking during a specific interval of time (the smoking-attributable fraction, or SAF). Prevalence-based analyses may be used by payers to determine how the mix of current, former, and never smokers will affect health expenditures in a given year. The prevalence-based approach is used when considering how changes in smoking rates would affect expenditures paid for by private health insurers, Medicare, and Medicaid.

A number of early U.S. studies used the prevalence approach (Hedrick 1971; Kristein 1977; Luce and Schweitzer 1978; Office of Technology Assessment

1985; Rice et al. 1986). Rice et al. (1986) were the first to estimate the SAF, focusing their efforts on health care utilization for three disease categories—cancer, vascular diseases, and respiratory diseases. More recent examples of the prevalence approach (Bartlett et al. 1994; Miller, Ernst, and Collin 1999; Miller et al. 1998a) use the 1987 National Medical Expenditures Survey (NMES) as the principal data source for estimating the SAF of medical expenditures. The NMES has extensive information on smoking history, medical conditions, and charges for medical care. Generally speaking, these studies used regression models to estimate expenditures as a function of smoking history, controlling for a number of factors. Spending was then predicted both under the observed scenario and under a counterfactual scenario in which all the current and former smokers were assumed never to have smoked. To calculate the SAF, the authors took the difference between the total expenditures under the observed and counterfactual scenarios and divided the difference by the total expenditures under the observed scenario.

These studies have generated a range of estimates for the SAF. Bartlett et al. (1994) estimated the SAF of medical expenditures by quantifying how smoking affects diseases—including heart disease, emphysema, arteriosclerosis, stroke, and cancer—and then incorporating those effects in to a model of health expenditures as a function of smoking and health status. They estimated a SAF of 6.3 percent. Building on this work, L. S. Miller et al. (1998a) used a complex, four-equation model linking smoking to disease, health status, and health care spending, controlling for age, race/ethnicity, marital status, education level, region of residence, use of seatbelts, and obesity to estimate age-sex-payer-specific SAFs. Using data on smoking prevalence from 1993, the authors estimated the SAF of medical expenditures for that year to be 11.8 percent. Two separate and related studies by L. S. Miller's group estimated the SAF of expenditures for Medicaid in 1993 to be 14.4 percent (Miller et al. 1998b) and for Medicare to be 9.4 percent (Zhang et al. 1999). Generally, SAF estimates are higher for Medicaid than for the general population because of the higher prevalence of smoking in low-income populations, and are higher for Medicare because many health consequences of smoking do not appear until individuals reach Medicare's age of eligibility. V. P. Miller and colleagues (Miller, Ernst, and Collin 1999) used a simpler two-part model of health expenditures as a function of smoking status, age, sex, race, ethnicity, region of residence, metropolitan area, education, marital status, pregnancy status, self-described propensity to take risks, physical activity, obesity, seatbelt use, HMO membership, and insurance type. They estimated a SAF of 6.5 percent. The widely used Smoking-Attributable Morbidity, Mortality, and Economic Costs (SAMMEC) model, published by the Centers for Disease Control and Prevention, is based on this latter study.

Our empirical strategy combines the incidence and prevalence approaches. Although we do not estimate smokers' lifetime costs under different policy scenarios, we are interested in how costs change over time as population demographics and smoking habits shift. We take changes in the distribution of smoking and projections of population size and demographics from the SimSmoke analysis outlined in chapter 2. We then apply estimates of health care expenditures by age, sex, and smoking status that are derived from prevalence-based analyses.

Our analysis addresses two main limitations of earlier prevalence-based studies. Most of these earlier studies estimated the effect of smoking on medical expenditures using a disease-specific approach. In other words, for a specified set of diseases, the proportion of cases attributable to smoking, or SAF of cases, is estimated. For each disease the SAF of cases is then applied to total health care spending for that disease, yielding the SAF of expenditures, or the fraction of expenditures attributable to smoking. For instance, if 80 percent of lung cancer cases are caused by smoking, then 80 percent of all medical care spending associated with lung cancer cases is assumed to be attributable to smoking. The overall effect of smoking on expenditures is the sum of these disease-specific estimates of smoking-attributable expenditures. This approach has two major limitations. First, one must completely enumerate all the health conditions that might be affected by smoking. Because most analyses using the disease-specific approach focus only on the major smoking-related diseases, they omit cases whose diagnoses are sequelae of smoking but are not considered smoking-related diseases in their own right, for example, peptic ulcers, arthritis, allergies, and back pain (Musich et al. 2003; Parasher and Eastwood 2000). They also omit more minor associations between smoking and health and health expenditures, for example, sinusitis (Lieu and Feinstein 2000). Second, by applying a smoking-attributable fraction of disease to the total expenditures for that disease, one assumes that the cost of treating the disease is the same for smokers and nonsmokers, an assumption that may not be true for all conditions.

Later studies (Bartlett et al. 1994; Miller, Ernst, and Collin 1999; Miller et al. 1998a, 1998b; Zhang et al. 1999) employed a more flexible and inclusive approach that models health expenditures directly as a function of smoking, eliminating the need to explicitly enumerate all smoking-related conditions and their costs. In other words, these models compare the medical expenditures for current smokers and former smokers with estimates of what their expenditures would have been had they never smoked. Our analysis of the adult, noninstitutionalized population, who generate the bulk of health expenditures, uses this more inclusive approach.

A second disadvantage that earlier studies face is their reliance on imperfect and obsolete data. Until recently, the 1987 NMES was the only survey of health expenditures that included detailed measures of smoking. Substantial changes in medical technology and health care financing have occurred since this survey was conducted more than 20 years ago. Recent developments such as interventional cardiology and new cancer drugs from biotechnology have significantly changed the treatment of smoking-related diseases. The 1980s and 1990s also saw the rise of managed care and the subsequent backlash against it, increases in the use of prospective payment, and increasing attention to the quality of medical care, all of which may have changed the costs of treating smoking-related illnesses. Particularly for projecting health care expenditures over the next 20 years, a more recent data source is preferable. The NMES has other limitations as well. As Cutler and colleagues (2000) point out, much of the smoking data in the NMES are imputed (i.e., estimated based on other information rather than measured directly), a problem for analyses in which smoking is a central variable. Moreover, the NMES lacks data on alcohol consumption, which is associated with smoking and is also likely to affect health care costs.

Fortunately, beginning in 1996, the Agency for Healthcare Research and Quality (AHRQ) began to field the Medical Expenditures Panel Survey (MEPS), a follow-up to the NMES. This survey is conducted annually and follows respondents for two years. The MEPS is designed to be representative of the civilian noninstitutionalized population. Each MEPS cohort is drawn from the previous year's National Health Interview Survey (NHIS), so that data from the two surveys can be linked. In 2000 the MEPS began collecting its own measures of smoking. The MEPS smoking data are not comprehensive, but by combining measures from the MEPS and the NHIS, we can estimate health expenditures in the context of relatively rich information on smoking. We use the MEPS in much of the analysis that follows.

METHODS AND DATA

To project expenditures based on SimSmoke's estimates of future smoking, we estimate per-capita spending by age, sex, and smoking status for each of the three study populations: the adult noninstitutionalized population, the neonatal population, and the nursing home population. Our results, however, are dominated by the results for noninstitutionalized adults, so readers mainly interested in our results may want to skim the methods we use for the other two populations.

Projecting health expenditures into the future is then a matter of combining the U.S. Census Bureau's population projection, the SimSmoke smoking prevalence projections, and our estimates of per-capita health expenditures for each age-sex-smoking status-payer group in each population for each year through 2025. Although the policy-driven reductions in smoking that are projected by

SimSmoke are likely to increase the longevity of the population somewhat, this effect will be small in this time frame, as Apelberg and Samet discuss; thus, we do not adjust the Census Bureau's population projections for survival differentials across our policy scenarios.

To project the effect of changes in tobacco policy on health expenditures into the future, we must estimate the causal effect of smoking on expenditures for people with a wide range of individual characteristics and across all permutations of smoking history (Rubin 2001). For example, to quantify the effect of reducing smoking initiation, we must estimate expenditure trajectories for individuals who smoke and for otherwise identical individuals who do not. To quantify the effect of smoking cessation on health expenditures, we need to know the expenditures of quitters as well as what quitters' expenditures would have been had they continued smoking.

In our analyses we applied a real annual discount rate of 3 percent, and all results are reported in present discounted values. This allows readers to weigh the opportunity costs of current investment in tobacco control against the downstream benefits of reductions in health expenditures. All dollar amounts were adjusted for inflation to year 2002 dollars using the All Items Consumer Price Index. Below, we discuss in detail the data components and analytical strategies used to generate projections in each of the three populations.

ADULT NONINSTITUTIONALIZED POPULATION

We projected future health expenditures for the adult noninstitutionalized population in several steps. Using the 2000–2002 MEPS linked with the 1998–2001 NHIS, we estimated individuals' average annual health expenditures and the SAF of health expenditures by age, sex, and payer. We then combined these figures to estimate excess expenditures attributable to smoking for each age-sex-payer cell. We generated separate estimates of excess spending attributable to smoking for current smokers and former smokers, with the latter subdivided based on the number of years since quitting. From these estimates, we calculated per-capita annual health expenditures by age, sex, smoking history, and payer. Below we provide more information on our methods; full details are available in appendix 11.1.

ESTIMATING THE SAF OF EXPENDITURES   We used multivariate regression to estimate the SAF separately for men and women in each of the SimSmoke age categories and for each payer. Private purchasers, Medicare, Medicaid, and out-of-pocket expenditures are defined in the MEPS. Other expenditures are those that do not fall into the first four categories and include those paid for by the Department of Veterans Affairs and TRICARE (for individuals not on active military duty), other government sources (e.g., the Indian Health Service or local governments), Worker's Compensation, and insurers covering medical liability (e.g., auto insurers or property insurers). In our first step, we estimated expenditures controlling for smoking history, demographics (age, sex, race, and ethnicity), socioeconomic status (education and income), alcohol consumption, body mass index, pregnancy status, risk-taking behavior as measured by seatbelt use and receipt of flu shots, geography (census region and Metropolitan Statistical Area designation), and insurance status. Smoking history was defined as current heavy smoking (> 15 cigarettes per day), current light smoking (≤ 15 cigarettes per day), former smoker for 15 or fewer years, former smoker for more than 15 years, or never smoker; current and former smokers were also identified based on the number of years they smoked, categorized as ≤ 10, 11–20, 21–30, or ≥ 31 years. Evidence suggests that further controls would not affect our estimates substantially (Malarcher et al. 2000; Thun, Apicella, and Henley 2000; Vollset, Tverdal, and Gjessing 2006). Next, we used the model to predict expenditures based on observed smoking patterns. Then we predicted expenditures anew, assuming that all current and former smokers had never smoked. The SAF is the difference between the predicted expenditures (based on observed smoking) and those based on the counterfactual assumption of no smoking, divided by the predicted expenditures based on observed smoking. Confidence bounds on the SAFs are derived using the bootstrap method.

As discussed above, our estimates of the effect of smoking on health expenditures control statistically for a variety of other factors relevant to health, including health behaviors such as alcohol consumption and risk-taking behavior as well as background factors such as income or place of residence. We included these controls in order to better isolate the effect of smoking status on health expenditures. Our projections assume that the distribution of these factors is constant within gender and age categories over the course of the simulation and that the distribution of payers within an age-sex-smoking status cell also remains constant over time.

ESTIMATING PER-CAPITA EXPENDITURES After calculating the SAFs, we estimated expenditures that were attributable to smoking for each age-sex-payer group by applying the SAF to the average expenditures for that group.

Estimating health care expenditures for former smokers required a more complex approach. We found a discrepancy between the pattern of results calculated with the MEPS data and evidence in the epidemiology literature. In the MEPS data, where smoking status and health expenditures are measured at the same time, former smokers have higher medical expenditures than current smokers. Epidemiological data, on the other hand, suggest that quitting smoking should decrease health expenditures because disease risks begin to decline almost immediately following smoking cessation (U.S. Department of Health and Human Services 1990). There is evidence that the higher spending among former smokers in the MEPS data appears because smokers often quit when they become sick (Martinson et al. 2003). Thus, quitting is not causing high health expenditures; rather, high medical expenditures—a proxy measure for illness—are causing quitting. We reconcile the MEPS data with the epidemiological data by forcing expenditures of former smokers to follow the decline observed in mortality following smoking cessation. This strategy is more applicable to our focus on the situation in which people are induced to quit because of policy factors such as higher excise taxes, clean air laws, or media campaigns rather than individual health events.

In other words, we accomplish reconciliation with the epidemiological data by disaggregating the excess spending attributable to smoking, assuming that with each year following smoking cessation, expenditures for former smokers would decline relative to current smokers in proportion to the decline in all-cause mortality risk. We assigned weights to current smokers, former smokers, and never smokers such that current smokers got a weight of one, former smokers were assigned weights that declined from one as a function of years since smoking cessation at the same rate as all-cause mortality risk declines following smoking cessation, and never smokers were assigned a weight of zero. Excess smoking-attributable expenditures were thus calculated for each person in the data according to age, sex, payer, and smoking status. Adding average expenditures not attributable to smoking and excess spending attributable to smoking gave us average per-capita expenditures specific to age, sex, smoking status, and payer.

NEONATAL POPULATION

Neonatal care is more expensive for infants born to mothers who smoke. We used several data sources to generate estimates of these smoking-attributable costs. The first is the CDC's Maternal and Child Health Smoking-Attributable Mortality, Morbidity, and Economic Costs (MCH-SAMMEC) model. MCH-SAMMEC calculates the SAF of neonatal intensive care unit (NICU) admissions and hospital days, assigning excess costs based on a weighted average of NICU costs and hospital day costs for infants born to smokers versus nonsmokers. Second, we gathered baseline age-specific maternal smoking rates from the 2002 Natality Detail File published by the National Vital Statistics Service (National Center for Health Statistics 2002). To project prenatal smoking rates through 2025 under the different policy scenarios, we assumed that age-specific smoking would change at the same rate for pregnant women as for all women of childbearing age (15–44 years old). We applied the relative changes in smoking rates projected by SimSmoke for women of these ages to our baseline maternal smoking rates from the Natality Detail File. The Census Bureau's Web site projects the number of births each year through 2025 (published January 1, 2000). Because smoking-attributable mortality is negligible for women of childbearing age, we took the Census Bureau's estimate of births to be the same in each policy scenario we simulated. We estimated the cost of prenatal smoking in each year as the product of the number of pregnancies per year, the proportion of pregnant women who smoke, and the excess neonatal health care cost per pregnant smoker. Our analyses assume that the proportion of pregnant women in each age group is constant over time, although the size of the age groups may change, and that the proportion of pregnant women with a given payer is constant within age groups over time. We were not able to assign statistical confidence bounds to our estimates.

The resulting estimates of smoking-attributable neonatal health care costs may be an underestimate. MCH-SAMMEC considers only the costs of NICU admissions and infant length of stay immediately following delivery. Any increases in infants' health care utilization that occur beyond the initial hospital stay following delivery are not counted here.

NURSING HOME POPULATION

We used a disease-specific approach to estimate the SAF of nursing home expenditures using the 1999 National Nursing Home Survey (NNHS) discharge file and various published data; this approach was necessary because the NNHS did not include person-specific information on smoking. We assumed that the SAF of disease for each NNHS respondent's diagnosis (his/her reason for being in a nursing home) was the SAF of the respondent's days in the nursing home and therefore the SAF of expenditures. For instance, if the SAF of lung cancer is 80 percent, then 80 percent of nursing home costs for patients admitted with lung cancer would be considered to be smoking attributable.

Each NNHS respondent was assigned a diagnosis based on his or her primary admitting diagnosis. This method is not perfect; it is possible that a respondent had a smoking-related disease that affected the duration of the nursing home stay, even if it was not the primary diagnosis leading to admission. The NNHS contains information on an additional five admitting and six ongoing diagnoses for each respondent. We conducted an alternative analysis in which the assigned diagnosis was the first diagnosis of a smoking-related disease listed in a respondent's record. This alternative analysis is likely to bias the SAF of nursing home expenditures upwards and so helps to set an upper bound for savings resulting from each policy scenario.

For the nursing home analysis, the SAF was calculated using the relative risk of dying from a specific smoking-related disease (a proxy for the relative risk of developing the disease) for current and former smokers, together with the probability of current and former smoking. An individual respondent's SAF of disease was ascertained by combining the relative risk of his/her assigned diagnosis for current and former smokers with the probability that the individual was a current or former smoker as estimated by SimSmoke given the respondent's age and sex. This procedure assumes that smoking rates for those admitted to nursing homes are the same as those in the general population and that the proportion of, for example, stroke patients entering nursing homes because of smoking is the same as the proportion of stroke cases attributable to smoking. The action of SimSmoke on the projections of nursing home expenditures is through changes in the SAF of disease.

Nineteen smoking-related disease categories and their relative risks were identified in the 2004 Surgeon General's report, "The Health Consequences of Smoking" (U.S. Department of Health and Human Services 2004a), including cancers of the mouth, esophagus, stomach, pancreas, larynx, lungs, cervix, bladder, and kidney; acute myeloid leukemia; ischemic and other heart diseases; cerebrovascular disease; atherosclerosis, aortic aneurysm, and other arterial diseases; pneumonia, influenza, bronchitis, emphysema, and chronic airway obstruction. Recall that the analysis does not assume all cases of these diseases are caused by smoking but simply estimates the increased risk of these diseases among current and former smokers. Conditions not deemed smoking-related by the Surgeon General's report were assumed to impart no additional risk of disease for individuals who smoked relative to those who did not. We applied a SAF to the number of days each NNHS respondent reported staying in the nursing home, according to the respondent's assigned diagnosis. Aggregating by age and sex, we generated overall age-sex-specific SAFs of nursing home days. These SAFs were made payer-specific by calculating the SAF of nursing home days separately according to the respondents' self-reported primary source of payment at admission.

We applied the SAFs to per-capita estimates of nursing home expenditures published by the Centers for Medicare and Medicaid Services (CMS) for 1999 (Centers for Medicaid and Medicare Services 2006). Per-capita nursing home expenditures were made payer-specific based on CMS's reports of the proportions of expenditures covered by each payer in each age group. Finally, we multiplied the per-capita estimates of smoking-attributable nursing home expenditures by the U.S. Census Bureau's population projections. As with the neonatal population, we had no basis on which to construct confidence bounds for our estimates of smoking-attributable nursing home expenditures.

EXPENDITURES NOT INCLUDED IN OUR PROJECTIONS

Some smoking-related health expenditures could not be considered in our projections due to lack of data. We do not have any data on non-civilian or institutionalized individuals other than those in nursing homes. Thus, members of the military, residents of state mental hospitals or rehabilitation hospitals, and individuals who are incarcerated are not included in our estimates. We also do not measure the effects of secondhand smoke on health spending because we lack data on passive exposure to tobacco smoke.

Perhaps most importantly, none of our data sources has adequate information on the number of cigarettes smoked per day, so our model cannot measure the effects of reductions in quantity smoked on health expenditures. Epidemiological research indicates a dose-response relationship between smoking intensity and smoking-related disease risk (U.S. Department of Health and Human Services 2004a), so that reductions in the number of cigarettes consumed per smoker will have some effect on health expenditures. The MEPS has data only on whether a respondent is a current smoker or not, while information on past smoking is taken from the NHIS. Although the NHIS does include a measure of the intensity of recent cigarette consumption, a better measure would be pack-years of cigarette exposure. Neither the MEPS nor the NHIS provides sufficient data to estimate this exposure. Nevertheless, the 100 percent cessation scenario gives an upper bound for the effect of reduced smoking prevalence and consumption on health care expenditures.

RESULTS

Taking together smoking-attributable health expenditures for the adult noninstitutionalized population, the nursing home population, and the neonatal population, we project savings of tens to hundreds of billions of dollars in health care costs between 2006 and 2025 under the three alternate policy scenarios relative to the status quo (figure 11.1). By 2015, cumulative health expenditures would be $24 billion lower under the IOM recommendations and $54 billion lower under the high-impact scenario than would be the case if current tobacco policy remained unchanged. By 2025, cumulative savings are projected to reach $59 billion under the IOM recommendations and $122 billion under the high-impact scenario. Because the health care sector is so large, these savings amount to only 0.43 percent and 0.88 percent, respectively, of total projected health expenditures under the status quo. Under the 100 percent cessation scenario, we project savings of $211 billion relative to the status quo by 2025, or 1.52 percent.

The savings resulting from a decline in smoking rates will not fall equally on all payers (figure 11.2). In absolute terms, private purchasers save the most

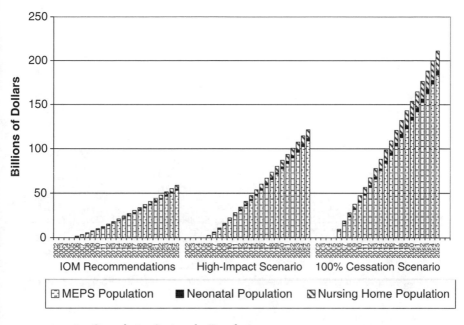

FIGURE 11.1 Cumulative Savings by Population

Note: Data in this figure are based on final equations in appendixes 11.1, 11.2, and 11.3.
Source: Authors' calculations.

money, which is not surprising because they pay for the bulk of health expenses. Private payers would save $26 billion under the IOM scenario and $54 billion under the high-impact scenario. Medicaid and other payers would see a drop in expenditures by roughly $12 billion and $22 billion, respectively, compared with the status quo for the IOM recommendations and the high-impact scenario. Medicare spending and out-of-pocket expenditures would be reduced by less than $6 billion under the IOM recommendations and less than $15 billion under the high-impact scenario.

The largest percentage reductions in spending through 2025 are achieved by the Medicaid program because of the disproportionate concentration of smoking in that population. We project that Medicaid expenditures would be 0.86 percent lower than the status quo under the IOM scenario and 1.74 percent lower under the high-impact scenario. We project other payers would reduce expenditures by 0.54 percent and 1.00 percent, respectively, under the IOM and high-impact scenarios. Private payers are projected to save 0.52 percent and 1.08 percent relative to the status quo under the IOM recommendations and the high-impact scenario, respectively. Medicare and out-of-pocket payers are expected to save less than 0.22 percent under the IOM recommendations and less than 0.53 percent under the high-impact scenario.

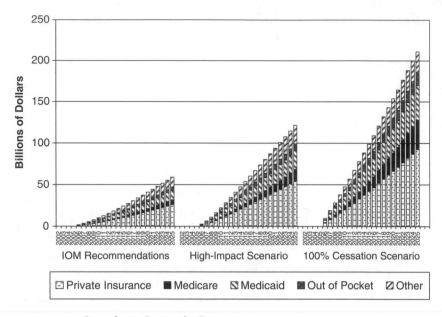

FIGURE 11.2 Cumulative Savings by Payer

Note: Data in this figure come from focusing the final equations in appendixes 11.1, 11.2, and 11.3 on specific payers and summing across populations. In this figure, private insurance includes the neonatal private payer category, which actually consists of private purchasers and other third-party payers. There was no out-of-pocket category in the neonatal population, though there were certainly out-of-pocket costs. Neonatal expenditures are sufficiently small that any misclassification of payers in that population will have a negligible effect on our conclusions.

Source: Authors' calculations.

ADULT NONINSTITUTIONALIZED POPULATION

As noted above, noninstitutionalized adults account for the vast majority of total health expenditures as well as most smoking-attributable spending. In the MEPS population, we estimate an overall SAF of expenditures of 5.11 percent (see table 11.1), which is slightly lower than the values reported in earlier studies. SAFs are higher for men than for women and generally increase with age. The overall SAFs of expenditures for Medicare and Medicaid are higher than for private purchasers, out-of-pocket expenses, or other payers. Though the SAFs are higher for the two public programs, they are less precisely estimated because the Medicare and Medicaid populations account for only 22.5 percent and 11.8 percent, respectively, of the 26,073 observations in our MEPS sample. The higher SAF for Medicaid is consistent with the higher smoking prevalence of Medicaid enrollees, and the higher SAF for Medicare reflects the appearance of most smoking-related diseases later in life.

TABLE 11.1 SAF of Total Expenditures by Age, Sex, and Payer for the Adult Noninstitutionalized Population

PAYER/SEX	AGE	SAF	95% CONFIDENCE BOUND	
All payers				
Overall		5.11%	(2.54,	7.90)
Male	18–44	2.53	(−0.46,	5.41)
	45–64	7.10	(3.66,	10.62)
	65–74	8.82	(4.74,	13.31)
	≥75	9.19	(4.24,	14.76)
Female	18–44	1.78	(−0.78,	4.28)
	45–64	5.05	(2.50,	7.75)
	65–74	5.79	(2.91,	9.13)
	≥75	3.84	(1.71,	6.37)
Private insurance				
Overall		6.38%	(3.11,	9.74)
Male	18–44	0.62	(−2.83,	4.13)
	45–64	11.13	(6.55,	15.61)
	65–74	16.89	(11.82,	21.82)
	>75	20.64	(14.92,	26.08)
Female	18–44	0.45	(−2.54,	3.41)
	45–64	8.38	(4.76,	12.17)
	65–74	12.50	(8.42,	16.56)
	≥75	9.97	(6.66,	13.35)
Medicare				
Overall		10.13%	(3.78,	16.99)
Male	18–44	12.73	(−1.10,	26.88)
	45–64	18.32	(6.38,	29.46)
	65–74	13.68	(5.53,	22.32)
	≥75	13.21	(3.93,	22.02)
Female	18–44	7.28	(−3.07,	18.79)
	45–64	13.19	(2.55,	23.08)

TABLE 11.1 *(Continued)*

PAYER/SEX	AGE	SAF	95% CONFIDENCE BOUND	
	65–74	9.25	(3.10,	15.76)
	≥75	5.43	(1.36,	9.93)
Medicaid				
Overall		11.19%	(3.57,	18.87)
Male	18–44	13.90	(4.82,	24.11)
	45–64	13.99	(2.33,	25.38)
	65–74	13.77	(−6.88,	29.85)
	≥75	10.42	(−6.77,	26.59)
Female	18–44	11.35	(2.99,	19.19)
	45–64	12.21	(2.68,	21.68)
	65–74	7.62	(−3.00,	18.64)
	≥75	4.39	(−1.95,	10.65)
Out of pocket				
Overall		1.50%	(−2.17,	5.06)
Male	18–44	−0.42	(−3.00,	1.98)
	45–64	1.78	(−2.72,	6.12)
	65–74	3.60	(−3.98,	11.28)
	≥75	4.61	(−4.21,	13.54)
Female	18–44	−0.17	(−2.58,	1.95)
	45–64	1.28	(−2.15,	4.49)
	65–74	2.23	(−2.48,	7.03)
	≥75	1.63	(−1.73,	5.34)
Other				
Overall		3.46%	(−7.99,	14.13)
Male	18–44	1.42	(−11.36,	13.87)
	45–64	5.83	(−7.97,	19.60)
	65–74	3.34	(−16.24,	19.36)
	≥75	−0.02	(−20.41,	15.77)

TABLE 11.1 *(Continued)*

PAYER/SEX	AGE	SAF	95% CONFIDENCE BOUND	
Female	18–44	3.32	(–7.34,	14.62)
	45–64	6.06	(–5.37,	16.38)
	65–74	4.30	(–9.04,	17.33)
	≥ 75	2.64	(–6.54,	12.26)

Source: Authors' calculations (see appendix 11.1).

There are several possible explanations for the difference between our overall SAF estimates and those previously published. First, using the MEPS we were able to explicitly and directly control for alcohol consumption, an important potential confounder in analyses of smoking-related health expenditures. This was not possible in the NMES, so some of the costs attributed to smoking may actually have been due to alcohol consumption since smoking and alcohol consumption are positively correlated. Second, we compared a variety of regression models for estimating health expenditures, including the two-part models typically used in NMES analyses as well as generalized linear models, which were not commonly used in health expenditure analyses when the NMES analyses were conducted. Thus, we were able to choose the statistical model that best fit the data. Last, a small proportion of the difference in estimated SAFs reflects the reduction in smoking rates between the 1990s, when many of the earlier studies were conducted, and the early 2000s, when the MEPS data were collected.

Private purchasers in the MEPS population stand to gain the most from vigorous tobacco control policies, with cumulative savings through 2025 of $53 billion under the IOM recommendations and up to $109 billion under the high-impact scenario (table 11.2, figure 11.3). Medicaid is projected to save fewer dollars, but the model projects a larger percentage reduction in spending relative to the status quo through 2025: savings were 0.75 percent under the IOM recommendations and 1.45 percent under the high-impact scenario. In both absolute and relative terms, out-of-pocket spending is the least affected expenditure category in the MEPS population.

In analyses reported in figure 11.4, we assess the sensitivity of our findings to our procedure for estimating the medical expenses of former smokers. As an alternative, we assumed that expenditures would fall in proportion to the decline in mortality from cardiovascular disease, lung cancer, and all smoking-related cancers. Although we analyzed these alternative assumptions for each

TABLE 11.2 Cumulative Savings Through 2025: Adult Noninstitutionalized Population

	IOM RECOMMENDATIONS		HIGH-IMPACT SCENARIO		100% CESSATION SCENARIO	
	ABSOLUTE ($ BILLION)	% STATUS QUO SPENDING	ABSOLUTE ($ BILLION)	% STATUS QUO SPENDING	ABSOLUTE ($ BILLION)	% STATUS QUO SPENDING
All payers	$53	0.40%	$109	0.81%	$183	1.37%
Private purchasers	25	0.52	52	1.09	88.7	1.84
Medicare	6	0.21	14	0.51	34	1.28
Medicaid	8	0.75	16	1.45	28	2.52
Out of pocket	3	0.11	6	0.23	10	0.39
Other	12	0.53	21	0.96	33	1.50

Source: Authors' calculations (see appendix 11.1).

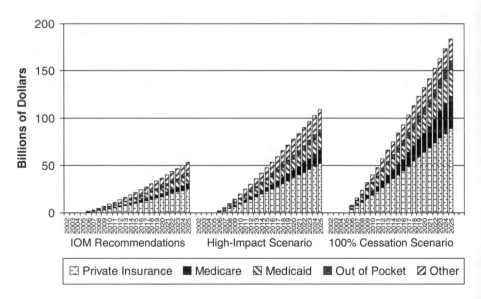

FIGURE 11.3 Cumulative Savings for Adult Noninstitutionalized Population, by Payer

Note: Data in this figure come from focusing the final equation in appendix 11.1 on specific payers.

Source: Authors' calculations.

policy scenario, we present only the IOM recommendations scenario in the figure because the sensitivity under the other scenarios is qualitatively similar. Our base-case assumption that expenditures fall at the same rate as all-cause mortality following smoking cessation is conservative relative to the other mortality models we considered. The greatest projected savings occurred under the assumption that expenditures fall along with lung cancer mortality (savings through 2025 of $69 billion for the IOM scenario and $145 billion for the high-impact scenario), followed by cardiovascular disease mortality and then by all smoking-related cancer mortality. Thus, more aggressive assumptions regarding the benefits of smoking cessation would increase savings through 2025 by $16 billion to $36 billion relative to our base-case assumption. These comparisons should be thought of as a means of assessing the upper bound of possible savings rather than representing a plausible range of savings.

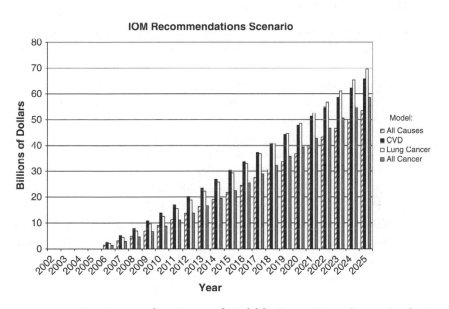

FIGURE 11.4 Sensitivity Analysis: Impact of Model for Former Versus Current Smokers' Expenditures on Cumulative Savings

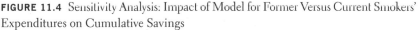

Note: Data in this figure come from appendix 11.1 with values of q (from chapter 10) adjusted to alternate assumptions about how expenditures decline following cessation.

Source: Authors' calculations.

NEONATAL POPULATION

On the basis of the MCH-SAMMEC model, we estimate that the average additional cost of neonatal care due to smoking is $810 per pregnant smoker, which is within the range of previously published estimates (Adams, Solanki, and Miller 1997; Miller et al. 2001; Oster, Delea, and Colditz 1988). Expenditures attributable to prenatal smoking are only a small portion of overall smoking-attributable health expenditures. Through 2025, we estimate savings of $1.5 billion (IOM recommendations) to $2.9 billion (high-impact scenario) compared to the status quo (table 11.3, figure 11.5). Because only current smoking affects smoking-attributable spending among neonates, the 100 percent cessation scenario would completely eliminate excess neonatal health expenditures attributed to smoking, a savings of $4.5 billion through 2025.

NURSING HOME POPULATION

Projections of the change in nursing home spending over the alternate policy scenarios derive from the changing SAF of nursing home expenditures as smoking rates change and from the changing age distribution of the population. If NNHS respondents are assigned their primary admitting diagnoses, the baseline SAF of nursing home expenditures is 4.7 percent under all scenarios (table 11.4, panel A). By 2025, the model predicts the SAF of nursing home expenditures under the status quo would be 4.8 percent compared to 4.4 percent under the IOM recommendations and 4.1 percent under the high-impact scenario. Under the 100 percent cessation scenario, the SAF falls to 3.4 percent. These estimates are substantially lower than most previously published SAFs of nursing home expenditures, which range from 6.6 percent to 22.1 percent. Assigning NNHS respondents the first diagnosis of a smoking-related disease that appeared on their records increased the overall baseline SAF to 11.2 percent, more in line with previous estimates (table 11.4, panel B). Under either analysis strategy, Medicaid and out-of-pocket payers have higher initial and final SAFs of expenditures than either private purchasers or Medicare.

When the primary admitting diagnosis is used in our SAF calculations, the model predicts reductions in nursing home spending by 2025 totaling $4.1 billion (4.1 percent of status quo nursing home spending) under the IOM recommendations and $9.7 (9.7 percent of status quo spending) billion under the high-impact scenario compared to the status quo by the year 2025 (table 11.5, panel A, and figure 11.6). Projections under the 100 percent cessation scenario predict savings of $23.0 billion, or 23.1 percent of status quo spending. When

Cumulative Savings Through 2025: Neonatal Population

	IOM RECOMMENDATIONS		HIGH-IMPACT SCENARIO		100% CESSATION SCENARIO	
	ABSOLUTE ($ BILLION)	% STATUS QUO SPENDING	ABSOLUTE ($ BILLION)	% STATUS QUO SPENDING	ABSOLUTE ($ BILLION)	% STATUS QUO SPENDING
payers	$1.49	0.41%	$2.94	0.80%	$4.5	1.23%
Private purchasers/ other purchasers	0.49	0.24	0.99	0.49	2.02	0.78
Medicaid	0.93	0.64	1.80	1.23	3.53	1.87
Other	0.07	0.38	0.15	0.77	0.30	1.19

rce. Authors' calculations (see appendix 11.2).

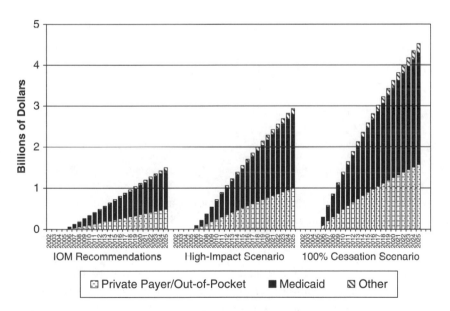

FIGURE 11.5 Cumulative Savings for Neonatal Population, by Payer

Note: Data in this figure come from focusing the final equation in appendix 11.2 on specific payers.

Source: Authors' calculations.

TABLE 11.4 Smoking-Attributable Fraction of Nursing Home Days, 2002 and 2025

YEAR	STATUS QUO		IOM RECOMMENDATIONS		HIGH-IMPACT SCENARIO		100% CESSATION SCENARIO	
	2002	2025	2002	2025	2002	2025	2002	2025
Panel A: Using Primary Admitting Diagnosis								
All payers	4.7%	4.8%	4.7%	4.4%	4.7%	4.1%	4.7%	3.4%
Private insurers	4.0	4.1	4.0	3.8	4.0	3.5	4.0	2.8
Medicaid	4.7	4.7	4.7	4.4	4.7	4.1	4.7	3.4
Medicare	4.0	4.0	4.0	3.8	4.0	3.6	4.0	3.0
Out of pocket	4.5	4.7	4.5	4.4	4.5	4.1	4.5	3.4
Other	9.2	8.9	9.2	8.0	9.2	7.0	9.2	5.1
Panel B: Using First-Listed Smoking-Related Diagnosis								
All payers	11.2%	11.4%	11.2%	10.6%	11.2%	9.8%	11.2%	8.1%
Private insurers	8.1	8.3	8.1	7.7	8.1	7.1	8.1	5.8
Medicaid	10.9	11	10.9	10.2	10.9	9.4	10.9	7.8
Medicare	11.6	11.9	11.6	11	11.6	10.2	11.6	8.5
Out of pocket	12.7	13.2	12.7	12.7	12.7	12.1	12.7	10.7
Other	14.2	13.7	14.2	12.3	14.2	10.9	14.2	8.2

Source: Authors' calculations (see appendix 11.3).

we use the more liberal criterion to assign diagnoses (first smoking-related disease diagnosis in the patient's record) in our SAF calculations, we predict a $10.7 billion reduction in nursing home spending by 2025 under the IOM recommendations and a $24.6 billion reduction under the high-impact scenario (table 11.5, panel B). In the 100 percent cessation scenario, we predict spending reductions of $56.7 billion. Payer-specific savings from reductions in smoking rates largely reflect the shares each payer contributes to nursing home spending. In absolute terms, the majority of savings fall to Medicaid and out-of-pocket payers. In percentage terms, we project the greatest savings will be realized by other payers, though other payers account for a very small portion of overall nursing home spending, and their savings are imprecisely estimated due to the small number of observations in that category.

TABLE 11.5 Cumulative Savings Through 2025: Nursing Home Population

	IOM RECOMMENDATIONS		HIGH-IMPACT SCENARIO		100% CESSATION SCENARIO	
	ABSOLUTE ($ BILLION)	% STATUS QUO SPENDING	ABSOLUTE ($ BILLION)	% STATUS QUO SPENDING	ABSOLUTE ($ BILLION)	% STATUS QUO SPENDING
Panel A: Using Primary Admitting Diagnosis						
All payers	$4.09	4.09%	$9.68	9.69%	$23.03	23.05%
Private purchasers	0.42	3.81	0.98	8.76	2.15	19.27
Medicare	0.30	3.18	0.67	7.14	1.56	16.55
Medicaid	1.94	4.33	4.68	10.44	11.10	24.77
Out of pocket	1.04	3.69	2.37	8.40	5.89	20.88
Other	0.38	6.06	0.98	15.48	2.34	36.87
Panel B: Using First-Listed Smoking-Related Diagnosis						
All payers	$10.67	4.31%	$24.57	9.92%	$56.74	22.91%
Private purchasers	0.78	3.90	1.80	8.98	4.22	21.06
Medicare	0.93	3.69	2.08	8.24	4.81	19.01
Medicaid	5.65	4.95	13.14	11.51	29.31	25.67
Out of pocket	2.07	2.55	4.79	5.91	12.82	15.79
Other	1.24	17.84	2.75	39.55	5.58	80.32

Source: Authors' calculations (see appendix 11.3).

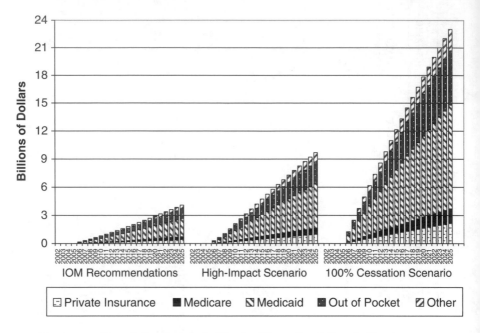

FIGURE 11.6 Cumulative Savings for Nursing Home Population, by Payer

Note: Data in this figure come from focusing the final equation in appendix 11.3 on specific payers. Admitting diagnoses are the basis for estimating the SAF.

Source: Authors' calculations.

DISCUSSION

How great an impact tobacco control policies will have on health expenditures is a matter of perspective. Estimates of the SAF of health expenditures—5 percent based on our estimates from the MEPS and from 6 percent to 14 percent based on earlier literature—are derived by comparing observed health expenditures to a counterfactual world where no one smokes and thus are an overall upper bound on the effect of tobacco control policies on health expenditures. Our projections indicate that plausible tobacco control measures will have a much smaller effect on health care spending than the upper bound indicated by the SAF. Even the more high-impact scenarios cannot achieve that level of spending reduction because the damage smoking has inflicted on the nation's health will continue to affect health care spending for decades. It follows, however, that the 100 percent cessation scenario is a more realistic and informative upper bound for the effect of tobacco control policies on health expenditures than the SAF because it takes account of the stock of smoking-related damage already present in the population's health as well as the downward secular trend in smoking rates under the status quo. Our projections suggest that the IOM recommendations would garner nearly 30 percent of the savings possible under the 100 percent cessation scenario. This is a much greater effect than is suggested by comparing savings from the IOM recommendations to the SAF.

Two principal avenues of change will operate to alter health expenditures following policy changes such as the IOM recommendations or the high-impact scenario. First, each scenario will reduce smoking initiation. However, few disease cases among the young are attributable to smoking because many smoking-related conditions do not arise until later in life, beyond the time horizon of our simulation. Second, the scenarios in question will increase smoking cessation. This is particularly relevant for older individuals both because older cohorts had higher ever-smoking prevalence and because they are of an age when smoking-related diseases become clinically apparent. Nevertheless, it may take five years (for cardiovascular and cerebrovascular diseases) to 20 years (for some cancers) for the risk of disease to revert to that of never smokers (U.S. Department of Health and Human Services 1990). So over 20 years, reductions in smoking initiation may have a large effect on a small number of young people, and increases in smoking cessation may have a small effect on large numbers of older people. Our projections suggest that the former would drive the changes in health expenditures through 2025. We see relatively small reductions in health expenditures among the Medicare population compared to the status quo. However, if the model were to extend far enough into the future, we would expect to see greater reductions in Medicare spending as those potential smokers who never started smoking reach old age. In other words, the argument that tobacco policy change can importantly reduce Medicare expenditures must take a very long-term perspective.

A few caveats and limitations are worth noting. The first concerns the limitations of existing data for estimating causal relationships between tobacco policy and health expenditures. Most changes in health expenditures caused by a change in tobacco policy follow a specific causal pathway: tobacco policy affects cigarette use, which in turn affects the prevalence and/or progress of smoking-related illnesses, which in turn affects health care usage, which in turn affects health expenditures. Each link in this chain may operate differently depending on its policy, environmental, and demographic context. The most precise assessment of how a tobacco policy affects health expenditures would explicitly and accurately take each step of this causal pathway into account, paying close attention to the timing of events. Our analysis, like others before it, has insufficient data to model such pathways in great detail. Instead, we extrapolated estimates of the effect of smoking on health expenditures and combined those results with an estimate of a policy change's effect on smoking in order to generate a first approximation of a tobacco policy's effect on health expenditures.

Second, although we know that tobacco control policies can have different effects on different groups of smokers, the analysis does not always reflect this heterogeneity. SimSmoke does incorporate the fact that cigarette price sensitivity diminishes with age, and because SimSmoke and our expenditure models incorporate stratification by age and sex, this heterogeneity is incorporated in our projections. However, an important limitation in our models is our inability to account for other factors affecting the impact of tobacco control policies. If, for example, the effectiveness of the tobacco control policies modeled in SimSmoke is higher for lighter smokers than for heavier smokers, and lighter smokers are healthier with fewer health expenditures, we have overstated the savings attributable to those policies. The problem of heterogeneous policy effects is eliminated when modeling the 100 percent cessation scenario because we assume all smoking is eliminated for all people.

Finally, although to some extent we can assess the impact of statistical uncertainty on our estimates, there are far greater unknowns that we are unable to incorporate into our models. The two largest are improvements in medical technology and changes in health care financing. Over the last 20 years, improvements in the treatment of heart disease and cancer have increased both life expectancy and medical expenditures. It is certain that medical innovation will increase expenditures in the future, but the extent to which technological improvements will also streamline care is not clear. Changes in health care financing will shift the burden of tobacco use from payer to payer and may change the efficiency with which health care funds are spent. For example, the Medicare Part D prescription drug benefit has likely increased Medicare's share of the cost of treating smoking-related diseases. By the same token, using pharmaceuticals to improve secondary and tertiary prevention for smoking-related diseases may reduce the number of smoking-related hospitalizations and improve the efficiency of medical care for smoking-related illnesses. Enactment of the Patient Protection and Affordable Care Act of 2010 will certainly have implications for smoking-associated medical care expenditures, but it is too soon to anticipate the scale and direction of its impact.

CONCLUSION

Given our estimates, it is unlikely that changes in tobacco policy will have a dramatic impact on overall health spending in the short or medium term, although we do anticipate some reduction in health expenditures. Enacting the IOM recommendations would go a substantial way toward achieving the upper bound savings in health expenditures indicated in the 100 percent cessation scenario.

However, from society's perspective the economic efficiency of tobacco control measures cannot be gauged by their effect on health expenditures alone. Rather, decisions should be considered in the context of the other issues addressed in this volume. The two factors that, in addition to health expenditures, will be the largest determinants of economically efficient tobacco control policy are improvements in population health and, to a lesser degree, changes in the obligations of the Social Security trust fund. As discussed in the next chapter, Hurd and colleagues estimate that reductions in smoking will increase the obligations of Social Security. On the other hand, Apelberg and Samet estimate substantial improvements to population health. In assessing whether or not the Master Settlement Agreement was a move toward economic efficiency for Massachusetts, Cutler et al. (2002) point out that although savings in health expenditures were relatively small, the greatest benefit came in the form of improved health, and Gruber and Köszegi (2001, 2004) have estimated large gains to smokers from increased cigarette taxes. When they consider tobacco control measures, policy makers should take reductions in health expenditures as one beneficial piece of a complex puzzle.

APPENDIX 11.1: PROJECTING HEALTH EXPENDITURES FOR THE NONINSTITUTIONALIZED ADULT (MEPS) POPULATION

OVERVIEW

SimSmoke projects future smoking prevalence disaggregated by age, sex, and smoking status. There are seven smoking status categories: current smokers, never smokers, and former smokers that have quit for 0–2, 3–5, 6–10, 11–15, and ≥ 16 years. To project future expenditures, we need to estimate average expenditures by age, sex, and smoking status.

Because cross-sectional analyses cannot directly account for the fact that many smokers quit when they are sick, one cannot just use the coefficient on former smokers in a regression of expenditures on smoking status and covariates to estimate expenditures for former smokers relative to current or never smokers. Therefore, we describe a model that assumes expenditures for former smokers decline relative to current smokers in proportion to the decline in all-cause mortality for former smokers relative to current smokers as a function of number of years since smoking cessation. Our analysis proceeded in three major steps. In the first, we estimated the SAF of expenditures by age, sex, and payer. Second, we disaggregated smoking-attributable expenditures to estimate health expenditures by age, sex, payer, and smoking status. Third, we combined these expenditure estimates with smoking estimates from SimSmoke and population estimates from the U.S. Census Bureau to project health expenditures into the future under each policy scenario.

ESTIMATING THE SAF

To estimate the SAF, we began with a data set linking the 1998–2001 NHIS with the 2000–2002 MEPS. All analyses with this linked data set were conducted accounting for the surveys' complex designs using the sampling data and weights from the MEPS 1996–2002 Pooled Estimation File (H36U02).

Next, we constructed regression models describing the relationship between cigarette smoking and health expenditures. As discussed briefly in the main body of the chapter, we estimated expenditures as a function of smoking history; demographics such as age, sex, race and ethnicity; socioeconomic status as measured by education and income; alcohol consumption; body mass index and its square; pregnancy status; risk-taking behavior as measured by seatbelt use and receipt of flu shots; geography (census region and Metropolitan Statistical Area designation); and insurance status. Age was coded in four groups and interacted with sex to account for different baseline expenditures along those dimensions. We assumed that the effects of the other covariates (except pregnancy) were consistent across age and sex. Smoking history was defined as current heavy smoking (> 15 cigarettes per day), current light smoking (≤ 15 cigarettes per day), former smoker for 15 or fewer years, former smoker for more than 15 years, or never smoker and separately as 0, 1–10, 11–20, 21–30, or ≥ 31 years as a smoker.

It is well known in the health economics literature that analysts using regression modeling to predict health expenditures face methodological challenges because traditional regression modeling assumptions are violated by health expenditure data. Specific characteristics of the data that complicate analyses are that many individuals will have no health expenditures at all and that the distribution of expenditures for those who do is highly positively skewed. Methods such as two-part regression models, smearing estimators, and/or generalized linear models (GLMs) have been developed to account for this data structure (Manning 1998; Manning and Mullahy 2001; Mullahy 1998). Not all of these techniques work equally well with all data sets. We followed the methods of Buntin and Zaslavsky (2004) to assess which of the four modeling options described in table 11.6 best fit the data. Ultimately, the best fit was achieved using GLM models with a log link and the Poisson distribution.

To calculate the SAF, we estimated our regression model and predicted health expenditures (E) for individuals indexed i given covariates (X) using first the observed smoking data (K) and then assuming all subjects were never smokers (K_0). The SAF is then:

TABLE 11.6 Regression Models Under Consideration for Estimating the SAF of Expenditures

1. One-part least-squares regression model of expenditures (untransformed) as a function of smoking and other covariates.

2. Two-part model in which the first part is a logistic regression of the probability of having positive medical expenditures as a function of smoking and covariates and the second part is a least-squares model of log expenditures given that expenditures are greater than zero as a function of smoking and covariates. Predicted expenditures for each individual in the data are then given by the product of the expected values from each part of the model. The predictions incorporate two separate smearing factors (Duan et al. 1983), one estimated for the top decile of predicted log expenditures and another for the bottom nine deciles of predicted log expenditures.

3. One-part generalized linear model of expenditures as a function of smoking and other covariates using a log link and the Poisson distribution.

4. One-part generalized linear model of expenditures as a function of smoking and other covariates using a log link and the gamma distribution.

$$SAF = \frac{\sum_i E(E_i \mid K_i, X_i) - E(E_i \mid K_0, X_i)}{\sum_i E(E_i \mid K_i, X_i)}$$

Separate SAFs were calculated for each age/sex group, though these estimates were based on a single regression model. To estimate confidence bounds on the SAF we used the bootstrap method, taking into account the complex sampling design of the data set when resampling. Payer-specific SAF estimates were made by using payer-specific expenditures as the dependent variable in the regression models and confining the regression sample to those survey respondents that had positive expenditures paid by that payer.

AGE/SEX/SMOKING STATUS-SPECIFIC HEALTH EXPENDITURES

Having estimated SAFs by age, sex, and payer, we now want to disaggregate age/sex-specific expenditures by smoking status. We begin by estimating mean annual expenditures (E) for respondents indexed i by age (a) and sex (s) using the survey weights (w). Then, we estimate mean smoking-attributable expenditures (SAE) and mean expenditures not attributable to smoking (NSAE). Next, we disaggregate smoking-attributable expenditures according to smoking status to get individual-level excess expenditures due to smoking. To do this, we assume that the ratio of excess expenditures for former smokers relative to current smokers tracks the mortality risk of former versus current smokers, q. Data for estimating q were provided by Samet and Apelberg based on all-cause mortality for males in the American Cancer Society's Cancer Prevention Study II. In the equation below, a is an indicator for the age range (denoted in the superscript) during which the individual quit smoking, and e_i is the number of years elapsed since smoking cessation. By definition, $q=1$ for current smokers and $q=0$ for never smokers. In addition, we estimate person-specific expenditures not attributable to smoking. The person-specific sums (E_i^*) of smoking-attributable expenditures and expenditures not attributable to smoking can thus be used to estimate mean per-capita expenditures by age, sex, and smoking status (E_{ask}). Estimates of E_{ask} are made separately for each payer.

$$E_{as} = \frac{\sum_i E_i w_i}{\sum w_i} \mid Age = a, Sex = s$$

$$SAE_{as} = E_{as}SAF_{as}$$

$$NSAE_{as} = E_{as}(1 - SAF_{as})$$

$$q_i = 0.6842 - 0.0226e_i + 0.0004e_i^2 + 0.0940a^{40-49} + 0.1488a^{50-59}$$
$$+0.2092a^{\geq60} + .0001a^{40-49}e_i + 0.0030a^{50-59}e_i + 0.0065a^{\geq60}e_i$$
$$+0.00001a^{40-49}e_i^2 + 0.00005a^{50-59}e_i^2 + 0.00007a^{\geq60}e_i^2$$

$$SAE_i = \frac{q_i w_i}{\sum q_i w_i} SAE_{as} \mid Age = a, Sex = s$$

$$NSAE_i = \frac{NSAE_{as}}{\sum w_i} \mid Age = a, Sex = s$$

$$E_i^* = SAE_i + NSAE_i$$

$$E_{ask} = \frac{\sum_i E_i^* w_i}{\sum w_i} \mid Age = a, Sex = s, SmokingStatus = k$$

PROJECTING HEALTH EXPENDITURES THROUGH 2025

With estimates of age/sex/smoking status-specific expenditures, projections are straightforward. The present (2002) discounted value of total expenditures in any given year y and policy scenario p are as follows:

$$E_{yp} = \frac{\sum\limits_{a}\sum\limits_{s}\sum\limits_{k} \Pr(K = k \mid y, p) n_{asy} E_{ask}}{1.03^{(y-2002)}}$$

ADDITIONAL NOTABLE ASSUMPTIONS

We assume that the distribution of regression covariates (except smoking) remains constant within age and sex over the course of the simulation. Furthermore, the projections assume the distribution of payers within an age-sex-smoking-status cell remains constant over time.

APPENDIX 11.2: NEONATAL SPENDING

Estimates of smoking-attributable spending on neonatal care are based on SimSmoke smoking prevalence projections, data on prenatal smoking from the National Vital Statistics Service Natality Detail Files, data on the projected number of births from the U.S. Census Bureau, and estimates of the excess health care costs due to smoking by pregnant women from the CDC's MCH-SAMMEC model.

PROJECTED PRENATAL SMOKING

We assume that smoking by pregnant women in a given age group changes proportionally to changes in smoking by women of childbearing age overall. For example, under the high-impact scenario, SimSmoke predicts that smoking prevalence among women ages 35–44 will decrease from 23.7 percent to 22.8 percent from 2002 to 2003, a relative reduction of 3.8 percent. Thus, given that prenatal smoking prevalence among 35- to 44-year-olds was 8.0 percent in 2002, it is projected to be 7.7 percent in 2003. For payer-specific estimates of smoking prevalence, we assumed the relative differences in age-specific prenatal smoking rates by payer in 1997 (according to MCH-SAMMEC) were constant going forward. We present the relative differences in table 11.7. For example, we estimate overall prenatal smoking prevalence for women 20–34 years old in 2007 under the IOM recommendations is 9.1 percent. Therefore, we estimate the prenatal smoking prevalence among women covered by Medicaid is 9.1 percent × 1.57 = 14.3 percent.

TABLE 11.7 Relative Differences in Prenatal Smoking Rates by Payer

SMOKING PREVALENCE	ALL PAYERS	PRIVATE/ OTHER PAYER	MEDICAID
All ages	1.00	0.66	1.52
15–19	1.00	0.82	1.06
20–34	1.00	0.66	1.57
35–44	1.00	0.71	2.12

Source: Authors' calculations.

PROJECTED NUMBER OF BIRTHS

We begin with the U.S. Census Bureau population projections for women of childbearing age (i.e., 15–44 years old) (U.S. Census Bureau 2006). This is used to project the distribution of women 15–19, 20–34, and 35–44 years old within the group that is 15–44 years old. Then, assuming the birth rate within each age group is constant over time, we apply the distribution of these age groupings to the projected number of births (U.S. Census Bureau 2000) in each year of the simulation to get age-specific estimates of the numbers of births.

EXCESS SPENDING PER BIRTH TO SMOKERS

To project smoking-related expenditures for neonatal care, we began by estimating the excess cost associated with a birth to a smoker. For each age group and payer we used MCH-SAMMEC to estimate the total excess spending due to prenatal smoking, smoking prevalence, and total number of births (see table 11.8). Excess spending per birth to a smoker is then given by:

$$ExcessSpendingPerBirth_{ap} = \frac{TotalExcessSpending_{ap}}{SmokingPrevalence_{ap} * Births_{ap}}$$

Excess health expenditures due to prenatal smoking for a given year and policy scenario are as follows:

$$ExcessExpenditures_{yk}$$
$$= \sum_{a} \Pr(smoke_{yka}) \Pr(a_y) TotalBirths_y \, ExcessSpendingPerBirthtoSmoker_a$$

TABLE 11.8 Excess Spending per Birth to Smokers

	TOTAL EXCESS SPENDING	SMOKING PREVALENCE	BIRTHS	EXCESS SPENDING PER BIRTH
		All Payers		
All Ages	$419,808,605	13%	3,880,862	$810
15–19	$62,467,803	18%	485,102	$733
20–34	$304,964,081	13%	2,913,150	$803
35–44	$52,376,721	11%	482,610	$986
		Private Payer		
All Ages	$138,567,418	9%	2,193,720	$719
15–19	$9,151,522	14%	102,205	$621
20–34	$104,108,384	9%	1,725,046	$698
35 44	$25,307,512	8%	366,469	$883
		Medicaid		
All Ages	$261,034,879	20%	1,482,082	$871
15–19	$50,779,324	19%	358,142	$760
20–34	$186,734,003	21%	1,034,541	$880
35–44	$23,521,552	23%	89,399	$1,125

Note: Numbers do not match perfectly, as values for smoking prevalence in this table are rounded.
Source: Authors' calculations.

APPENDIX 11.3: NURSING HOME CALCULATIONS

We project nursing home expenditures using the 1999 National Nursing Home Survey and a disease-specific approach. For each respondent in the survey, we calculate the SAF of the diagnosis responsible for the nursing home stay. We assume that the distribution of diagnoses is constant over time, but the SAF of each diagnosis changes as smoking prevalence changes in the response to the policies enacted in each of our scenarios. Then, assuming the SAF of disease is equal to the SAF of nursing home days and that expenditures are proportional to length of stay, we are able to project expenditures through 2025 by applying the SAF to per-capita nursing home expenditures and age/sex-specific population projections.

The distribution of smoking status (current, former, never) is determined using SimSmoke by age and sex for each year under each scenario. Then, for each respondent in the 1999 NNHS, we calculate the SAF of the nursing home stay based on the person's diagnosis, the distribution of smoking status for a person of the respondent's age (a) and sex (s) (where $k \cdot c$, $k \cdot f$, and $k \cdot n$ indicate current, former, and never smoking status) and the relative risk of the person's diagnosis given smoking status, age, and sex. First, we gathered the relative risk of dying for 19 smoking-related disease categories from the Surgeon General's 2004 report (U.S. Department of Health and Human Services 2004a). These conditions included cancers of the mouth, esophagus, stomach, pancreas, larynx, lungs, cervix, bladder, and kidney; acute myeloid leukemia; ischemic and other heart diseases; cerebrovascular disease; atherosclerosis, aortic aneurysm, and other arterial disease; pneumonia, influenza, bronchitis, emphysema, and chronic airway obstruction. The three-digit International Classification of Diseases, ninth revision (ICD9) codes deemed smoking-related and their relative risks were taken from the Surgeon General's 2004 report. Diagnoses not listed in the report were assigned relative risks of 1. Smoking-attributable nursing home days were estimated as the product of the population smoking-attributable fraction of the diagnosis and the length of the nursing home stay in days.

$$ \mathrm{SAF}_i = \frac{(p_{k \cdot n_{as}} + p_{k \cdot c_{as}} RR_{k \cdot c_{as}} + p_{k \cdot f_{as}} RR_{k \cdot f_{as}} - 1)}{(p_{k \cdot n_{as}} + p_{k \cdot c_{as}} RR_{k \cdot c_{as}} + p_{k \cdot f_{as}} RR_{k \cdot f_{as}})} $$

In the base case NNHS analysis, the diagnosis of interest for each respondent in the NNHS is the primary admitting diagnosis. We use this diagnosis to estimate the smoking-attributable fraction of each respondent's nursing home stay according to the relative risk of the diagnosis for current and former smokers compared to never smokers.

We also examine the SAF of each stay by assigning the respondent's diagnosis using one of three alternative algorithms in order to test the sensitivity of our nursing home results to how diagnoses are assigned. The algorithms are as follows: (1) assign the first diagnosis for a smoking-related disease from the list of six admitting diagnoses; (2) assign the first diagnosis for a smoking-related disease from the list of six current diagnoses; (3) assign the first diagnosis for a smoking-related disease, first from the list of six admitting diagnoses, then from the list of six current diagnoses.

Upon assigning a SAF for each respondent, we calculate the average SAF of nursing home days by age and sex, weighted by the NNHS survey weights. The age/sex-specific SAFs are calculated for each policy scenario (p) and each year (y) of the simulation. We are able to project nursing home spending for each year in each policy scenario according to the equation below by combining the

SAF, the U.S. Census Bureau's population projections (n), and data on age-specific per-capita nursing home spending (C) from CMS's 1999 National Health Accounts. Per-capita nursing home spending figures were inflated to 2002 dollars using the all-items Consumer Price Index. All projected expenditures were discounted to their 2002 present values using a 3 percent discount rate.

$$NursingHomeSpending_{yp} = \frac{\sum_{as} (SAF_{asyp} n_{asy} C_a)}{1.03^{y-2002}}$$

Payer-specific estimates are different in two ways. First, the sample used to estimate the aggregate SAFs is restricted to respondents whose primary source of payment for their nursing home stays was a given payer. Thus, the age/sex-specific SAF of nursing home days (and thus expenditures) for Medicaid reflects the distribution of admitting diagnoses for 1999 NNHS respondents whose primary source of payment was Medicaid. Second, CMS reports the percentage of per-capita nursing home spending that was covered by private third-party payers, Medicare, Medicaid, out-of-pocket payments, and other public/private payers. For example, CMS reports that average per-capita nursing home expenditures for individuals aged 55–64 years old were \$191 in 1999, and 59.2 percent of that was covered by Medicaid. Thus, per-capita nursing home expenditures covered by Medicaid are estimated to be \$113. Two major assumptions of these payer-specific projections are that (1) we take no account of potential differences in smoking prevalence by payer, and (2) we assume the distribution of primary payers by age and sex is constant into the future.

12

THE EFFECTS OF TOBACCO CONTROL POLICY ON THE SOCIAL SECURITY TRUST FUND

MICHAEL HURD, YUHUI ZHENG, FEDERICO GIROSI, AND DANA GOLDMAN

Smoking cessation will reduce mortality, and this reduction in mortality will affect Social Security in two main ways. First, more people will survive to retirement age, and these additional survivors will pay taxes, thus benefitting the Social Security trust fund. Second, because more people will reach retirement, and life expectancy following retirement will be higher, the outflow from the Social Security trust fund will also increase. Tobacco control policy may also affect Social Security in other ways. Because workers will be in better health and thus more productive, their earnings will be greater and they will retire somewhat later, thus increasing the inflow of taxes. In addition, because fewer workers will die, there will be a reduction in survivor benefits to underage children and their caretakers. The overall effect of a reduction in smoking on the Social Security trust fund is an empirical question that requires evaluation of these offsetting effects.

Given the concern about the future of Social Security, it is critical to understand how a significant decline in smoking might affect the Social Security trust fund. Previous analyses have found that smokers receive less in Social Security benefits than nonsmokers because of their shorter life expectancies. For instance, Shoven, Sundberg, and Bunker (1990) found that a typical single male worker received $20,000 less than his nonsmoking counterpart in Social Security benefits net of taxes; the individual smoker's loss was substantial, about 25 percent of lifetime benefits. For couples, the loss depended on whether both spouses qualified for Social Security based on their earnings records and whether one or both smoked. Generally the loss by couples was smaller than the loss by singles: for example, if only one spouse had worked and only the husband smoked, the loss would be about 15 percent of the couple's lifetime benefits net of taxes. This early study has some limitations. It was based on life tables from the early 1960s, when a much greater fraction of the population smoked than is the case today. The relationship between smoking and mortality may have changed since that time. In addition, the study assumed all of the mortality difference between smokers and nonsmokers was due to smoking, when other differences between smokers and nonsmokers might be responsible for part of the mortality differential. In a more recent analysis, Sloan et al. (2004) used the Health and Retirement Study—a newer data set with better measures of health, smoking, and economic status—to estimate the effect of smoking on Social Security benefits net of taxes. Their study, which addressed many of the limitations of Shoven, Sundberg, and Bunker (1990), found similar results. Other research on the effect of smoking on Social Security and other pension or retirement plans has also found that smokers cost less and derive less benefit from these plans (Armour and Pitts 2006; Viscusi 1995).

By reducing smoking rates and thus increasing the net benefits received, these studies suggest, tobacco control policies could be very costly for the Social Security program. However, studies like those by Shoven, Sundberg, and Bunker (1990) and Sloan et al. (2004) identify the effects of smoking for the individual worker, not for the Social Security trust fund as a whole. The aggregate impact is likely to be smaller than these studies might imply because Social Security taxes paid and benefits received would change primarily for the minority of Americans who smoke. In addition, as the two previous chapters indicate, even under extreme assumptions about how quickly smoking rates might fall, the consequences for health and mortality—and thus for Social Security outlays—appear only gradually because the elevated disease risk associated with smoking persists for years after cessation and because a decline in initiation among the young would not affect health among older adults for several decades.

In contrast to previous studies, which focus on individuals, this chapter estimates the effects of tobacco control policy for the Social Security trust fund as a whole. We consider the same four policy scenarios discussed earlier in this volume. To understand the effects of these scenarios, we use a dynamic model of health and labor market economic activity, the Future Elderly Model (FEM) (Goldman et al. 2004, 2005). The FEM is a microsimulation model of health status transitions that is estimated on seven waves of panel data of the Health and Retirement Study (HRS). Using this model, we simulate the health and economic transitions made over time by a population of older adults, using the HRS to understand how the likelihood of these transitions varies by smoking status as well as other individual characteristics. For any given year, we can use these simulated values to calculate the total Social Security taxes paid, total Social Security benefits received, and participation in the Social Security Disability Insurance (SSDI) program.

Consistent with other research in this volume, we develop near-term projections for Social Security outlays over 20 years. Because the Health and Retirement Study data are collected in even-numbered years, our near-term projections run from 2004 to 2024, rather than from 2005 to 2025 as in previous chapters. In addition, given policy concern about the long-term financial viability of Social Security, we extend our projections to the year 2050. Because our model is based on the Health and Retirement Study, which includes individuals aged 51 and older, our estimates of Social Security taxes paid and benefits received are for the population aged 51 and older. Because the health effects of smoking—and thus the impacts on Social Security—are concentrated among older adults, exclusion of individuals aged 50 and younger is expected to have little impact on the conclusions we draw from these results.

THE FUTURE ELDERLY MODEL

The FEM begins with a representative sample of over 80,000 individuals aged 51 or over. The initial FEM sample comes from the 1998, 2000, 2002, and 2004 waves of the HRS. (See appendix 12.1 for a brief introduction to the HRS data and relevant measures.) Characteristics of each individual are given by the HRS data and include age, gender, race (black, white, and other), ethnicity (Hispanic origin), educational level (less than high school, high school graduate, some college but no degree, college degree and above), marital status (married, divorced, or single), smoking (smoking now, ever smoked), BMI status, chronic disease conditions, functional status, and economic situations (receipt of earnings and/or benefits from Old-Age and Survivors Insurance [OASI]). We have augmented the FEM model to include additional transitions and states including smoking status, labor force status, earnings, Social Security taxes, Social Security benefits, and participation in the SSDI. We pooled multiple years of data to increase the sample size and to obtain a smoother joint distribution of the characteristics. Each individual is replicated three times to further increase the sample size for Monte Carlo simulation. Each sample member has a sampling weight specified by HRS. The magnitude of the sampling weight is adjusted so that the sum is equal to the Census population in year 2004. The relative magnitude of the sampling weight is also adjusted to reflect the Census population distribution in year 2004 by gender, race/ethnicity, and age group. The population health status, behavioral risk factors, and economic situations, however, reflect a weighted average level over the period from 1998 to 2004.

A population-representative cohort enters the model at age 51 or 52 and makes transitions as it ages into the various health and economic states, via Monte Carlo simulation. Probabilities of transitioning into various health and economic states were estimated over actual transitions in the HRS data. Whether an individual enters a certain health or economic state is determined by comparing the predicted transitioning probability with a random draw from a uniform distribution; if the predicted probability exceeds the corresponding random draw, we project that the transition takes place. In each health and economic state, individuals receive earnings, pay Social Security taxes, and receive Social Security benefits at levels based on earnings, taxes, and benefit levels observed in the data, possibly modified by covariates. In any year we can calculate total Social Security taxes paid and benefits received by the population 51 or older. As the simulations continue, members of the cohort die, with probabilities determined from mortality estimations in the HRS until the last member of the cohort has died.

To keep the simulated population representative of those aged 51 years or older, every two years we add a simulated cohort of 51- and 52-year-olds. We call this cohort the "incoming cohort." Although the incoming cohort is assigned ages 51 or 52, we actually draw them from the sample of 51- to 54-year-olds of the pooled HRS data from 1998 to 2004. We include multiple years of data as well as those 53–54 years old to increase the sample size and to obtain a smoother joint distribution of characteristics; we adjusted the demographics of the 51- to 54-year-old sample to reflect the demographics of the 51- to 52-year-olds. The population size of the incoming cohort is predicted using Census population projections up to year 2050. As we discuss below, the smoking status and history of these incoming cohorts are manipulated based on smoking projections for the tobacco control policy scenarios.

Initially the model was populated at each age by individuals from the HRS; in 2004, therefore, it represents the actual population aged 51 and over. Every two years, a new (simulated) cohort of 51- and 52-year-olds enters the model. Over time, the characteristics of the population are increasingly determined by the characteristics of these incoming cohorts and by the transition rates from one health and economic status to another. By 2050, the entire original HRS population has almost been entirely replaced by the survivors of the incoming cohorts.

MODELING TRANSITION PROBABILITIES

We model the transition probabilities based on the longitudinal experience of HRS respondents, assuming a first-order Markovian process (second-order Markov models are used to model transitions in functional status). Because the HRS data are collected every other year, we estimated two-year transition probabilities. We estimated the probabilities of the following transitions: developing one or more of six chronic conditions (including the major illnesses associated with smoking), quitting or initiating smoking, between four functional states, between the joint status of any earnings and receiving any OASI, and of dying. Covariates that may influence these transition probabilities include smoking status and smoking history, BMI status, and socioeconomic status. We treated all six chronic health conditions as "absorbing": a person who gets an illness is assumed to have it forever and therefore cannot get it again. (See appendix 12.1 for more details and for model estimates.)

MODELING ECONOMIC OUTCOMES

Economic outcomes included annual Social Security taxes paid, OASI benefits received, and SSDI benefits received. Social Security taxes paid are calculated using self-reported earnings that are subject to Social Security payroll taxes. Because a large proportion of the population has zero values for each item, we used a two-step procedure for estimation.

We used a multinomial logit regression to model a first-order Markov transition for the joint status of receiving (positive) earnings and receiving (positive) OASI benefits. Next we used least-squares regression to estimate the amount of OASI benefits received, if any. Among those with earnings, we took another two-step estimation to estimate the probability of earning more than the maximum taxable amount for Social Security payroll taxes and, for those who earn less than the maximum taxable limit, the amount of earnings.

Smoking status (smoking now and ever-smoked) and health conditions were covariates in all but one model for economic outcomes. The one exception is the model for the amount of OASI benefits received, if any, because smoking only enters the benefit calculation via earnings and labor force participation, which themselves depend on smoking. (See appendix 12.1 for more details and for model estimates.)

IMPLEMENTATION OF TOBACCO CONTROL POLICY SCENARIOS

In our model, current smoking status and smoking history (ever smoked) affect almost all health transitions and many economic states. We estimated the effects of changes in current smoking status and smoking history with two simulations. In the first, we simulated a population to 2024 and to 2050 using our baseline estimates of the smoking status and smoking history of the incoming cohorts. In the second, we altered the smoking status and smoking history of the incoming cohorts consistent with smoking prevalence rates associated with the tobacco policy scenarios. We attributed the differences in outcomes such as health status and economic status to changes in smoking behavior.

We analyzed the impact of the four scenarios discussed earlier in this volume. Under the status quo scenario, tobacco control policies are frozen in place as of the beginning of 2006, with excise tax rates assumed to be adjusted for inflation. The Institute of Medicine (IOM) scenario assumes a $2 increase in tobacco excise taxes as well as other policy changes recommended by the IOM. The high-impact scenario assumes that the IOM policy changes are adopted and that these changes combined with other (unspecified) medical and policy changes result in no new initiation under the age of 18, a doubling of the quit rate for adults under 40, and a 50 percent drop in prevalence by 2010. Finally, the "100 percent cessation" scenario assumes that all smoking ceases beginning in 2006 with no new initiation at any age. (Hereafter we will refer to the latter three scenarios as "intervention scenarios.")

The predicted smoking prevalence and prevalence of ever smokers (both ex-smokers and current smokers) by age group under the four scenarios from 2005 to 2025 are shown in figures 12.1 and 12.2. In the short term, scenarios 2 through 4 lead to a rapid decrease in smoking prevalence between 2006 and 2010. After 2010, the trends in prevalence are similar across the first three scenarios. In the long run, scenarios 2 through 4 affect prevalence of ex-smokers and current smokers in the older population by lowering the initiation rates of smoking among the younger population (ages 15–24). (All four scenarios assume no smoking initiation after age 24.)

We implemented these scenarios in four runs of FEM simulations by adjusting the prevalence of former smokers and current smokers in the incoming cohorts of 51- to 52-year-olds based on the SimSmoke projections reported in chapter 2. Because SimSmoke predictions after year 2025 are unavailable, we extrapolated the smoking history and current smoking status from 2026 to 2050. For current smoking status, because the predicted prevalence in year 2025 for the incoming cohort is low, especially for the three intervention scenarios, we assumed that current smoking prevalence in the incoming cohorts would stay at the same level between 2026 and 2050. We did a robustness check by assuming that smoking prevalence continued to decrease at the same rate it did between 2004 and 2025; this adjustment made little difference to the results.

Figure 12.3 shows the projected prevalence of current smoking in the population aged 51 and over. Differences in the prevalence of current smokers begin to appear after the interventions begin in 2006, although the drop in prevalence for scenarios 2 and 3 is less marked for older than for younger populations. In 2024, the prevalence of current smokers in the incoming cohort (those aged 51–52 years old) is 16.55 percent under the status quo scenario, 11.69 percent under the IOM scenario, 6.09 percent under the high-impact scenario, and 0.00 percent under the 100 percent cessation scenario. In the total population aged 51 and over in the same year, the variation across scenarios in smoking

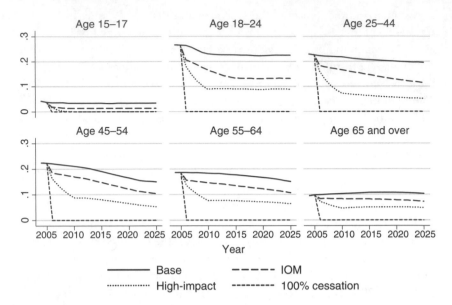

FIGURE 12.1 Trends in Current Smoking Prevalence Under Tobacco Control Policy Scenarios

---

Notes: In figures 12.1 and 12.2, the x axis indicates year of prediction. The y axis presents the proportion of current smokers within the specified age group, under various tobacco control policy scenarios.

"Base" refers to the status quo scenario, in which tobacco control policies are frozen in place as of the beginning of 2006, with excise tax rates adjusted for inflation.

"IOM" refers to an intervention scenario assuming a $2 increase in tobacco excise taxes as well as other policy changes recommended by the Institute of Medicine (IOM).

"High-impact" refers to a second intervention scenario. It assumes that the policies recommended by IOM are adopted, and that these changes combined with other (unspecified) medical and policy changes results in no new initiation under the age of 18, a doubling of the quit rate for adults under 40, and a 50 percent drop in prevalence by 2010.

"100% cessation" refers to a third intervention scenario, which assumes that all smoking ceases beginning in 2006 with no new initiation at any age.

Data source: Chapter 2.

prevalence is smaller: 11.32 percent under the status quo scenario, 10.09 percent under the IOM scenario, 8.53 percent under the high-impact scenario, and 0.0 percent under the 100 percent cessation scenario.

We also projected the prevalence of "ever smokers," a category that includes both current and former smokers. Because the scenarios assume no initiation after age 24, the predicted prevalence of ever smokers among 45- to 54-year-olds in 2035 should equal the prevalence for 35- to 45-year-olds in 2025, and the predicted prevalence among 45- to 54-year-olds in 2045 should equal that for

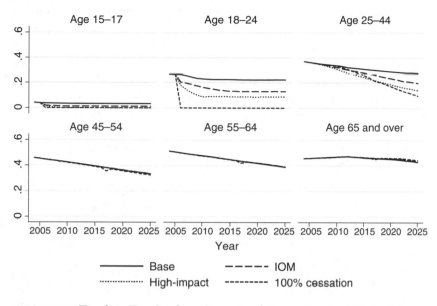

FIGURE 12.2 Trends in Ever Smokers (Current and Former Smokers) Under Tobacco Control Policy Scenarios

Data source: chapter 2.

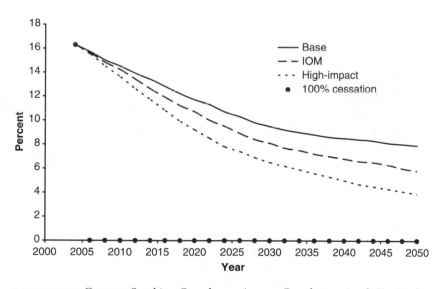

FIGURE 12.3 Current Smoking Prevalence Among Population Aged 51+ Under Tobacco Control Policy Scenarios

Data source: Predictions from the Future Elderly Model.

25- to 34-year-olds in 2025, setting aside differences in mortality between smokers and nonsmokers. Using these figures, we estimated the annual reduction rates in ever smokers from year 2025 to 2045 and assumed the trends would stay the same between 2045 and 2050.

Although there were differences in cessation rates across the scenarios, all the scenarios assume no smoking initiation after age 24. However, until 2033, there are virtually no differences across the four scenarios in the prevalence of ever smokers (see figure 12.4). Individuals who are aged 18–24 when the scenarios begin will also exhibit differences in initiation, and this cohort begins to reach age 51 in 2033. At that point, because initiation rates vary across the policy scenarios, the trends in prevalence of ever smokers begin to diverge. After 2033, under the 100 percent cessation scenario, all individuals aged 51 and 52 are never smokers; the prevalence of ever smokers in the population aged 51 and older declines as the incoming cohorts make up a successively larger fraction of this older population (see table 12.1).

We assumed that the prevalence of ever smokers in the incoming cohort would decrease at the same rate across scenarios until 2032. Therefore, in 2024, the prevalence of ever smokers in the incoming cohort is the same across the four scenarios: 42.75 percent. However, because quitting smoking reduces

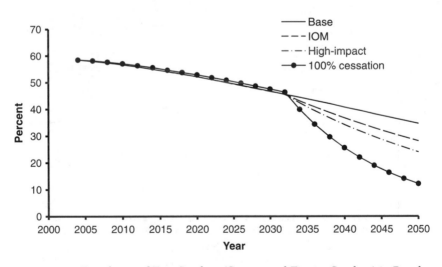

FIGURE 12.4 Prevalence of Ever Smokers (Current and Former Smokers) in Population Aged 51+ Under Tobacco Control Policy Scenarios

Data source: Predictions from the Future Elderly Model.

TABLE 12.1 Annual Rate of Reduction in the Prevalence of Current Smokers and Ever Smokers Among Those Aged 51–52 Years

	FEMALE				MALE			
	BASE	IOM	HIGH-IMPACT	100% CESSATION	BASE	IOM	HIGH-IMPACT	100% CESSATION
Current smokers								
2004–2025	-1.8%	-3.5%	-5.6%	-100.0%	-2.0%	-3.7%	-6.8%	-100.0%
2026–2032	0.0%	0.0%	0.0%	0.0%	0.0%	0.0%	0.0%	0.0%
2033–2050	0.0%	0.0%	0.0%	0.0%	0.0%	0.0%	0.0%	0.0%
Ever smokers								
2004–2025	-1.3%	-1.3%	-1.3%	-1.3%	-1.7%	-1.7%	-1.7%	-1.7%
2026–2032	-1.2%	-1.2%	-1.2%	-1.2%	-2.0%	-2.0%	-2.0%	-2.0%
2033–2050	-1.2%	-3.7%	-5.4%	-100.0%	-2.0%	-4.5%	-6.1%	-100.0%

Source: Data from chapter 2 and authors' calculations.

mortality, more individuals with smoking history survive under the intervention scenarios. For example, the prevalence of ever smokers under the 100 percent cessation scenario is 1.7 percent higher than that under the status quo.

CHARACTERISTICS OF SMOKERS AND NONSMOKERS

We manipulated the characteristics of the original incoming cohort to yield the smoking prevalence figures for future incoming cohorts by the four scenarios. We changed the smoking status of the original incoming cohort by randomly moving people in or out of three possible states: never smokers, ex-smokers, and current smokers. For each relevant outcome, we moved individuals in or out of a given category based on the differences between the original cohort (the status quo) and predicted prevalence. We aimed to retain the original joint distribution of characteristics by changing status only for those who were at the margin—those who had the highest probability to be in a given category but originally were not or those who were originally in a certain category but have the smallest predicted probability to be in that category—depending on whether the predicted prevalence is higher or lower than the original prevalence for a certain category. For example, because smoking is less common for individuals with higher education, when we moved individuals from currently smoking to never-smoking status, those with higher education were more likely to be reassigned as never smokers.

Smoking rates decline for the future incoming cohorts across all scenarios, and because smoking is associated with chronic disease conditions (cancer, lung disease, heart disease, and stroke), the incoming cohorts are expected to be healthier. Their lower smoking rates may also have implications for their functional status and labor force participation. Therefore, we adjusted the health status, functional status, and labor force participation of those whose smoking status was reassigned. To make this adjustment, we first estimated the marginal distributions of health status and labor force participation among never smokers, controlling for gender, race/ethnicity, and educational levels. Next, we applied these estimates to current or former smokers who were reassigned to be never smokers to obtain the distributions of health and labor force participation for them after eliminating smoking history. The method assumes that, conditional on gender, race/ethnicity, and education, there are no differences in these distributions between never smokers and the current or former smokers reassigned to be never smokers. In some cases, current smokers will be reassigned to be former smokers, but in these cases we do not alter their health status because any immediate effect on health is likely to be small.

This method is not without weakness: we assume the cross-sectional association between smoking and outcome variables reflects a causal relationship, and we do not consider the joint distribution of health, functional status, and economic outcomes. But because the adjustments are in the expected directions (people with demographic characteristics of smokers are healthier if they never smoke), and there are only minor differences among the unadjusted and adjusted distributions, the simulation results are not sensitive to the degree of adjustments we make.

IMPACTS OF TOBACCO CONTROL POLICIES ON THE SOCIAL SECURITY TRUST FUND

We focus our discussion on the outcomes in 2024 and 2050. Comparing outcomes in the year 2024 helps us to understand the dynamic effect of higher quit rates among older Americans; outcomes in the year 2050 reflect the longer-term effects of reducing initiation among those who are young adults in 2006.

The FEM allows both direct and indirect effects of smoking status on the Social Security trust fund (hereafter, the "trust fund"). Changing smoking status could directly affect the trust fund by influencing the probability of having earnings or of receiving any OASI or DI benefits or by influencing the amount of taxable earnings or amount of DI benefits received. As shown in appendix 12.1 (see tables 12.6 and 12.7), being a current smoker did not have a statistically significant association with the probability of working or receiving OASI or DI benefits, but it was negatively associated with the amount of taxable earnings and DI benefits, conditional on receipt of that type of income. Ever smoking had a statistically significant association with the probability of receiving any DI benefits: compared with never smokers, those who had ever smoked were 40 percent more likely to receive DI benefits.

In addition, smoking could have indirect effects on Social Security outlays by affecting the probability of poor health, functional limitations, or mortality. Differential mortality rates due to changing smoking status will affect the size of the population as well as the characteristics of those who survive. Appendix 12.1 (see table 12.4) shows the effects of smoking status on the probability of developing six chronic conditions. Ever having smoked was significantly associated with increased risks of the incidence of heart disease, lung disease, and cancer. Being a current smoker added additional risks to stroke, heart disease, and lung diseases but was not significantly associated with the risk of incident cancer; given the extensive epidemiological evidence connecting smoking with cancer risk, we expect this insignificant result may reflect the small sample size. (Just 11 percent of those 51 or older are current smokers.) Appendix 12.1 (see table 12.5) shows that being a former smoker was associated with increased risk of mortality but not with the onset of functional limitations. Current smoking, however, was significantly associated with higher risk of both mortality and functional limitations.

Summaries of key outcomes are shown in tables 12.2 (for 2024) and 12.3 (for 2050). Because a decline in smoking rates reduces mortality, the tobacco

TABLE 12.2 Population, Earnings, Social Security Benefits, and Taxes Under Four Scenarios of Smoking Status, 2024

	OUTCOMES UNDER DIFFERENT SCENARIOS				% CHANGE RELATIVE TO STATUS QUO		
	STATUS QUO	IOM	HIGH-IMPACT	100% CESSATION	IOM	HIGH-IMPACT	100% CESSATION
Population 51 and over (millions)	117.58	117.64	117.72	119.66	0.05%	0.13%	1.77%
Population 65 and over (millions)	59.66	59.68	59.70	61.44	0.03%	0.08%	3.00%
% Working among aged 51–65	58.03	58.06	58.10	58.18	0.06%	0.12%	0.26%
Average taxable earnings among aged 51–65 (if any)	39,510	39,610	39,710	40,021	0.25%	0.51%	1.29%
Total taxable earnings among aged 51–65 (billions)	1,418	1,423	1,429	1,448	0.39%	0.82%	2.15%
Total Social Security taxes paid (billions)	191.54	192.22	192.97	195.98	0.35%	0.75%	2.32%

Total outlay of OASI benefits (billions)	656	656	657	674	0.03%	0.08%	2.70%
% Receiving DI among aged 51–65	4.68	4.66	4.65	4.62	−0.35%	−0.60%	−1.29%
Average DI benefits received (if any)	10,606	10,628	10,654	10,747	0.20%	0.45%	1.33%
Total outlay of DI benefits (billions)	32.74	32.72	32.76	32.96	−0.07%	0.03%	0.65%
% Smoking among aged 51 and over	11.32	10.09	8.53	0.00	−10.87%	−24.62%	−100.00%
% Ever smoked among aged 51 and over	49.97	49.99	50.03	50.83	0.05%	0.13%	1.74%
% Smoking among aged 51–52	16.55	11.69	6.09	0.00	−29.33%	−63.19%	−100.00%
% Ever smoked among aged 51–52	42.75	42.75	42.75	42.75	0.00%	0.00%	0.00%
Net Social Security outlay (billions)	497.25	496.73	496.34	510.75	−0.10%	−0.18%	2.71%

Source: Authors' calculations (see appendix 12.1).

TABLE 12.3 Population, Earnings, Social Security Benefits, and Taxes Under Four Scenarios of Smoking Status, 2050

	OUTCOMES UNDER DIFFERENT SCENARIOS				% CHANGE RELATIVE TO STATUS QUO		
	STATUS QUO	IOM	HIGH-IMPACT	100% CESSATION	IOM	HIGH-IMPACT	100% CESSATION
Population 51 and over (millions)	144.41	144.87	145.29	147.23	0.32%	0.61%	1.96%
Population 65 and over (millions)	80.89	81.23	81.56	83.33	0.42%	0.82%	3.02%
% Working among aged 51–65	58.01	58.17	58.35	58.91	0.27%	0.59%	1.55%
Average taxable earnings among aged 51–65 (if any)	39,159	39,321	39,431	39,542	0.41%	0.70%	0.98%
Total taxable earnings among aged 51–65 (billions)	1,533	1,547	1,559	1,583	0.89%	1.66%	3.23%
Total Social Security taxes paid (billions)	208.58	210.52	212.19	215.61	0.93%	1.73%	3.37%
Total outlay of OASI benefits (billions)	857	860	862	879	0.34%	0.67%	2.60%

% Receiving DI among aged 51–65	4.56	4.33	4.22	3.85	−5.09%	−7.45%	−15.64%
Average DI benefits received (if any)	10,414	10,480	10,538	10,651	0.63%	1.19%	2.27%
Total outlay of DI benefits (billions)	34.07	32.61	32.03	29.61	−4.28%	−5.97%	−13.09%
% Smoking among 51 and over	8.18	6.01	4.08	0.00	−26.47%	−50.07%	−100.00%
% Ever smoked among aged 51 and over	34.28	27.65	24.66	18.91	−19.33%	−28.07%	−44.84%
% Smoking among aged 51–52	16.33	11.00	5.73	0.00	−32.63%	−64.88%	−100.00%
% Ever-smoked among aged 51–52	27.88	14.69	9.56	0.00	−47.30%	−65.73%	−100.00%
Net Social Security outlay (billions)	682.20	681.75	682.27	693.01	−0.07%	0.01%	1.58%

Source: Authors' calculations (see appendix 12.1).

control policy scenarios influence the size of the population aged 51 and older. Differences across scenarios are small, however, except for the 100 percent cessation scenario, in which the elderly (65+) population increases by 3 percent by 2024. Taxable earnings are slightly higher under the intervention scenarios, and Social Security taxes paid also increase.

The effect of quitting smoking on total DI benefits is uncertain. Quitting smoking improves health status, thus decreasing the probability of receiving any DI benefits. On the other hand, because individuals are healthier, their productivity is higher, and so is their wage. Therefore, the amount of DI benefits they received, if any, will be higher than before. The net effect is very small across the three intervention scenarios in 2024. Quitting smoking does not have a direct effect on receiving DI benefits, but eliminating smoking itself significantly decreases the probability of receiving DI benefits. As a result we observe a net drop of total DI benefits in all three intervention scenarios in year 2050. Under the status quo, DI benefits for people aged 51 and over are $34.07 billion, while under the 100 percent cessation scenario, the total is $29.61 billion, 13 percent lower than under the status quo.

To determine the implications of these changes for the Social Security trust fund, we examine the net Social Security outlay, defined as the sum of OASI and DI benefits, minus the total Social Security taxes paid, among the population aged 51 and older. These figures are shown in the last rows of tables 12.2 and 12.3. In 2024 the net outlay is projected to be $497.25 billion for the status quo scenario, $496.73 billion for the IOM scenario, $496.34 billion for the high-impact scenario, and $510.75 billion for the 100 percent cessation scenario. Only under the 100 percent cessation scenario is the difference of an important magnitude, about 2.7 percent.

In 2050 (table 12.3), some effects of earlier tobacco control policies are magnified because the differences in smoking history across policy scenario are much greater. Among adults aged 51 and older, rates of ever smoking are predicted to be 34.3 percent under the status quo compared with 18.9 percent under the 100 percent cessation scenario. The net Social Security outlay would be $682.20 billion, $681.75 billion, $682.27 billion, and $693.01 billion for the status quo, IOM, high-impact, and 100 percent cessation scenarios, respectively. In 2050, as in 2024, the predicted effects of the IOM and high-impact scenarios on net outlays are very small. Under the 100 percent cessation scenario, the net outlay in 2050 is 1.58 percent higher than in the status quo scenario. Notably, this increase is smaller than the increase in the elderly population (3.02 percent). It is also smaller than the difference in 2024, mostly because predicted Social Security tax receipts are higher and outlays for disability benefits are lower in 2050.

CONCLUSION

From 2006 to 2050, under the two most likely intervention scenarios—the IOM and high-impact scenarios—the net Social Security outlays are predicted to change little relative to the status quo. Even under the extreme assumption that all smoking ceased in 2006, the long-term impact on the Social Security trust fund is expected to be small. Under that scenario, Social Security obligations rise because of a growth in the elderly population, but this increase is partly offset by higher labor participation and taxable earnings and by lower disability benefits. We project a net increase in outlays of only 1.58 percent.

These added costs are far smaller than we might have expected based on calculations at the individual level, which find that workers who smoke (and the spouses of men or women who smoke) derive substantially less benefit than non-smokers from the Social Security program. The differences between our estimates and previous work are due primarily to the difference between estimating the effects of smoking at the individual level rather than the aggregate level.

We note several limitations of the simulations reported here. First, we have assumed that smoking is causal for health and functional status and that its effect can be quantified by our methods. Although it is not controversial that smoking qualitatively affects health, quantifying its effect may be controversial because of comorbidities and unobserved tastes and health. In our implementation we have accounted for a large number of comorbidities, but we acknowledge that there could remain unobservables that have led less healthy individuals to smoke. If that is the case, smoking cessation would reduce health improvements leading to smaller changes in the Social Security trust funds than the already small changes we have estimated.

A second limitation is that we did not take into account how reducing smoking would affect the costs of the Social Security Survivors Insurance program by lowering mortality rates among parents of underaged and adult dependent children. Leistikow, Martin, and Milano (2000) estimated that smoking-attributable deaths among those aged 15 to 54 resulted in additional costs of $1.89 billion for Survivors Insurance in the United States in 1994. In 2050, we project, smoking-attributable deaths would account for $2.27 billion under the status quo scenario—a cost that would be largely eliminated under the 100 percent cessation scenario (see appendix 12.1 for details). Taking account of savings in the Survivors Insurance program would obviously reduce our estimates of the Social Security costs of a tobacco control policy. In 2050, for instance, taking account of savings from Survivors Insurance would reduce the increase in net outlays under the 100 percent cessation scenario from 1.58 percent to about 1 percent.

In addition, we did not consider the impact of smoking cessation/elimination on disability benefits received by individuals aged younger than 51. Here, the direction of the impact is uncertain. Although reducing smoking could lower the probability of receiving benefits, it could also increase the amount of disability benefits paid to qualified individuals because they may have had higher productivity before becoming disabled. Nor did we estimate the effects on Social Security of reduced mortality among those 51 and younger. Again, the direction of the impact is uncertain. The net effect depends on relative magnitudes of the additional Social Security taxes paid compared with the additional outlay of OASI and DI benefits.

More generally, like the other analyses found elsewhere in this volume, the results reported here depend on a number of contingencies. New medical treatments could reduce mortality from smoking-attributable diseases, for instance. We might also see changes in key features of the Social Security program, such as tax rates, benefit levels, or retirement age. Adjusting for these contingencies would certainly alter our projections of the size and characteristics of the elderly population and of Social Security outlays over the next several decades.

These adjustments, however, are unlikely to change the central point of this chapter: although a significant reduction in smoking may increase the financial burden on the Social Security program, the magnitude of this increase is expected to be small even in the unlikely scenario that all smoking ceased immediately. To underline this point: according to the 2007 Social Security Trustees Report, spending by OASDI is expected to be about 26 percent higher than tax revenue in 2050.[1] Under the 100 percent cessation scenario, taking into account the savings from reductions in Survivors Insurance noted above, the increase in net Social Security outlays would be only about 1 percent. In other words, this increase is just 4 percent of the Social Security deficit in 2050. We find no evidence that tobacco control policy would significantly increase the financial problems facing Social Security over the next half century.

APPENDIX 12.1

Details of the HRS can be found at http://hrsonline.isr.umich.edu/. Here we briefly summarize. The HRS is a longitudinal biennial survey of individuals aged 51 or older and their spouses. It is representative of the U.S. population except for oversamples of African Americans and Hispanics. Its main domains are health, economic status, labor market activity, and family linkages. It was initially fielded in 1992, and the latest wave, the seventh, was fielded in 2004. There are approximately 20,000 interviews in each wave, most of which are by telephone. Most important for this project are the extensive health measures, present and prior smoking status, complete measures of income and wealth including Social Security income, earnings (which can be used to calculate Social Security contributions), and vital status. We use the RAND version of the HRS data (St. Clair et al. 2006). Key variables are briefly discussed below.

HEALTH MEASURES

We include six self-reported doctor-diagnosed chronic conditions: (1) high blood pressure or hypertension; (2) diabetes or high blood sugar; (3) cancer or a malignant tumor of any kind except skin cancer; (4) chronic lung disease except asthma, such as chronic bronchitis or emphysema; (5) heart attack, coronary heart disease, angina, congestive heart failure, or other heart problems; (6) stroke or transient ischemic attack (TIA). Respondents are asked questions in the form of "Has a doctor ever told you that you have . . ."

SELF-REPORTED FUNCTIONAL STATUS

We examine two summary measures of functional status. One is the number of limitations for Instrumental Activities of Daily Living (IADL), including using the phone, managing money, and taking medications. The other is the number of limitations in Activities of Daily Living (ADL), including dressing, bathing, eating, getting in and out of bed, and walking across a room. Based on the two measures we generate a variable of functional status with four mutually exclusive categories: no limitations, IADL limitations only, one or two ADL limitations, and three or more ADL limitations.

PRESENT AND PRIOR SMOKING STATUS

HRS asks about prior smoking status during the first interview of each respondent. The question is: "Have you ever smoked?" and the answer is yes or no. Present smoking status is asked to all respondents except in wave 7, fielded in 2004. In that year those who were previously identified as nonsmokers are no longer asked if they smoke. Other respondents are asked: "Do you smoke cigarettes now?"

BMI STATUS

HRS asks the respondent's weight in pounds at each wave. The respondent's height in feet and inches is generally only asked during the first interview. Based on self-reported weight and height, the measure of body mass index (BMI) was generated. We then construct a measure of BMI status with four exclusive categories: underweight (BMI $< 18.5\,\text{kg/m}^2$), normal weight ($18.5\,\text{kg/m}^2 \le \text{BMI} < 25\,\text{kg/m}^2$), overweight ($25\,\text{kg/m}^2 \le \text{BMI} < 30\,\text{kg/m}^2$), and obese (BMI $\ge 30\,\text{kg/m}^2$).

TRANSITION PROBABILITIES

We estimated the probabilities of the following transitions: developing one or more of six chronic conditions (including the major illnesses associated with

TABLE 12.4 Probability of Developing Various Health Conditions as a Function of Individual Characteristics

RISK FACTOR	STROKE	HEART DISEASE	HYPERTENSION	DIABETES	LUNG DISEASE	CANCER
Age						
Age 51 to 55			(reference category)			
Age 56 to 59	1.564**	1.062	0.912	1.073	0.929	1.253
Age 60 to 64	1.944***	1.294**	1.147*	1.264*	1.044	1.794***
Age 65 to 69	2.401***	1.850***	1.452***	1.633***	1.766***	2.438***
Age 70 to 74	3.394***	2.263***	1.488***	1.587***	1.724***	2.712***
Age 75 to 84	5.762***	3.017***	1.688***	1.372**	1.983***	2.967***
Age 85 or above	8.554***	4.485***	1.389**	0.958	1.768**	2.429***
Male	1.080	1.291***	0.847***	1.263***	0.908	1.480***
Black	1.180	0.728***	1.256***	1.311***	0.753**	0.837
Hispanic	0.838	0.735**	1.125	1.666***	0.505***	0.489***
Education						
Less than high school	1.245**	1.225***	1.078	1.265***	1.288***	1.028
High school graduate			(reference category)			
Some college and above	0.918	1.008	0.914*	0.947	0.734***	1.110

Marital status						
Widowed	1.192*	1.028	1.072	1.227**	1.127	1.037
Married				(reference category)		
Single	1.081	1.086	1.097	1.097	1.345***	1.227*
Body mass index (BMI)						
Obese (BMI ≥30)	0.927	1.290***	1.901***	6.154***	1.348***	1.120
Overweight (25 ≤ BMI < 30)	0.886	1.057	1.417***	2.556***	0.973	1.064
Normal weight (18.5 ≤ BMI < 25)				(reference category)		
Underweight (BMI < 18.5)	0.973	1.425*	0.850	0.823	1.466*	1.258
Smoking						
Ever smoked	1.060	1.148**			1.999***	1.244***
Current smoking	1.698***	1.352***			2.768***	1.160
Health conditions						
Hypertension	1.511***	1.570***				
Diabetes	1.768***	1.692***	1.461***			
Heart disease	1.554***					

Notes: Models are logit models. Results are reported in odds ratios.
*p < 0.05; **p < 0.01; ***p < 0.001.
Data source: Health and Retirement Study, 1992–2004.

TABLE 12.5 Probability of Dying or Developing Functional Limitations

RISK FACTOR	MORTALITY	ONE OR MORE IADLS	ONE OR MORE ADLS	THREE OR MORE ADLS
Age				
Age 51 to 55	(reference group)			
Age 56 to 59	1.429*	0.905	0.992	0.975
Age 60 to 64	1.903***	0.918	1.002	1.085
Age 65 to 69	2.953***	0.997	1.015	1.050
Age 70 to 74	4.050***	1.329***	1.357***	1.442**
Age 75 to 84	7.273***	1.892***	1.784***	1.963***
Age 85 or above	17.179***	2.615***	2.585***	3.634***
Male	1.667***	0.895**	0.804***	0.817***
Black	1.157**	1.176***	1.146**	1.296***
Hispanic	0.894	1.193**	1.185**	1.299**
Education				
Less than high school	1.106*	1.158***	1.069	1.130
High school graduate	(reference group)			
Some college and above	0.926	0.876***	0.894**	1.071
Marital status				
Widowed	1.195***	1.123**	1.189***	1.178*
Married	(reference group)			
Single	1.305***	1.243***	1.248***	1.154
Body mass index (BMI)				
Obese (BMI ≥ 30)		1.544***	1.677***	1.029
Overweight (25 ≤ BMI < 30)		1.124**	1.121**	0.886
Normal weight (18.5 ≤ BMI < 25)	(reference group)			
Underweight (BMI < 18.5)		0.838	0.816	0.817

TABLE 12.5 (*Continued*)

RISK FACTOR	MORTALITY	ONE OR MORE IADLS	ONE OR MORE ADLS	THREE OR MORE ADLS
Smoking				
Ever smoked	1.197***	1.059	1.072	0.995
Current smoking	1.741***	1.165***	1.205***	1.224*
Health conditions				
Cancer	2.096***	0.976	1.005	0.866
Hypertension	1.198***	1.109**	1.125***	1.009
Diabetes	1.731***	1.312***	1.303***	1.289***
Heart disease	1.625***	1.157***	1.178***	1.097
Lung disease	2.135***	1.206***	1.219***	0.970
Stroke	1.371***	1.303***	1.279***	1.466***
Functional status				
No functional limitations		(reference group)		
IADL only	1.893***	4.941***	2.410***	3.686***
ADL 1 or 2	2.078***	5.037***	5.578***	6.450***
ADL 3 or more	3.938***	5.991***	7.300***	18.760***
Living in nursing home				
Lag of IADL only		2.458***	1.528***	1.819***
Lag of ADL 1 or 2		2.931***	3.098***	1.853***
Lag of ADL 3 or more		3.012***	3.255***	3.095***

Notes: The HRS wave 1 data are not used because the IADL and ADL measures are different from those in waves 2–7.
*p < 0.10; **p < 0.05; ***p < 0.01.
Data source: Health and Retirement Study, 1994–2004.

smoking), quitting or initiating smoking, among four functional states, between the joint status of any earnings and receiving any Old-Age and Survivors Insurance (OASI), and of dying. As noted above, all six chronic health conditions are treated as "absorbing": a person who gets an illness is assumed to have it forever and therefore cannot get it again; this assumption is consistent with the way the data were obtained and with the course of most of the chronic conditions. Model estimates for transitional probabilities are shown in tables 12.4 and 12.5.

INCOME FROM EARNINGS AND SOCIAL SECURITY

Questions are asked in each wave about various components of respondents' income in the last calendar year. Individual earnings include the sum of the respondent's wage/salary income, bonuses/overtime pay/commissions/tips, second job or military reserve earnings, professional practice, and trade income. We then apply the historical maximum taxable earnings to obtain taxable earnings for each respondent in each wave. Multiplying the sum of taxable earnings by Social Security payroll tax rates in the corresponding year, we can estimate the amount of Social Security taxes paid by the respondent. The two measures of Social Security income are income from Social Security disability insurance (DI) and from Social Security retirement, spouse, or survival benefits (i.e., OASI). We constructed a variable indicating the joint status of receipt of any earnings and receipt of any OASI. We also generated an indicator of whether a respondent receives any DI. Missing values or brackets for income measures are imputed in RAND HRS using a method described in St. Clair et al. (2006).

Because a large proportion of the population has zero values for income from DI and from OASI, we used a two-step procedure for estimation. We used a multinomial logit regression to model a first-order Markov transition for the joint status of receiving (positive) earnings and receiving (positive) OASI benefits. Possible states are: (1) income from earnings and no OASI benefits, (2) income from both earnings and OASI benefits, (3) no income from earnings and no OASI benefits, and (4) no income from earnings and receipt of OASI benefits. Next we used least-squares regression to estimate the amount of OASI benefits received, if any. Among those with earnings, we used another two-step procedure to estimate the probability of earning more than the maximum taxable amount for Social Security payroll taxes and, for those who earned less, the amount of earnings.

Because SSDI benefits convert to retirement benefits when people turn 65, we modeled SSDI benefits received only for individuals aged 51 to 65. We used a logit model to estimate the probability of receiving any SSDI benefits, and then a least-squares regression for the amount of benefits received, if any. Model estimations are in tables 12.6 and 12.7. All dollar values are in 2005 dollars.

TABLE 12.6 Probability of Receiving Positive Earnings, Receiving OASI, and Receiving DI Benefits

	RECEIVED POSITIVE EARNINGS	RECEIVED OASI	RECEIVED DI
Age			
Age 51 to 55	(reference category)		
Age 56 to 59	0.796***	1.962***	1.196
Aged 60	0.654***	12.755***	
Aged 61	0.437***	55.844***	
Aged 62	0.363***	57.821***	
Aged 63	0.396***	48.861***	
Aged 64	0.359***	116.736***	
Age 60 to 64			1.321
Aged 65			0.900
Age 65 to 69	0.421***	101.161***	
Age 70 and above	0.216***	46.653***	
Male	1.272***	0.839***	1.579***
Black	1.031	0.780***	1.318
Hispanic	1.054	0.642***	0.647*
Education			
Less than high school	0.754***	0.923	0.947
High school graduate	(reference category)		
Some college and above	1.128***	0.750***	0.477***
Marital status			
Widowed	1.148**	1.263***	1.523*
Married	(reference category)		
Single	1.202***	0.856**	1.215
Body mass index (BMI)			
Obese (BMI ≤ 30)	1.054	1.176***	1.338
Overweight (25 ≤ BMI < 30)	1.119***	1.123**	1.149
Underweight (BMI < 18.5)	0.845	0.877	1.079

TABLE 12.6 (*Continued*)

	RECEIVED POSITIVE EARNINGS	RECEIVED OASI	RECEIVED DI
Smoking			
Ever smoked	0.945	1.076	1.406**
Current smoking	0.991	1.015	0.984
Health conditions			
Cancer	0.983	1.121	1.018
Diabetes	0.915*	0.899	1.335*
Heart disease	0.813***	1.050	2.091***
Hypertension	0.949	1.088*	1.336*
Lung disease	0.805***	0.802**	1.766***
Stroke	0.637***	1.164	2.227***
Functional status			
Healthy	(reference category)		
IADL only	0.578***	0.993	4.043***
ADL 1 or 2	0.495***	0.982	5.492***
ADL 3 or more	0.205***	0.939	6.842***
Labor participation and OASI benefits in previous period			
Received any earnings and no OASI	(reference category)		
No earnings nor OASI	0.040***	1.295***	
Received any earnings and OASI	0.711***	63.702***	
No earnings and received OASI	0.025***	75.907***	

Notes: Models are logit models. Results are reported in odds ratios. The HRS wave 1 data are not used because the IADL and ADL measures are different from those in waves 2–7.
$*p < 0.05$; $**p < 0.01$; $***p < 0.001$.
Data source: Health and Retirement Study, 1994–2004.

TABLE 12.7 Least-Squares Estimations of Taxable Earnings and OASI and DI Benefits (If Any)

	ANNUAL TAXABLE EARNINGS IF > 0	ANNUAL OASI BENEFITS IF > 0	ANNUAL DI BENEFITS IF > 0
Age			
Aged 51 to 55	(reference category)		
Age 56 to 59	−1,417.49*** (273.72)	594.95** (294.28)	28.92 (296.85)
Aged 60	−3,198.55*** (483.24)	1,818.24*** (393.95)	
Aged 61	−3,362.62*** (495.08)	569.73* (333.60)	
Aged 62	−3,675.58*** (523.14)	−2,537.97*** (270.69)	
Aged 63	−712.10 (611.62)	−710.42*** (248.93)	
Aged 64	−2,323.91*** (689.13)	957.78*** (248.21)	
Age 60 to 64			119.62 (300.28)
Aged 65			237.49 (361.82)
Age 65 to 69	−680.76 (585.09)	1,241.97*** (231.13)	
Age 70 or above	−5,742.32*** (635.78)	1,584.01*** (228.77)	
Male	11,355.15*** (224.44)	3,543.58*** (41.51)	3,996.95*** (278.71)
Black	−1,486.87*** (367.00)	−1,299.47*** (71.55)	−1,128.14*** (310.26)
Hispanic	−5,242.10*** (446.39)	−1,750.60*** (92.00)	−1,206.04*** (459.69)
Education			
Less than high school	−5,213.29*** (338.19)	−987.10*** (48.69)	−1,197.92*** (301.36)

TABLE 12.7 (*Continued*)

	ANNUAL TAXABLE EARNINGS IF > 0	ANNUAL OASI BENEFITS IF > 0	ANNUAL DI BENEFITS IF > 0
High school graduate		(reference category)	
Some college and above	6,682.25***	762.54***	570.31
	(231.74)	(45.96)	(350.05)
Marital status			
Widowed	1,414.55***	2,266.40***	331.37
	(403.50)	(46.66)	(368.44)
Married		(reference category)	
Single	450.41*	628.77***	−478.05
	(262.37)	(61.36)	(308.66)
Smoking			
Ever smoked	−333.95		−146.72
	(242.02)		(309.31)
Current smoking	−2,437.90***		−667.12**
	(295.15)		(302.94)
Health conditions			
Cancer	−575.55		−111.37
	(399.61)		(373.83)
Diabetes	−546.74		−126.52
	(351.27)		(288.73)
Heart disease	−1,203.42***		277.80
	(331.11)		(267.17)
Hypertension	157.97		93.39
	(224.27)		(269.36)
Lung disease	−2,358.70***		−164.86
	(475.28)		(301.31)
Stroke	−818.70		432.43
	(693.36)		(347.95)
Functional status			
IADL only	−5,378.29***		−792.64
	(713.29)		(485.25)

TABLE 12.7 (*Continued*)

	ANNUAL TAXABLE EARNINGS IF > 0	ANNUAL OASI BENEFITS IF > 0	ANNUAL DI BENEFITS IF > 0
ADL 1 or 2	−4,449.78*** (495.62)		−27.07 (273.03)
ADL 3 or more	−5,484.18*** (1,241.79)		−522.68 (348.10)
Any OASI benefits	−16,981.72*** (505.97)		
Any earning		520.71*** (55.02)	
Constant	29,875.06*** (301.96)	6,869.04*** (230.62)	9,125.65*** (486.04)

Notes: The HRS wave 1 data are not used because the IADL and ADL measures are different from those in waves 2–7.
All dollars are converted to year 2005 dollar values.
$*p < 0.10$; $**p < 0.05$; $***p < 0.01$.
Data source: Health and Retirement Study, 1994–2004.

ACCOUNTING FOR SOCIAL SECURITY BENEFITS FOR SURVIVING DEPENDENTS AND CARETAKING PARENTS

The FEM does not model Social Security benefits for surviving dependents and parents who take care of them. Therefore, we resort to other information to infer how smoking policies would impact these benefits. An article by Leistikow, Martin, and Milano (2000) estimated smoking-attributable deaths among people aged 15–54 and the resulting Social Security costs for Survivors Insurance in the United States in 1994. They found that the Social Security costs of supporting U.S. children who lost a parent due to smoking were $1.86 billion (sensitivity range: $0.789–$5.05 billion). These costs include payments to children under age 18, disabled adult children, students aged 18 to 19, and parents who took care of them. According to the Annual Statistical Supplement (Social Security Administration 1996), Social Security paid $11.64 billion in support of bereft children and their caregivers in 1994, accounting for 4 percent of the total OASI benefits. Therefore, 0.64 percent (4 percent × 1.86/11.64) of the OASI benefits could have been avoided if no one aged 15 to 54 ever smoked. In 1994, the prevalence of ex- or current smokers among those aged 15–54, as reported by the National Health Interview Survey (NHIS), was 48.70 percent.

Smoking prevalence has been declining over time, and this trend is expected to continue in the near future. In year 2004, NHIS reported that 40.15 percent of those aged 15 to 54 are former or current smokers. The SimSmoke simulation reported in chapter 2 projected the prevalence of former and current smokers aged 15 and 54 between 2006 and 2025 under alternative tobacco control policy scenarios. Under the status quo scenario (no further change in smoking policy), the prevalence of former and current smokers among those aged 15 to 54 would decline from 35.00 percent in 2004 to 26.40 percent in 2025. We assume that the prevalence will continue to decline and that in 2050 it will be 17.60 percent, two-thirds of that in 2025. Under the 100 percent cessation scenario, there is no new smoking initiation (among those aged 15 to 24) beginning year 2006; therefore, in year 2036, when those aged 24 in year 2006 survive to age 54, all individuals between ages 15 and 54 will be free of smoking history. Therefore, in 2050, payments for Social Security benefits to support children who lost a parent due to smoking would be very low; these payments won't be exactly zero because some might receive benefits for more than 14 years.

To estimate how smoking policy under the 100 percent cessation scenario would impact the outlay of survivors' benefits in year 2050, relative to payments under the status quo scenario, we perform the following calculation: In year 1994 NHIS reported the prevalence of former or current smokers among persons aged 15 to 54 to be 48.70 percent, whereas in year 2050 the figure is down to 17.60 percent. Taking into account the discrepancy in estimates between NHIS and the data source used by Levy and Mumford (in 2004 the prevalence is 40.15 percent in NHIS and 35.00 percent in Levy and Mumford's model), we estimate that in 2050, the prevalence of former and current smokers among those aged 15 to 54 will decline by 58.5 percent $[1 - (17.6/48.7) \times (40.15/35)]$, relative to that in year 1994. We assume that if there were no decline in prevalence of ex- or current smokers among those aged 15–54 from year 1994 to 2050, the same proportion of OASI benefits (0.64 percent) will be paid out due to smoking-attributable deaths between ages 15 and 54 in 2050 as in 1994. Since we predict that there will very likely be a decline in smoking, we estimate that under the status quo, in year 2050, the proportion of OASI benefits attributed to smoking-attributable deaths between ages 15 and 54 will be 0.64 percent $\times (1 - 58.5$ percent$) = 0.265$ percent. Based on FEM simulation results, the total of OASI benefits is $857 billion in year 2050. Therefore, the costs due to smoking-attributable deaths between ages 15 and 54 will be $2.27 billion ($857 \times 0.265$ percent$= 2.27$). This amount of cost will be mostly eliminated under the 100 percent cessation scenario.

These calculations also assume that most of the deceased parents whose children receive Social Security survivors benefits died under age 54 and that the fraction of survivors benefits attributable to smoking is proportional to the prevalence of smoking.

NOTE

1. See http://www.ssa.gov/OACT/TRSUM/trsummary.html, accessed May 23, 2007.

PART 3

LAW AND SOCIETY

13

ENHANCING COMPLIANCE WITH TOBACCO CONTROL POLICIES

FRANK J. CHALOUPKA, PHILIP J. COOK, RICHARD M. PECK,
AND JOHN A. TAURAS

Achieving compliance is necessary if tobacco taxes and regulations are to improve the public health. These measures are not self-enforcing. High tax rates coupled with lax enforcement create profitable opportunities for tax evasion, which has indeed been a growing problem over the last decade. The financial incentive to violate youth access laws is strong enough to require systematic policing. Even clean air regulations, for which social pressure by nonsmokers does much of the work, at least initially require some backup from enforcement. Enforcement efforts use public resources and must be budgeted as part of a comprehensive plan to improve compliance.

The prospect of more vigorous tobacco control policies, such as the measures recently recommended by the Institute of Medicine (IOM), heightens these concerns about enforcement. On the one hand, these new policy measures might require significantly higher expenditures to ensure compliance, deterring states from adopting or enforcing them. There is also concern that these measures—particularly the tobacco tax increases—could promote criminal activity such as large-scale cigarette smuggling. This chapter addresses these concerns with a detailed discussion of enforcement of three IOM-recommended policies: excise tax increases, stronger youth access laws, and more extensive clean air regulations. (The other three IOM policies—media campaigns, school-based interventions, and cessation programs—aim at changing attitudes toward smoking or supporting cessation and do not involve law enforcement.)

Although we present some evidence about the cost of enforcement, this chapter focuses primarily on issues of regulation. As we will show, enforcement costs are not fixed but depend heavily on regulation. There are efficient methods for improving compliance, especially compliance with excise taxes, that involve relatively modest costs. A well-designed system of regulations would allow federal, state, and local governments to adopt more vigorous tobacco control measures while avoiding both an increase in criminal activity and an inordinate burden in enforcement costs.

The discussion that follows examines the enforcement first of excise taxes, then of youth access laws and clean air laws. Of these three, we give the most attention to excise tax enforcement, which is distinctive in several ways. First, tax enforcement is more important to public health outcomes; raising prices through higher taxes is at the forefront of the current efforts to reduce smoking. Second, unlike enforcement of clean air or youth access regulations, tax enforcement tends to pay for itself many times over in the form of increased collections. Last, the regulatory framework is far more important to tax compliance than to the other two policies and thus requires more extensive treatment.

TAX COMPLIANCE AND ENFORCEMENT

The IOM-based policy scenario used in this volume calls for every state to raise its excise tax on a pack of cigarettes by $2. This tax increase is intended to raise cigarette prices and reduce consumption, but it would also increase the financial incentive to evade state cigarette taxes. To the extent that tax evasion and avoidance undercut the effects of the tax increase, the reduction in smoking would be smaller than projected. The SimSmoke model discussed earlier in this volume makes no explicit assumptions about regulations or the extent of tax evasion. The price-elasticity parameters used in its estimates are based on historical data, reflecting past methods for combating tax evasion. In looking to the future, it is important to note that tax-enforcement regulation is not static and that the actual effects of the recommended tax increase would depend on the regulatory regime. There have been a number of innovations in recent years to combat tax evasion and avoidance, and it is safe to say this trend will continue as states seek to improve their tax collections.

This section describes the main channels of cigarette excise-tax evasion and discusses the evolution of the regulatory structure designed to curtail this evasion. After a general discussion of tax evasion and avoidance, we discuss measures intended to address four types of activities: Internet or "direct" purchases, purchases from Native American reservations, other individual efforts to evade or avoid taxes, and large-scale smuggling. We close the section with a discussion of enforcement costs under alternative regulatory frameworks.

TAX EVASION AND AVOIDANCE

Tax evasion and avoidance differ in their legal status: tax evasion involves illegal activities, whereas avoidance involves legal activities such as purchases in lower-tax jurisdictions or from a duty-free shop. Most tax evasion and avoidance activities channel cigarettes from low-tax or tax-exempt sources to smokers in higher-tax jurisdictions. Federal and state excise taxes account for over 40 percent of cigarette prices on average.[1] The federal government imposes a uniform excise tax on cigarettes, but state and local taxes are far from uniform, and the resulting cost differences are substantial. As of early 2010, state cigarette taxes ranged from a low of 7 cents per pack in South Carolina to a high of $3.46 per pack in Rhode Island. In addition, some localities apply sizable additional excise taxes; notable examples include New York City ($1.50 per pack), Chicago (68 cents per pack), and Cook County, Illinois ($2.00 per pack). These differences in tax rates create large geographic differences in cigarette prices, sometimes across nearby juris-dictions. For example, the combined state and local taxes in Chicago are $3.66 per pack, over two and a half times higher than taxes in Indiana (99.5 cents per pack) and substantially higher than in Wisconsin ($2.52 per pack). Moreover, Indian reservations are typically exempt from state and local excise taxes and hence can sell cigarettes at a discount. Further differentiation results from gen-eral sales taxes. Sales tax rates differ widely across jurisdictions, and in some ju-risdictions cigarettes are exempt.[2] Variation in sales taxes adds to the differences in the final price smokers pay for cigarettes.

Although jurisdictional differences have existed for many years, the magni-tude of these differences, both absolutely and as a share of cigarette prices, has increased sharply in recent years. These differences create incentives for tax evasion and avoidance, both for individual smokers and criminal organizations. The growth of the Internet over the past decade and the emergence of hun-dreds of online cigarette vendors have facilitated evasion.

Measuring tax avoidance and tax evasion is difficult, but estimates indicate that they accounted for a significant share—one-eighth or more—of total ciga-rette consumption in the United States in the early 2000s (Stehr 2005). The extent of the problem differs by jurisdiction and is most severe in high-tax ju-risdictions with ready access to low-tax or untaxed cigarettes. In addition, smok-ers differ in their likelihood of engaging in these activities, with heavier smok-ers and those with higher incomes more likely to report purchasing from low-tax or untaxed sources (Hyland et al. 2006). Tax evasion and avoidance reduce but do not negate the revenue and public health impact of cigarette excise tax in-creases (Farrelly, Nimsch, and James 2003; Merriman, Yurekli, and Chaloupka 2000; Yurekli and Zhang 2000).

The major forms of tax evasion or avoidance can be differentiated by the scale of the activity and its legal status. First, individuals make Internet, telephone, or mail-order purchases from vendors based in low-tax states or in tax-exempt locations. Although purchasers are generally liable for paying the taxes in their state of residence, they rarely do so in practice.[3] Second, individuals may buy cigarettes for personal consumption from reservations. Nonnatives buying from reservation stores are liable for excise taxes, but compliance is low for reservation purchases as well. Third, individuals purchase cigarettes for personal use from other tax-exempt sources such as military commissaries or duty-free shops, or from lower-tax jurisdictions. Last, criminal enterprises purchase large quantities of cigarettes from low-tax jurisdictions or divert cigarettes from distribution before any taxes are paid and smuggle these cigarettes to high-tax jurisdictions for sale to scofflaw retailers. As we discuss, governments at all levels have tried to curb each of these means of tax evasion or avoidance.

DIRECT OR INTERNET PURCHASES

The growth of the Internet and the emergence of hundreds of Internet cigarette vendors have helped smokers avoid state cigarette taxes (Ribisl, Kim, and Williams 2007).[4] Although surveys suggest that relatively few smokers buy regularly from Internet vendors, one widely cited study projected that Internet sales of tobacco products would be as high as $5 billion in 2005, with states losing $1.4 billion in tobacco tax revenues as a result (Forrester Research, Inc. 2001).[5]

Smokers purchasing cigarettes from direct channels are generally required to pay the applicable state taxes on these cigarettes, although the specific requirements differ from state to state. For example, in Illinois the "use tax" is 98 cents per pack plus 6.25 percent of the purchase price less the sales tax per pack (if any) paid where purchased; this use tax is equivalent to the sum of the state's cigarette excise and general sales taxes.[6] Some states mandate interest or penalties on unpaid or overdue taxes. Without active enforcement, however, virtually no one complies with these requirements. Enforcement is hampered by the fact that states cannot identify who is buying cigarettes from out-of-state vendors or measure the quantities purchased.

As tax revenue losses from Internet sales increased, states began exploring options for dealing with this problem. Particularly important in early efforts was the Jenkins Act (15 USC 376a), a federal statute adopted in 1949. The Jenkins Act was intended to curb tax evasion resulting from the interstate sale of mail-order cigarettes. The Act requires vendors who market or ship cigarettes across state lines to register with the tobacco tax administrator of the destination states and to send this office monthly statements or copies of invoices documenting the names and addresses of recipients and the quantities of cigarettes shipped.

This information would allow states to collect excise taxes from recipients of cross-state shipments.

The Jenkins Act applies to Internet cigarette sales as well as to other direct (mail and telephone) sales. States' initial efforts to apply the Jenkins Act met resistance from Internet cigarette vendors, however, and received no support from the U.S. Department of Justice (DOJ), the federal agency with primary enforcement authority for the Act.[7] Washington State has moved ahead with efforts to apply the Jenkins Act to Internet sales. In October 2002 the Washington Department of Revenue filed a complaint against Dirtcheap Cigarettes (www .dirtcheapcig.com) asserting the state's authority to enforce the Jenkins Act and requiring the online vendor to provide reports on sales to Washington residents (*State of Washington v. D.C. Inc.*, No. CV02-2438L). The Federal District Court agreed, concluding that the state's right to enforce the Jenkins Act was implied given that Congress's intent in adopting the Act was to help states crack down on cigarette tax avoidance (Banthin 2004). Given the ruling, Dirtcheap settled with the state before going to trial, agreeing to provide the information required by the Jenkins Act.

Washington State's success in applying the Jenkins Act led to similar efforts in many other states. Those obtaining customer lists from online vendors have often shared these lists with other states. Comprehensive information on the extent of these efforts, their costs, and the revenues generated from them is not available.[8] However, newspaper reports suggest that the revenues derived from these efforts are a large multiple of the costs. For example, Michigan reported collecting $5.9 million from about 9,000 residents based on lists provided by 13 online vendors (Christoff 2006).

Washington State continues to provide leadership among the states, becoming the first state to obtain a customer list from a reservation-based online vendor. In January 2005, the Washington State Department of Revenue sued one of the largest reservation-based Internet vendors, Smokesignals.com, run by a member of the Seneca Nation and located on the Seneca reservation in New York. In a stipulated judgment reached in July 2005 in U.S. District Court, the company agreed to provide the information required under the Jenkins Act (Washington State Department of Revenue 2005). The resolution of this lawsuit suggests that tribal sovereignty does not exempt reservation-based Internet cigarette vendors from the Jenkins Act. As a result, the Smartsmoker.com Web site (an alternative name for Smokesignals.com) stated:

> As part of the Seneca Nation of Indians and the Iroquois Confederacy, Smart-Smoker is currently not required to collect state sales tax for products sold on Tribal land. Nonetheless, we are required under federal law to report all sales and shipments of cigarettes to the state taxing authority within your home state. You should

contact the taxing authority within your state to determine your tax obligation on the use of these products within your state.[9]

One result of these efforts may be a growth in sales by foreign-based Internet vendors, a group that has received little attention to date. Hundreds of foreign-based Internet sites sell cigarettes (including American brands) directly to smokers in the United States (Ribisl, Kim, and Williams 2007). To our knowledge, no enforcement actions have been taken against foreign-based Internet cigarette vendors under the Jenkins Act or other applicable federal or state statutes. A limited review of the Web sites of foreign-based Internet vendors suggests that many of the same issues that arose in efforts targeting domestic vendors are likely to arise in enforcement actions targeting foreign vendors. For example, with respect to the legality of shipping internationally and the payment of applicable taxes, one such vendor—SimplySmoke.com, apparently based in Russia—cited the 1999 Universal Postal Convention in support of the legality of shipping cigarettes through the mail and placed the responsibility for tax compliance squarely on the purchaser:

> U.S. consumers who buy goods from foreign sources become the importer. Payment terms on this site: cash before delivery. Once the goods are paid, title of the product is transferred, and SimplySmoke no longer owns the product, once it leaves the stock—the buyer, which is the importer, then owns the product. The importer is responsible for assuring that the shipments comply with a variety of both state and federal government import regulations. To avoid misunderstandings we highly recommend you consult your local tax office.[10]

Some foreign vendors have stated more or less explicitly that they will not comply with Jenkins Act requests:

> All orders are processed and shipped from out of the US. Therefore We don't report tax or customer information to any government agency or other entity. (Cigoutlet.net, based in Moldova)

> SimplySmoke.com does not distribute, sell or rent your name, email address, or other personal information to any third party. (SimplySmoke.com)[11]

Both of these sites (and likely most sites of other foreign vendors) indicate that they ship cigarettes in small quantities, regardless of the quantity purchased. For example, Cigoutlet.net splits larger orders into shipments of no more than two cartons. These smaller shipments appear designed to avoid the attention from U.S. Customs authorities that larger shipments might attract.

Enforcement actions against off-shore vendors would be more difficult than comparable actions against domestic vendors. However, the federal government has a greater incentive to become involved because foreign vendors are evading federal taxes, not just state and local taxes. Targeting these sites may become increasingly important in coming years given the success states have had in targeting domestic vendors.

In addition to their efforts to collect applicable taxes from smokers buying directly, states have also tried to curtail Internet and other direct cigarette sales. State Attorneys General (AGs) have been at the forefront of many of these efforts. In 2005, state AGs reached agreements with major shipping companies (including Federal Express, United Parcel Service, and DHL) to ban direct tobacco product shipments to U.S. residents, leaving the U.S. Postal Service as the only major delivery option. (In 2010, the Prevent All Cigarette Trafficking Act [PACT] banned delivery of cigarettes through the Postal Service.) In early 2005, state AGs also negotiated agreements with major credit card companies (including Visa, MasterCard, American Express, and Discover) to prohibit the use of credit cards for online cigarette purchases; PayPal, the online payment service, agreed to do the same.[12] Smokers can still pay for online purchases with checks or money orders. In early 2006, Philip Morris reached an agreement with state AGs not to provide its cigarettes to vendors who do not comply with policies governing Internet and other direct sales. These agreements cost states little or nothing and are likely to be highly effective in reducing Internet and other direct purchases and in generating new revenues.

Many states have passed legislation that targets Internet and other direct cigarette sales. In 2000, New York became the first state to ban Internet and other direct sales to state residents; the law was eventually upheld after a legal challenge brought by Santa Fe Natural Tobacco Company and Brown & Williamson Tobacco Company and went into effect in 2003. A few other states have adopted similar bans. More common are measures limiting Internet and other direct sales. Maine, for example, prohibits delivery services from delivering tobacco products from vendors either not licensed by the state or not in compliance with the state's policies regarding direct shipments; other states have adopted similar policies. California and some other states require Internet vendors either to pay the state taxes on cigarettes shipped to the state or to inform customers that they are required to pay these taxes. Arizona law stipulates that out-of-state shippers are liable for paying the state's excise tax on cigarettes, which raises interesting constitutional issues; the Supreme Court has held that out-of-state shippers are *not* liable for paying sales and use taxes, but the Court might take a different view of excise taxes serving a state regulatory purpose, such as improving public health (Graff 2006).

Finally, two major bills addressing Internet and other direct sales of tobacco products were introduced in Congress in the early 2000s. In June 2003, Senators Hatch and Kohl introduced the Prevent All Cigarette Trafficking Act (PACT). Among other provisions, the bill required that all applicable taxes in the state to which cigarettes are being shipped be paid in advance, banned delivery by mail or common carrier of tobacco products not labeled as being in compliance with the Act, required all Internet and other direct vendors (including those located on reservations) to comply with the Jenkins Act, raised Jenkins Act violations from misdemeanors to felonies, and granted states explicit authority to enforce the Jenkins Act. A companion bill—the Internet Tobacco Sales Enforcement Act (ITSE)—introduced in the House in July 2003, contained similar provisions designed to strengthen the Jenkins Act. The PACT Act passed the Senate in December 2003, while the ITSE Act was unanimously approved by the House Judiciary Committee in January 2004. Provisions strengthening the reporting requirements of the Jenkins Act were subsequently adopted as part of legislation extending the USA Patriot Act (PL-109-177, enacted March 9, 2006), and the PACT Act was finally signed into law on March 31, 2010.

In sum, while Internet sites continue to offer direct shipment of cigarettes on which state and local taxes have not been paid, those offers are less attractive to potential customers than they used to be: transactions costs have increased (no credit cards allowed) and customers face a greater risk of being identified and forced to pay the taxes. The ban on delivery of cigarettes through the U.S. Postal Service is expected to curtail further sales by mail. Site operators are under increasing legal pressure. With or without federal action, there is good reason to think that this channel for excise tax evasion is becoming less profitable.

RESERVATION SALES

There are approximately 275 Native American reservations located in the United States. About two-thirds of states include reservation land, with some reservations located near large population centers. The sovereign-nation status of tribes located on reservations has implications for state taxation and regulation of businesses based on these reservations. Sovereignty has meant that cigarettes and other tobacco products sold on reservations have been exempt from state cigarette excise taxes and sales taxes applied to cigarettes. This exemption does not extend to nonnatives who purchase these products on reservations. Historically, however, there has been little compliance with state policies requiring the payment of applicable taxes on tobacco products purchased on reservations.

Until recently, states did little to address this problem because of uncertainty about their right to collect taxes on reservation sales. As discussed below, a U.S.

Supreme Court decision involving Kansas's efforts to collect state gasoline taxes may lead to a resolution of this question. In the meantime, however, states have taken other approaches to collecting cigarette taxes from nonresident smokers who buy cigarettes from reservation outlets. The first involves "tribal taxes" levied on cigarettes sold on reservations, with most or all of the tax revenue remaining with the tribe. Some of these tribal taxes are enacted in response to state efforts to minimize the difference between prices on and off reservations, so as to reduce the incentive for nonreservation residents to purchase cigarettes at reservation outlets. Perhaps a third or more of states have entered into over 200 such agreements with various tribes. For example, an agreement reached between Washington State and the Puyallup tribe, effective January 2005, called for a tribal tax of $11.75 per carton for cigarettes sold on the reservation.[13] This agreement requires that tax stamps reflecting payment of the tribal tax be applied to all cigarettes sold on the reservation and that 30 percent of the tax revenues go to the state, with the remainder staying with the tribe (RCW 43.06.564). The agreement notes that the "tribal tax is in lieu of the combined state and local sales and use taxes, and state cigarette taxes" and that the tribal tax will be increased when the state tax increases (as was the case in July 2005 when the state tax was increased by 60 cents per pack). Most such agreements, often called "compacts," are negotiated separately with individual tribes, and their terms may vary for tribes within the same state.

Second, states have sought to collect applicable excise and sales taxes for cigarettes sold on reservations. One of the more contentious of these efforts is that of New York State. For many years, a New York statute has required the collection of state taxes on cigarettes sold at reservation outlets to individuals not residing on the reservation. The state has generally not enforced the policy, however, despite a 1996 U.S. Supreme Court decision allowing it to do so. An enforcement effort in 1997 led to a Seneca Nation protest that closed a portion of the New York State Thruway, a highway that crosses tribal land. As New York's cigarette tax increased over time and the state lost more revenue to reservation purchases by nonresidents, the state legislature renewed calls for the policy to be enforced. In 2003, enforcement was mandated as part of a state budget bill. Despite this mandate, as well as subsequent legislation passed under governors Eliot Spitzer and David Paterson, New York State has not resolved the legal and political problems raised by collection of excise and sales taxes for cigarettes sold on reservations. If enforcement ever begins, the New York experience will provide valuable information about the costs and effectiveness of this type of policy.

Other states have adopted more straightforward methods for collecting cigarette taxes on reservation sales. These approaches generally involve state collection of taxes from wholesalers or distributors on cigarettes destined for reservations, and the return of a portion of these taxes to the tribe based on the share of reservation sales made to tribal members (Zello 2005). Nebraska, for example, allows reservation retailers to obtain a credit from wholesalers for the taxes paid on sales to reservation residents, while Wisconsin refunds to tribal councils the state tax on cigarettes consumed by tribal members. A related approach used in some states including Washington allows for a small number of untaxed cigarettes to be provided to registered tribes for sale to tribal members, with the number based on the tribal population and expected consumption. Nothing prevents these cigarettes from being sold to nonresidents, however. Other states require tax-exempt stamps to be attached to cigarettes sold to tribal members on reservations. Arizona, for example, requires a "green stamp" on these packs, in contrast to the "blue stamp" applied to cigarettes on which the state excise taxes have been paid.[14]

The final approach is least common but simplest administratively: collect state cigarette taxes from all cigarettes sold anywhere in the state, including those sold on reservations and to tribal members, with no refunds or credits. Kansas, for example, does not exempt from tax cigarettes or tobacco products that are sold on Indian reservations or land, or sold to retailers who are Indian tribes or tribal members (Notice 00-07 2000). The U.S. Supreme Court decision concerning Kansas's taxation of gasoline sold on reservations suggests this may be a viable option in other states (*Wagnon v. Prairie Band Potawatomi Nation*, 546 U.S. 95 [no. 04-631], 2005). Clearly, a uniform system applying state cigarette excise taxes to all cigarettes, without exceptions for tribal members, is the simplest option. It would eliminate an important channel for tax avoidance and would also mean that reservations in high-tax states like New York could no longer operate profitable Internet sales operations. The political feasibility of extending state tax laws to Indian reservations remains to be tested.

OTHER INDIVIDUAL TAX AVOIDANCE AND EVASION ACTIVITIES

Individuals can engage in other forms of tax avoidance and evasion, including cross-border shopping (purchase of cigarettes in lower-tax localities for consumption in their own higher-tax locality) or purchase of cigarettes from duty-free outlets. These behaviors may account for 1 to 2 percent of cigarette consumption nationally and more in populous areas near low-tax jurisdictions. The international Framework Convention on Tobacco Control (FCTC) calls for the elimination or restriction of duty-free cigarette sales; to the extent that countries ratify this treaty, duty-free options will be reduced for Americans traveling abroad.[15] Similarly, the voluntary agreements reached with shipping companies and credit card companies could serve as a model for similar agreements with international airlines for bans on the duty-free sale of tobacco products.

With respect to small-scale cross-border shopping by individual smokers, states have few, if any, cost-effective options for collecting taxes on these sales directly. Instead, regional approaches may be more effective in addressing this problem. For example, efforts to increase cigarette taxes regionally may help reduce interstate tax differentials and thus the incentive for small-scale cross-border shopping. Regional efforts to raise state cigarette taxes in the Northeast and in the South have been somewhat effective in this regard, although sizable differences remain among some states in each region. Likewise, limits on the quantity of cigarettes purchased would reduce the savings from a cross-border shopping trip; such limits would have the added benefit of discouraging larger-scale smuggling.

LARGE-SCALE CIGARETTE SMUGGLING

The large differences in state tobacco tax rates create profitable smuggling opportunities. Most commonly the smuggling pipeline is filled by large purchases of tax-paid cigarettes in low-tax states, which are then transported to high-tax states and sold by retailers as if they were legitimate. Smuggling from other countries in North America is also conceivable but has not been important in the past.

The key federal legislation targeting large-scale cigarette smuggling is the Contraband Cigarette Trafficking Act (CCTA). This law was enacted in 1978 in response to the increase in cigarette smuggling after interstate cigarette tax differentials rose sharply in the 1960s. The Act made it a felony for an unauthorized individual to ship, receive, sell, or possess contraband cigarettes, which were defined as quantities of more than 60,000 cigarettes (300 cartons) for which there was no evidence that taxes had been paid.[16] The act was amended as part of an extension of the USA Patriot Act; the most significant change was lowering the permissible quantity to 10,000 cigarettes (50 cartons).[17] This amendment was added to the USA Patriot Act after the identification of cigarette smuggling operations that generated funds for terrorist organizations.

The application of cigarette tax stamps is likely to be the most important state-level measure targeting large-scale smuggling.[18] Michigan's experiences in the 1990s provide a clear illustration. On May 1, 1994, Michigan's excise tax was raised from 25 cents to 75 cents per pack, making Michigan's tax the highest in the country. At the time, Michigan was one of very few states that did not apply a tax stamp to cigarette packs to indicate that the state tax had been paid. Although cigarette tax revenues more than doubled after the tax increase, the revenue increase was smaller than expected, with the gap attributed to a dramatic rise in smuggling of cigarettes from low-tax states. This smuggling was facilitated by North Carolina's decision to stop requiring tax stamps on cigarettes at almost the same time as the Michigan tax increase; South Carolina followed suit in 1996. Given state tax rates of five and seven cents, respectively, the elimination of the North and South Carolina tax stamps allowed fortunes to be made by smuggling cigarettes from these states to Michigan. Despite Michigan's enforcement efforts, smuggled cigarettes may have accounted for 15 percent or more of the market at its peak. The loss of revenue to the state prompted Michigan to require a tax stamp on all cigarettes sold in the state, with the new legislation fully implemented by September 1, 1998. The tax stamps strengthened the state's enforcement capacity by making it easier to identify smuggled cigarettes. The impact was dramatic; gross state cigarette tax collections rose by about 14 percent from fiscal year 1998 (ending June 30) to fiscal year 1999.

In early 2010, three states—North Carolina, South Carolina, and North Dakota (with excise taxes of 45, 7, and 44 cents, respectively)—did not require tax stamps. The lack of stamps on cigarettes from these states facilitates smuggling, while the large differences between taxes in these states and those in high-tax states create a significant incentive. Reinstating the stamping requirements in North and South Carolina and introducing this requirement in North Dakota would be a significant step in addressing this problem.

To avoid detection, smuggling operations often employ counterfeit tax stamps that are applied to unstamped packs or substituted for the stamps on packs from low-tax states. To address this problem, California adopted legislation in 2002 that called for a new, high-tech stamp that includes encrypted information identifying the name and address of the distributor who applied the stamp, when it was applied, and its value, along with other features making the stamp more difficult to counterfeit. In addition, the legislation strengthened licensing requirements, making it easier to track cigarettes through the distribution chain. Inspectors using hand-held scanners can quickly scan the stamps, identify packs being sold illegally, and track the sources of the illegal cigarettes. The new stamps were phased in with a target date of January 1, 2005. In late 2005, the *Los Angeles Times* reported that the new stamps had been highly effective in generating revenues and curbing cigarette smuggling. Over the previous 20 months, the state's revenues from tobacco taxes rose by more than $124 million, numerous smuggling rings were identified, and millions of illegal cigarettes were seized (Halper 2005). A report in *Convenience Store News* (2006) noted that 8,420 compliance checks were conducted in fiscal year 2005, leading to 523 citations.

The tactics used by California to crack down on cigarette smuggling, including prominent, difficult-to-counterfeit tax stamps, licensing of those involved in the distribution chain, pack-specific information identifying those in the distribution chain, and stricter recordkeeping requirements, combined with aggressive enforcement, have been suggested for many years (e.g., Joossens et al. 2000;

Sunley, Yurekli, and Chaloupka 2000). The FCTC calls for many of these elements, along with labeling provisions that would help identify packs being sold illegally. California's success shows that similar efforts in other states and at the federal level can be highly effective in reducing cigarette smuggling and increasing revenues generated from tobacco taxes.

EXCISE TAX COMPLIANCE AND REGULATORY REGIMES

Based on this discussion, we can make some qualitative judgments about the implications of a uniform $2 increase in state excise tax on tax compliance (see table 13.1). This tax increase is likely to have little effect on the most common means of avoidance—individual purchases from vendors in low-tax jurisdictions[19]—but would increase the incentive to evade state taxes altogether. Under the existing regulatory regime, direct Internet sales from reservation or foreign vendors are likely to increase, as are smuggling from foreign sources and individual purchases from reservations.

Whether evasion rates would actually increase, however, would depend on the loopholes in the regulatory framework and the intensity of enforcement. As we have seen, there are a variety of regulations that would reduce profits from tax evasion and curtail opportunities for avoidance. The table distinguishes outcomes under two regulatory frameworks—the patchwork of federal and state

TABLE 13.1 Change in Tax Evasion Resulting from Large Tax Increase

EVASION METHOD	REGULATORY FRAMEWORK AS IN 2006	REFORMED REGULATORY FRAMEWORK
Direct Internet sale from		
Reservation	+	0
Abroad	+	0
Low-cost state	0	0
Smuggling from		
Low-tax state	0	0
Foreign sources	+	0
Individual purchase in low-tax state	0	0
Individual purchase on reservation	+	0

Note: + indicates an increase in tax evasion; 0 indicates no change in tax evasion.

regulations that applied in 2006 and a framework that incorporates reforms suggested by the discussion above: (1) all reservations are subject to state cigarette taxes; (2) U.S. Postal Service joins other shippers in refusing to ship cigarettes to evade taxes; (3) embargo continues on use of credit cards to pay for mail-order cigarettes; (4) all states adopt high-tech tax stamps and tracking systems, with regular inspections of the supply chain.

The actual regulatory framework has evolved rather rapidly and may approach something like this new configuration in the near future. The result would be to close the principal loopholes by which cigarette taxes are currently evaded. Under this new regime, consumers could continue to avoid taxes by purchasing cigarettes in low-tax jurisdictions. As shown in the table, however, the incentive for individuals to purchase in other jurisdictions would be just the same after a uniform $2 increase in state taxes as it is now—all prices would be higher, but interjurisdiction price differences would remain approximately the same.

The costs of tax enforcement depend on the intensity of the enforcement effort chosen by the relevant government agencies. To the extent that enforcement budgets are influenced by the marginal payoff in terms of additional tax collections, we expect these expenditures to be influenced by both the regulatory framework and the tax rate. In other words, the effect of a tax increase on enforcement expenditures is indeterminate but will likely be influenced by the payoffs (in terms of increased tax collections) from additional enforcement efforts. Jurisdictions choose how much to spend on compliance efforts, and there is nothing about a $2 increase that would compel a change in these efforts. On the other hand the extra $2 per pack tax would ensure a greater payoff to compliance efforts for all but the relatively low-tax states, which might benefit even more from purchase for illegal sale elsewhere. There is no good way to predict states' budget priorities in this new regime.

YOUTH ACCESS

A number of regulations aim to reduce youth access to tobacco and lower smoking initiation among teenagers. These youth access laws include state laws prohibiting sale to minors, prohibitions on self-service displays, and restrictions on placement of vending machines. Most states also sanction minors for purchasing, using, or possessing tobacco products (the so-called PUP laws). Although laws prohibiting the sale of cigarettes to minors have been on the books since the 1890s, these laws were rarely enforced. For example, in 1988 minors are estimated to have purchased about 1 billion cigarettes, yet there were only 32 reported violations of youth access laws in all 50 states (Centers for Disease Control 1990). The impact of PUP laws is debated among tobacco control experts, with some asserting that criminalization of purchase, use, and possession may glamorize tobacco products and heighten their appeal to teens (Wakefield and Giovino 2003).

The Synar Amendment passed by Congress in 1992 put a national youth-access policy into place. It stipulated that states would lose federal funding for mental health programs if they failed to adopt and adequately enforce stringent regulations. The law required states to set the minimum age for the legal purchase of tobacco products at 18 or higher. It also required states to enforce youth access tobacco laws by auditing retail tobacco outlets. A state agency (or a private concern under contract) was to conduct random, unannounced audits using decoy minors. States were required to reduce the retailer violation rate to below 20 percent by a deadline that depended on the rate of noncompliance in the base year, 1997. All states were to be in compliance by 2003. By 2005, Kansas was the only state with a noncompliance rate above 20 percent, at 38 percent.[20] In 2009, the average noncompliance rate among the states was 10.9 percent, and several states had noncompliance rates below 5 percent.[21]

Although most states' compliance rates meet federal standards, survey evidence indicates that youth access to cigarettes has changed little since 1992 (Centers for Disease Control and Prevention 2006; DiFranza, Savageau, and Bouchard 2001). One reason is that, with a noncompliance rate of 10.9 percent, minors can still purchase cigarettes at almost one in nine retailers. In addition, many teens get cigarettes from older friends and family members. There is evidence that for younger teens, access to cigarettes through retail purchase has declined, but access from social sources (family and friends) may have increased.[22]

The Synar compliance checks may not be very effective at identifying retailers who sell to minors. The usual audit procedure is to send a minor into a store to attempt to buy a pack of cigarettes. States are advised to follow the Substance Abuse and Mental Health Services Administration (SAMHSA) protocol for these underage purchases by decoys. However, this protocol does not capture the way in which most young people would actually try to buy cigarettes. Decoy minors are not allowed to lie about their age or use false identification; actual underage purchasers are likely to do both. Indeed, when minors presented a bona fide ID card upon request by a store clerk, they were six times more likely to be allowed to buy cigarettes, even though the ID card identified them as underage (Levinson, Hendershott, and Byers 2002). In addition, clerks are much more likely to sell cigarettes to minors who are frequent customers, but decoy minors are unlikely to have visited the store frequently enough to become familiar to store clerks (Landrine and Klonoff 2003).

Because the Synar Amendment penalizes states that record high rates of noncompliance, state agencies have little incentive to use more effective means of detecting youth access violations (DiFranza 2001; U.S. General Accounting Office 2001). For example, states have discretion regarding age and sex of decoys. Knowing that 14-year-old boys are probably more likely to be refused service than 17-year-old girls creates an incentive to use the former as decoys. Furthermore, Synar audits often lead to enforcement activity that tips off other stores in the area, temporarily raising compliance rates. Because both state agencies and retailers have an incentive to avoid successful purchases by decoys, the Synar noncompliance rates are likely to understate the number of retailers who sell cigarettes to minors. Indeed, underage smokers claim that purchasing cigarettes is relatively easy even in communities with high measured compliance rates (DiFranza and Coleman 2001).

In addition to these problems with compliance checks, the penalties available to states are weak. In 32 states, as of 2006, regulators could not impose civil or administrative penalties on retailers selling cigarettes to minors.[23] In these states, the only resort was criminal prosecution of a clerk, a cumbersome and unrewarding venture. Youth access laws structured in this way legally insulate owners and allow them to make underage sales with little risk of prosecution.[24]

Even when retailers can be fined, current sanctions may not be a sufficient deterrent. Fines are typically graduated but are rarely more than $1,000.[25] These fines are trivial compared with the profitability of convenience store sales to underaged teens. DiFranza and Librett (1999) estimated that underage smokers in 1996 spent about $1.9 billion (2006 dollars)—in other words, about $8,500 per store if distributed evenly among the roughly 221,000 retail outlets selling tobacco in 2002.[26] Underage smokers buy cigarettes mostly from convenience and liquor stores and gas stations; if all such purchases were made from these outlets, the annual revenue per store would be about $14,000, with a net revenue of $1,100 assuming a 10 percent markup. If the retailer is caught and fined $500 once a year, then profits net of the penalty are still positive. If only a small percentage of this subset of stores sell cigarettes to teens, then profit rates are higher. When only 20 percent of outlets are noncompliant and the detection rate is 50 percent, net profits rise to $6,800.

In some states, penalties for retailers selling cigarettes to minors can include suspension or revocation of retail tobacco licenses. Of the 40 states that required licenses in 2005,[27] 28 allow suspension of the licenses of stores selling to underage youths, and 12 allow revocation of retail licenses for repeated noncompliance with youth access.[28] License revocation is a severe penalty because about 25 percent of all convenience store revenues, an annual average of $206,000 or about $3,400 per week (2006 dollars), comes from cigarette sales.[29] But even in states that permit it, licenses are rarely revoked.

The IOM policy scenario calls for strengthening youth access laws by requiring four randomly timed compliance checks each year at each tobacco retailer, with penalties for noncompliance that are potent and well enforced, and with heavy publicity and community involvement. For the SimSmoke simulations, maximum civil penalties were set at $1,000 and suspension of the retailer's license to sell tobacco products,[30] with graduated civil penalties, universal licensure for tobacco retailers, and bans on vending machines and self-service displays. The SimSmoke youth access module also assumes "full community mobilization" and wide publicity.

In addition to these policies, other measures are considered "best practice" by the American Lung Association and industry sources on youth access.[31] One is electronic age verification. By 2010, all states except Wyoming issued driver's licenses with magnetic stripes or bar codes; licenses of young customers can be scanned into an electronic scanning device that verifies age.[32] This makes false identification easier to detect and records the purchase if it occurs. In Connecticut the use of ID scanners is the only affirmative defense for making an underage sale, providing an incentive to install and use the devices. (If the customer appears to be underage and presents an out-of-state driver's license, both the customer and license are photographed.) Finally, enforcement would be strengthened by establishment of a statewide agency charged with monitoring and enforcing compliance with youth access laws. Enforcement costs could, at least in part, be financed by the fines collected (U.S. Department of Health and Human Services 2000).[33]

What would be the direct cost of imposing these policies? One approach is to cost out specific policy measures. For instance, four compliance checks per year at each retail outlet selling tobacco, at an average cost of $170 per audit, yields a total cost of about $150 million.[34] Modifying the audit protocol to establish familiarity (two extra visits per establishment) might add $86 million to the cost of compliance checks.[35] The total national annual cost of ID scanners is likely to be about $110 million,[36] which would presumably be borne by the retailers. The cost of a bureau to issue and revoke licenses and administer fines would differ widely by state, but in any event, that cost is likely to be covered by the collection of fines and fees. These considerations suggest total costs of about $346 million, with almost a third of that cost borne by retailers. Because the states already conduct some compliance checks, the marginal cost of achieving the best practice level would be lower.

Alternatively, enforcement costs can be estimated using CDC best practice funding formulas (Centers for Disease Control and Prevention 1999, 4), which estimate the cost of a package of measures similar to those proposed by the IOM. The CDC enforcement formula (which includes enforcement of both youth access and clean air regulations) recommends expenditures between $0.53 and $0.98 per capita in 2006 dollars as well as fixed costs of administration and interagency cooperation of $187,000 to $367,000 per state. These financial guidelines place annual enforcement costs between $169 million and $314 million in 2006 dollars. The CDC also provides funding guidelines for other statewide programs that include grants to cities and local law enforcement agencies to aid in enforcing youth access laws.[37] The suggested range of expenditures for these programs is $146 to $366 million. Taken together, then, the estimated total cost of enforcing youth access laws would range from $313 to $680 million. Our estimate of $346 million for compliance checks is at the low end of this range—not surprising because the CDC best practice figures include other youth access enforcement measures as well as the cost of clean air enforcement.

With youth access laws, as with excise taxes, regulatory change could improve compliance at relatively modest cost. For instance, the minimum age of legal purchase could be raised to 19 (as it currently is in four states), or even 21; this would mean that very few high school students could legally obtain cigarettes from commercial outlets and would limit social sources of cigarettes for underage smokers. Second, allowing minor decoys to lie about their age and to use ID (both valid and fraudulent) would give a more accurate indication of teen access to cigarettes through retail outlets. Although these additional measures are not explicitly assumed by the SimSmoke model, they may be necessary to achieve the reduction in youth smoking assumed by the SimSmoke simulations.[38] The 2009 passage of the Family Smoking Prevention and Tobacco Control Act, which grants the Food and Drug Administration (FDA) authority to regulate the distribution of tobacco products, requires age verification with photo ID for purchase of tobacco products by anyone up to age 26. However, it is too soon to tell what implications FDA regulation of tobacco products will have for youth access enforcement mechanisms, costs, and effectiveness.

SMOKE-FREE AIR LAWS

The enactment of smoke-free air laws by federal, state, and local governments is an attempt to protect nonsmokers from exposure to the health and other effects of secondhand smoke. Although most such laws are enacted by states, counties, and municipalities, the federal government has intervened in several instances. In 1988 President Ronald Reagan signed the Federal Aviation Act into law, making all domestic flights lasting two hours or less smoke-free. In 1990, all domestic flights lasting six hours or less became smoke-free. In 2000, the Wendell H. Ford Aviation and Investment and Reform Act made all flights to and from the United States smoke-free. The Pro-Children's Act of 1994 prohibited smoking in facilities that receive federal funding for children's services on a regular or routine basis.

All 50 states and the District of Columbia have enacted laws restricting smoking in certain public places. Many states and hundreds of municipalities have legislated complete indoor smoking bans in various public places and private worksites. As of April 1, 2010, comprehensive bans on workplace smoking covered jurisdictions that included 57.2 percent of the total U.S. population, while restaurants were subject to comprehensive smoking bans for 68.1 percent and bars 57.1 percent (American Nonsmokers Rights Foundation 2010). Most other states had partial bans in place. For comparison, the IOM-based scenario used throughout this volume assumes that all states ban smoking in indoor worksites and restaurants and in three out of four other categories of places (government buildings, retail stores, public transportation, and elevators).

Several outdoor smoking bans have been enacted. In 2004, California prohibited smoking within 20 feet of all public building entrances, exits, operable windows, and air intakes. Moreover, a growing number of local-level ordinances have banned smoking in outdoor areas. Solana Beach, California, became the first city in the continental United States to enact a beach smoking ban in 2003. By 2010, 97 municipalities had prohibited smoking on public beaches.[39] In addition, many municipalities have enacted smoking bans in outdoor areas including arenas, stadiums, public parks, school grounds, and bus stops.

Through a series of detailed case studies, Jacobson and Wasserman (1997, 1999) were among the first to examine the process by which smoke-free air laws were enforced. They concluded that, with few exceptions, individuals voluntarily comply with smoke-free air laws in the absence of proactive enforcement efforts by either state or local agencies. The states that Jacobson and Wasserman studied spent few resources enforcing smoke-free air laws because the enforcement mechanisms were mainly complaint driven; in other words, enforcement agencies would respond to complaints made against individuals and establishments after violations had occurred.

Studies suggest that complaints of violations of clean air laws rise after a smoking ban is passed but then decline over time. For instance, when restaurants became smoke-free in New York City in 1995, there was initially a dramatic increase in complaints that subsided within two years (Hyland, Cummings, and Wilson 1999). Moreover, Massachusetts experienced a large number of complaints immediately following the enactment of its smoke-free workplace law. According to the Massachusetts Tobacco Control Program (2006), 742 calls were placed to the complaint and information phone line during the first month after the law went into effect (18 percent of them about alleged violations). The number of calls quickly declined; by the twelfth month following the enactment of the law, only 29 calls were received.

Several studies have found smoking bans to be highly effective despite limited enforcement. Skeer et al. (2004) found that the percentage of bars in Boston observed with smokers decreased from 100 percent before the implementation of a smoking ban to 2.5 percent within 3 months of the enactment of the ban. The smoking ban in Boston was supported by preimplementation outreach and educational campaigns by the Boston Public Health Commission. Skeer and colleagues speculate that the education and media campaign contributed to the high compliance rate.[40] Weber et al. (2003) examined long-term compliance by bar patrons with the California Smoke-Free Workplace Law in Los Angeles County. They found compliance rates increased in each of the four years after the California Smoke-Free Workplace Law was implemented. In particular, the percentage of free-standing bars in Los Angeles County that were observed to be smoke-free increased from 46 percent in 1998 (the year the smoking ban was implemented) to 76 percent in 2002. Among bars with restaurants, the percentage that were smoke-free rose from 92 percent in 1998 to 98.5 percent in 2002. Lee, Moore, and Martin (2003) examined compliance by patrons of free-standing bars five years after the California Smoke-Free Workplace Law began, using unobtrusive observation techniques in an unnamed California city. They found that smoking was observed at least once in half of the bars, suggesting a lower compliance rate for this California city than Los Angeles County. Interestingly, a one-year review of the law requiring smoke-free workplaces in the Republic of Ireland found compliance rates over 90 percent in workplaces, including hotels, restaurants, and pubs; a phenomenally high 93 percent of the public thought the law was a good idea, including 80 percent of smokers (Office of Tobacco Control 2005). Similarly, Fong and colleagues (2006) surveyed smokers in Ireland a few months before the ban was implemented and eight to nine months afterward, and found that the Irish law led to dramatic declines in smoking in workplaces (from 62 percent to 14 percent), restaurants (from 85 percent to 3 percent), and bars/pubs (from 98 percent to 5 percent). Moreover, 83 percent of smokers in Ireland thought that the smoking ban was a "good" or "very good" thing.

Why are these bans effective? Social pressure is doubtless much of the explanation. As social acceptance of smoking in public declines, smokers may be more likely to conform to clean air laws, and nonsmokers may be more willing to object when smokers violate the law. In general, these laws have been embraced by the public. Tang and colleagues (2003) found California bar patrons' approval and acceptance of the California smoke-free bar law increased steadily during the first two years. Similarly, two studies of workplace smoking bans found that employee approval increased substantially after smoking restrictions were introduced (Borland et al. 1990; Rosenstock, Stergachis, and Heaney 1986). Following enactment, both studies found, approval of workplace smoking bans increased significantly among both nonsmokers and smokers, with smokers increasing their level of approval more than nonsmokers.

To ensure high compliance rates, some states use random inspections of businesses. For example, in Massachusetts, local health departments funded by the Massachusetts Tobacco Control Program (MTCP) are required to randomly inspect businesses and follow up on reports of violations. Between July 5, 2004 and June 30, 2005, MTCP-funded local health departments conducted 5,356 random inspections yielding a compliance rate of 91 percent (MTCP 2006). Violations included active smoking, smoke odor, or missing signage. Another effort, as described in the aforementioned MTCP (2006) document, by the Massachusetts Association of Health Boards and MTCP-funded Community Mobilization Networks attempted to monitor compliance in bars and restaurants on weekend evenings. They observed 515 establishments and found an 88 percent compliance rate.

The direct costs of enforcing smoke-free air laws fall on state and local governments. Enforcement activities may include conducting inspections (either proactively or in response to complaints), processing complaints, and taking steps to sanction violators. The example of New York State is instructive. Enforcement of the state's smoke-free air laws—New York State Clean Indoor Air Act (CIAA) and New York City (NYC) Smokefree Air Act (SFAA)—is carried out locally by city or county health departments or by state health department district offices, and usually by the public health sanitarians or technicians who also enforce the youth access and sales-to-minors laws. Enforcement is funded by contractual agreement with the state at levels based on the number of tobacco retailers operating within the jurisdiction. Leftover funds from the sales-to-minors program have typically been used to support CIAA enforcement, which is an unfunded mandate. In program year 2006–2007, county health departments and the NYC Department of Health and Mental Hygiene received $5.8 million for tobacco enforcement activities. This represented a 45 percent increase in funding from the previous program year and was intended to enhance local CIAA/SFAA enforcement (personal communication, Brian M. Miner, October 16, 2006). In addition, staffing resources are provided to state district offices for enforcement of youth access laws and the CIAA. Although total funding cannot be broken down by tobacco enforcement program activities, time spent on enforcement activities can. In 2004, the state health department used 366.7 full-time-equivalent staff days for CIAA enforcement activities and conducted 434 inspections (Miner 2005). In the same year, county health departments used 1814.2 full-time-equivalent staff days for CIAA enforcement activities and conducted 4,748 inspections (Miner 2005). Comparable figures are not available for the NYC Department of Health and Mental Hygiene because SFAA inspections cannot be distinguished from other inspections that the agency conducts. The three entities combined issued 2,873 citations for violations of clean air laws, yielding penalties totaling $1,215,550 in 2004 (Miner 2005).

There is also limited evidence on the direct government costs of conducting compliance checks. The MTCP, for example, funds local health departments to conduct random inspections of businesses. Local departments of health receive allocations based on the number of tobacco retailers operating under their jurisdiction. The funds are used for youth access compliance checks, smoke-free-air compliance checks, and administration costs. During the 2005–2006 fiscal year, local health departments received a total of $1,600,000 from MTCP for tobacco control purposes, or $240 per tobacco retailer operating in each community (all figures in this paragraph from personal communication, Eileen M. Sullivan, August 8, 2006). The local health departments are expected to conduct three random smoke-free air and youth access inspections at each tobacco retailer as well as conduct random smoke-free air inspections of other businesses. Approximately $320,000 (20 percent of the funds for tobacco control) received by local health departments from the MTCP were used for smoke-free air compliance checks; the remaining $1,280,000 was used to cover youth access inspections and administrative costs. Businesses found not to be compliant with the Massachusetts Smoke-Free Air ordinance were issued either a ticket with a fine or a citation with no fine. In 2005, 122 tickets and 35 citations were issued for noncompliance with the smoke-free air law, generating revenue of $21,550. On several occasions, search warrants were required in order to conduct the inspections, raising costs by about $100 per site.[41]

As part of the best practice guidelines discussed above, the Centers for Disease Control and Prevention (CDC) (1999) recommended that states spend a minimum of $0.55 per capita in 2008 dollars to enforce youth access laws, retailer licensure provisions, and non–sales policy areas such as smoke-free air restrictions to implement and sustain comprehensive tobacco control programs. Thus, the CDC's minimum recommendation implies that the states should be spending a total of $176 million on tobacco control enforcement in 2008.[42] If we assume other states divide the budget as Massachusetts did, with 20 percent of tobacco funding spent on clean air enforcement, all states combined would spend $35.2 million to enforce smoke-free air laws as part of a minimally funded comprehensive tobacco control program.

Opponents of smoking bans argue that the imposition of such laws would inflict economic losses on bars and restaurants and have a negative impact on employment levels in localities that enact such laws. The chapter by Hyland and colleagues (chapter 7) examines the merit of this argument. Businesses operating in smoke-free air environments may actually reap cost savings. Potential operational cost savings include lower fire insurance premiums, reduced cleaning costs, lower capital replacement costs because of fewer burned materials, and reduced absenteeism of employees. Unfortunately, we have little evidence about these cost savings, and future research about their magnitude is warranted.

CONCLUSION

This chapter examined the enforcement of three tobacco control policies: excise taxes, youth access laws, and clean air laws. As we have discussed, there are efficient methods for improving tax compliance that require little in the way of additional government resources. Interstate smuggling could be greatly reduced if the low-tax states raised their rates. Barring that, any state could fend off illegal imports through measures such as improved tax stamps, licensing of those involved in the distribution chain, and better record-keeping requirements. Internet marketing from Indian reservations could be reduced simply by requiring that prices paid in tribal stores include state excise taxes (something the states could do, according to a Supreme Court ruling on a related matter). The Internet market has already been curtailed by state enforcement efforts coupled with agreements with shippers and credit card companies and will be limited further with the enactment of the PACT Act. These and other measures are not expensive and are likely to be effective. The scarce resource is political will.

We have not estimated the enforcement costs that would be associated with a $2 a pack increase in excise tax rates because states would not be obligated to spend more on enforcement as a result of the tax increase. There would, however, be some incentive for them to do so under the current regulatory regime, for two reasons. First, the higher tax rates would probably induce more tax avoidance and evasion activity, especially mail-order sales from Indian reservations and abroad, and in-person purchases from reservations and military installations. In addition, the loss of tax revenue for every pack for which the state tax was not paid would be $2 greater than otherwise. But we argue that if all the states adopted several simple reforms, such as taxing sales on reservations and using high-tech cigarette-tax stamps, those methods of evasion would be far less profitable and hence less prevalent, and thus, states would have correspondingly little incentive to increase enforcement expenditures. With those reforms in place, any given level of excise taxation would be more effective in promoting the public health.

Compliance with youth access and clean air laws can also be improved through change in the regulatory framework, but both also require regular compliance checks for the regulations to be effective. We provide some rough estimates of the costs of compliance checks for both tobacco retailers and other entities governed by clean air provisions. If every state conducted several inspections of tobacco outlets each year and ran a vigorous program of clean air inspections while supporting local community efforts with a grants program, the total cost could be between $176 million and $329 million.[43] Some part of that cost would be defrayed by income from fines. Because states are already funding compliance efforts, the marginal cost would be far less. To put these estimates in perspective,

total state expenditures for all aspects of tobacco control, prevention, and cessation programs were about $717 million in FY2008.[44]

NOTES

1. This section focuses on cigarette taxation, but the policies that are discussed generally apply to other tobacco products, including loose tobacco.
2. Alaska, Delaware, Montana, New Hampshire, and Oregon do not impose a general
sales tax, while the general sales tax is not applied to cigarettes in Minnesota and
Oklahoma (Orzechowski and Walker 2008).
3. Similarly, the Internal Revenue Code (chapter 52) requires that federal excise taxes are
to be paid on cigarettes sold by foreign-based vendors; to the extent that foreign vendors
are not compliant with this policy, they are also likely to be noncompliant with other
federal policies, including those requiring health warning labels (Cohen 2005).
4. The same applies with respect to payment of the federal cigarette tax on purchases
made from foreign-based vendors. To date, there is little evidence to indicate that
foreign-based Internet vendors account for more than a minimal share of online
cigarette sales. However, as efforts targeting domestically based vendors become increasingly successful, foreign-based vendors' share is likely to increase.
5. More recent data on the actual level of Internet sales and resulting lost tax revenues
are not available.
6. For details, see the "Illinois Cigarette Use Tax Return," available online at http://
www.revenue.state.il.us/taxforms/Misc/Cig/rc44.PDF.
7. The Bureau of Alcohol, Tobacco and Firearms, which until 2003 was part of the
Department of Treasury (and is now in the DOJ), has "ancillary" authority to enforce
the Act when the sales under investigation may be violations of the Contraband
Cigarette Trafficking Act (discussed below), for which it has primary enforcement
authority (U.S. General Accounting Office 2002).
8. An effort to systematically collect this information from states for use in this chapter
was unsuccessful.
9. www.smartsmoker.com/content/aboutus.asp, accessed March 12, 2006.
10. www.simplysmoke.com/faq.php#Legal, accessed March 15, 2006.
11. www.cigoutlet.net and www.simplysmoke.com/privacy.php, accessed March 15, 2006.
12. It appears that these agreements do not extend to the use of credit cards for purchases from foreign-based vendors. For example, the SimplySmoke.com and Cigout-
let.net sites discussed above indicate that they accept payment by credit card.
13. At the time of the agreement, the Washington State cigarette excise tax was $14.25
per carton, along with a state sales tax of 6.5 percent.
14. Arizona also uses a "red stamp" for cigarettes that are sold at reservation outlets to
non-tribal members, on which a lower tax is applied.
15. This would be true regardless of whether or not the United States ratifies the treaty.
16. There are exemptions in the Act for common carriers and in states where there are
no tax markings required.
17. Some states have limits below those set by the CCTA or the recent amendment to
the CCTA.
18. State tax stamps are applied by cigarette wholesalers, who generally receive a modest
commission from the state for the application of the stamp.

19. The uniform increase in state tax rates would leave the current disparities unchanged in an absolute sense—Chicago residents would save the same amount per carton by driving to Indiana. But the relative disparities would be reduced by raising all taxes, and that may make some difference in cross-border purchases.
20. The Synar data for years 1997–2009 can be found on the Substance Abuse and Mental Health Services Administration (SAMHSA) Web site at http://prevention.samhsa.gov/tobacco/01synarreport2009.pdf.
21. Authors' calculation from Synar data provided by SAMHSA Web site mentioned in note 20.
22. According to Monitoring the Future, a survey of a nationally representative sample of 50,000 8th, 10th, and 12th graders, the perception of the availability of cigarettes has declined for both 8th and 10th graders. See http://www.monitoringthefuture.org/data/05data/cfig05_1.pdf.
23. This number is extracted from the American Lung Association (2006), which provides the relevant text from state youth access laws.
24. Some retail outlets have very high turnover rates for their employees. On average, the staff of a convenience store turns over almost completely in a year. For full-time employees, turnover is about 102 percent annually, and for part-time employees the turnover rate is 138 percent (National Association of Convenience Stores press release December 12, 2002 at www.nacsonline.com/NACS/news/press_release.
25. American Lung Association (2006); ImpacTeen data at http://www.impacteen.org/tobaccodata.htm.
26. Authors' calculation; the number of retail outlets is from U.S. Department of Commerce (2006). Other figures on retail establishments cited here are also from U.S. Department of Commerce (2006).
27. This is for the fourth quarter of 2005 and obtained from the State Tobacco Activities and Tracking and Evaluation (STATE) System Web site, which is provided by the CDC. The Web site URL is http://apps.nccd.cdc.gov/statesystem/index.aspx.
28. American Lung Association (2006); ImpacTeen data at http://www.impacteen.org/tobaccodata.htm.
29. Authors' calculation using U.S. Department of Commerce (2006).
30. Personal communication with David Levy, September 15, 2006; also see Levy and Friend (2000).
31. Connecticut and New York received "A" from the American Lung Association for the design and enforcement of their youth access laws. The industry site WeCard.org recommends the purchase of electronic age verification devices as a best practice.
32. http://www.aamva.org/KnowledgeCenter/DLIDStandards/IDSecurityTechnologies/uslicensetechnology.htm.
33. Most of these recommendations are found in Centers for Disease Control and Prevention (1999). The American Lung Association (2006) recommends electronic ID scanning in its best practices report for 2005. DiFranza (2005) provides an updated list of best practices.
34. The cost per audit at the state level reported in DiFranza et al. (2001) is $150 (2001 dollars), which is $170 in 2006 dollars.
35. The figure is calculated by the authors assuming a cost of $170 (2006 dollars); see note 34 for details.

36. The cost of ID scanners ranges between $300 and $1,400, so complete coverage for the United States lies between about $60 million and $300 million. Assuming full depreciation in three years and using the upper price limit, this works out to an annual mean cost of $500 per retailer. Some retailers will of course require more than one scanner. Cost figures are from one manufacturer, Tokenworks, at http://www.cardvisor.com/shop/store/dynamicIndex.asp.

37. This includes funds for program evaluation, media advocacy, and grants to various nongovernmental organizations to inform various population subgroups about tobacco control.

38. Personal communication with David Levy, September 15, 2006; also see Levy and Friend (2000).

39. American Nonsmokers Rights Foundation, "Municipalities with Smokefree Beach Laws," April 1, 2010.

40. An earlier study of compliance with a local ordinance in Cambridge, implemented in 1986, found low compliance rates in stores. Employees reported that after two years, 38 percent of stores allowed customers to smoke (Rigotti et al. 1993).

41. Law student interns were used to obtain the search warrants.

42. These numbers are updated from the CDC's recommendations for 1999 on enforcement and administration expenditures. The recommended enforcement in 1999 was $0.43 (minimum) to $.80 (maximum) per capita. Those recommendations, updated to 2008 using the CPI inflation calculator, are $0.55 to $1.03. The U.S. population as of May 2008 is 304 million, so the total enforcement budget should be $167.3 to $313.3 million. The CDC specified 1999 administrative costs as 5 percent of program costs, yielding a total recommended enforcement plus administrative cost of $175.7 to $329.0 million.

43. See note 42.

44. Campaign for Tobacco-Free Kids, "Key State Specific Tobacco-Related Data and Rankings," at http://www.tobaccofreekids.org/reports/settlements/2008/execsum.pdf.

14

STIGMA AND SMOKING INEQUALITIES

JENNIFER STUBER, SANDRO GALEA, AND BRUCE LINK

In the last half century the cigarette has been transformed. The fragrant has become foul. . . . An emblem of attraction has become repulsive. A mark of sociability has become deviant. A public behavior is now virtually private. Not only has the meaning of the cigarette been transformed but even more the meaning of the smoker [who] has become a pariah . . . the object of scorn and hostility.

—ALLAN BRANDT (1998)

Few within the tobacco control community would disagree with Brandt's analysis that the social unacceptability of cigarette smoking has grown substantially over the last half century in the United States. What is perhaps more controversial in his analysis is whether smokers themselves have become the object of scorn and hostility.

Stigma, we suggest, is a double-edged sword. On the one hand, stigma may be a useful and underrecognized tool for reducing the prevalence of smoking. Concerns about stigma might discourage initiation of smoking or strengthen the motivation to quit. Between 2000 and 2004, the CDC estimates, smoking and exposure to tobacco smoke were associated with $96 billion in medical costs, $96.8 billion in lost productivity, and 443,000 premature deaths annually in the United States (Centers for Disease Control and Prevention 2008). If stigma did reduce smoking, there might be significant benefits for individual smokers and for society.

However, it is possible that stigma has unintended and potentially harmful or counterproductive effects (Bayer and Stuber 2006; Stuber, Galea, and Link 2009). Evidence from other public health epidemics such as tuberculosis and HIV/AIDS suggests that the use of stigma to control behavior can backfire. In these epidemics, stigmatization has promoted the spread of disease by erecting barriers between caregivers and those who are sick and by constraining those who would intervene to contain the spread of illness (Herek 1999; Jaramillo 1999). Among smokers, similar dynamics might occur: for example, smokers who perceive stigma might keep their smoking status a secret from doctors or others who could help them stop smoking (Stuber and Galea 2009) or may withdraw socially from nonsmoking peers, further entrenching their identity as smokers. Additionally, stigma may contribute to disparities in smoking prevalence. There are significant differences in smoking rates by race/ethnicity, gender, socioeconomic status, and sexual orientation. If the perception or effect of stigma differs by social group, these differences may have implications for disparities in smoking rates.

In this chapter we provide a historical perspective on how certain anti-tobacco policy interventions and media campaigns may contribute to the creation of smoking as a stigmatized social status, discuss how many smokers currently perceive stigma, and examine the potential consequences and patterns of the stigmatization of smoking. By stigma, we are following Link and Phelan's (2001) definition whereby stigmatization occurs when labeling, stereotyping, disconnection, status loss, and discrimination all exist within a power situation that allows stigma to occur.

BACKGROUND

We begin with a historical perspective on the U.S. tobacco control movement and the production of smoking as a stigmatized smoking status. The tobacco control movement began with the Surgeon General's 1964 report, which legitimized 15 years of growing evidence about the dangers of smoking to health. Initially, this report did little to shape the patterns of smoking in the United States. The limited impact was due in part to the aggressive marketing of tobacco products by the tobacco industry. A widespread libertarian ethic, which framed government involvement in the affairs of individuals as an unwanted intrusion, was another factor (Brandt 1990). The effort to discourage smoking by providing information about how cigarettes harm the health of smokers had only a modest effect.

This changed when mounting evidence of the health hazards posed by secondhand smoke to nonsmokers made it possible to reframe the debate about smoking in terms that legitimized government and nongovernmental action. What was once considered a matter of individual choice became an issue of nonsmokers' rights to lead healthy lives and hastened policy interventions to discourage smoking (Brandt 1998). Thus, despite intense opposition from the tobacco industry, the emerging scientific consensus on environmental tobacco smoke (ETS) became a powerful force to mobilize public opinion in favor of greater regulation of tobacco products and spawned numerous anti-tobacco media campaigns (U.S. Department of Health and Human Services 1986).

Three such anti-tobacco interventions may have contributed to the creation of smoking as a stigmatized social status by reifying negative stereotypes about smokers, generating social cleavages between smokers and nonsmokers, and creating power differentials between smokers and nonsmokers.

The first type of anti-tobacco intervention that may contribute to the formation of stigma includes policies that restrict the opportunities of smokers in important life domains such as employment and housing. Examples of such policies have emerged in the context of the tobacco epidemic. For example, a 1988 Administrative Management Survey estimated that 6,000 companies (e.g., Alaska Airlines, Union Pacific, and the World Health Organization) refused to hire smokers (National Workrights Institute 1994). Policies such as this make an "us" versus "them" distinction between nonsmokers and smokers, impose material disadvantages on smokers, and symbolically convey society's rejection and exclusion.

A second type of anti-tobacco intervention that may contribute to the formation of stigma is clean air laws in public places such as restaurants or workplaces. These laws convey a symbolic message of moral condemnation and belittlement and contribute to the "us" versus "them" distinction. Although clean air laws regulate the act of smoking, not smokers as a class of people, smokers become temporarily segregated and visible when they are required to smoke outdoors. In addition, one goal of the bans is to convince nonsmokers that they have a stake in enforcing policies that "penalize, isolate, and restrict the activities of smokers in the name of public health" (Gilpin, Lee, and Pierce 2004a). In effect, nonsmokers are deputized to monitor compliance with clean air laws. This allows these laws to be enforced at a trivial expense to the state. However, this strategy for enforcement also pits nonsmokers against smokers; individuals who smoke may face a confrontation with nonsmokers sharing the same venue.

Finally, some tobacco control media campaigns also convey messages of condemnation and belittlement aimed at smokers. A variety of anti-tobacco media strategies have been deployed including some that present graphic depictions of the adverse health consequences of smoking, convey moral arguments about smoking related to ETS, or highlight the deceptive and misleading conduct of the tobacco industry. The media campaigns that may contribute to the formation of stigma are those that belittle smokers or blame smokers for their own poor health and the poor health of others. For example, a 1998 poster from the Centers for Disease Control and Prevention shows the face of a teenage boy who looks into the camera as he is about to light up a cigarette; his face has been superimposed onto a cigarette butt. The message suggests that smoking makes one look like a "butthead"—a reference to stupidity or ridiculousness in the vernacular of teenagers. (We note, of course, that tobacco companies have generated images and messages to counteract these tobacco control media campaigns and to portray the smoker in positive and glamorous ways.)

We do not suggest that the intent of these anti-tobacco interventions is to stigmatize smokers, but rather that the intention is to change the social acceptability of smoking (Gilpin, Lee, and Pierce 2004a). Research suggests this strategy has been quite effective in reducing tobacco use in the United States (Alamar and Glantz 2006b). However, the mechanisms underlying the link between social unacceptability and tobacco use are not well understood and likely also include stigmatization. Tobacco control policies that segregate, alienate, or chastise smokers and depict them in negative ways may contribute to the formation of stigma. As a result, some nonsmokers may develop emotional reactions toward smokers (e.g., disgust), which amplifies discrimination. The embarrassment and shame that some smokers feel as a result of behavior now construed as deviant can further reinforce these sentiments.

Having discussed the possible connection between anti-tobacco interventions and stigma, we now turn to empirical evidence about stigma among current and former smokers. We provide some preliminary answers to the following questions: (1) How common are perceived stigma and perceptions of unfair treatment among smokers and ex-smokers? (2) Is perceived stigma associated with smoking cessation? (3) Among current smokers, is stigma associated with keeping one's smoking status a secret from a health care provider and with social withdrawal from nonsmoking peers? (4) Does the perception of stigma vary by gender, race/ethnicity, or socioeconomic status? (5) Are perceptions of anti-tobacco policies related to stigma?

METHODS

SAMPLE

This study is based on survey questions appended to the New York Social Environment Study (NYSES). The NYSES is a cross-sectional random-digit dial (RDD) telephone survey of 4,000 New York City residents aged 18 or older. It was conducted between June and December 2005 by the University of Michigan. It was designed to assess the relationship between neighborhood characteristics and drug use behavior—including tobacco, alcohol, and illicit drug use—and collected information on a range of demographic and social factors shown to be associated with drug use behavior as well as information on prevalence of use. The NYSES was administered in English, Spanish, Mandarin, and Cantonese and employed structured telephone-based interviews using closed-ended questions. The response rate among those persons eligible for the NYSES was 54 percent (American Association for Public Opinion Research 2003), which is typical for RDD telephone studies (Galea et al. 2003). Comparisons of the NY-SES sample to the U.S. Census indicate that the sample is representative of New York City residents.

The findings discussed in this chapter are based on responses from 915 current smokers and ex-smokers who stopped smoking after January 2002. We expected that ex-smokers who quit relatively recently would have better recall of stigma associated with smoking. The date January 2002 was chosen because this is when NYC began to enact aggressive tobacco control policies, including a $1.50 tax increase on a pack of cigarettes. A year later, the city's smoking ban was extended to all restaurants and bars (Frieden et al. 2005).

MEASURES

There were no extant measures of smoker-related stigma, perceived unfair treatment due to one's smoking, social withdrawal from nonsmoking peers, or keeping one's smoking a secret available in the literature. To aid in designing these new measures, we pretested the survey on 20 participants randomly selected from New York City and elicited from these participants commentary about the questions. We refined the survey after the pretesting phase of the study. Figure 14.1 shows the four items used to create a stigma index. Responses to each component question were on a four-point Likert scale that ranged from strongly disagree to strongly agree. We created a summary score of these four items ($\alpha = 0.61$) and divided it into tertiles representing low, medium, and high stigma.

Three items were used to measure perceived unfair treatment. We asked: Have any of the following things ever happened to you because of your smoking? Have you had difficulty renting an apartment? Were you turned down for a job for which you were qualified? Were you refused or charged more for your health insurance? Response categories were no (coded as 0) and yes (coded as 1). We created a measure from these three items, coded with 0 representing experiencing no events and 1 representing experiencing at least one event of unfair treatment. Three items were included in the survey to measure social withdrawal from nonsmokers: As a smoker, it is awkward to socialize with nonsmokers. As a smoker, I socialize more with smokers than with nonsmokers. As a smoker, I avoid people with negative opinions about smokers ($\alpha = 0.63$). Response categories ranged from 1 to 4 (strongly disagree, somewhat disagree, somewhat agree, strongly agree). We created a summary score of these three items (ranging from 1 to 10). To assess secrecy, respondents were asked three yes-or-no questions: Have you ever kept your smoking a secret from your doctor or other health care

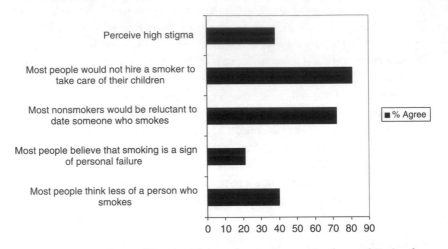

FIGURE 14.1 Prevalence of Perceived Stigma Among Current Smokers and Ex-Smokers (*N* = 915)

Source: New York Social Environment Study.

provider? Have you ever kept your smoking a secret from a close friend or family member? Have you kept your smoking a secret from an employer? A summary score of these three items was created based on the number of secrets told (0–3).

To assess current smoking status we coded current smokers as 1 and ex-smokers as 0. Socioeconomic status was assessed by educational level (coded as less than high school, high school or GED, some college or college graduate, and graduate school). Individual-level income was measured using the categories $40,000, $40,001–$80,000, $80,001+, and missing. Employment status categories included employed full-time, employed part-time, unemployed, and other (out of the labor force). Age was measured continuously and in three categories (18–34, 35–54, 55+). Race/ethnicity was self-reported using the following categories: white, Latino, black, and other. Self-reported health status (coded as excellent, very good, or good versus fair or poor); whether one is the parent of a child under the age of 21; tobacco dependence, measured using the World Mental Health Comprehensive International Diagnostic Interview (CIDI) (Kessler and Ustun 2004); and the number of major stressors (0, 1, 2, 3, or 4+) experienced in the last 12 months are other variables included in the analyses.

To measure perceived enforcement of smoke-free air laws in bars, we asked respondents which statement best describes smoking in bars in their neighborhood: people smoke in all bars (coded as 1); people smoke in some bars (coded as 2); people do not smoke in any bars (coded as 3); don't know or not relevant because I don't go to the bars in my neighborhood. Those who indicated that people do not smoke in any bars were coded as exposed to smoke-free air laws in bars as compared to everyone else. The same question and coding scheme was used to assess exposure to smoke-free air laws in places of employment.

STATISTICAL ANALYSES

We report the prevalence of stigma and self-reported unfair treatment. To assess the consequences of stigma, in bivariate analyses we assess the relationship between stigma and current smoking status. In a multivariate logistic regression model predicting current smoking status, we regress stigma on current smoking status while controlling for race/ethnicity, employment status, socioeconomic status, age, gender, parental status, self-reported health status, life stressors, and tobacco dependence. Among current smokers, we also examine the correlations among stigma, secrecy, and social withdrawal from nonsmoking peers.

Next, we examine patterns in terms of who perceives stigma utilizing our stigma index as a polychotomous outcome (low, medium, and high). We examine bivariate relations between stigma and race/ethnicity, socioeconomic status, age, gender, current smoking status, perceived unfair treatment due to one's tobacco use, and perceived enforcement of smoke-free air laws in bars and places of employment. We then construct a polychotomous regression model to examine the predictors of stigma including race/ethnicity, socioeconomic status, age, gender, current smoking status, and perceived unfair treatment due to one's tobacco use. Analyses were completed using SAS and SUDAAN to account for complex survey weighting.

RESULTS

PREVALENCE OF STIGMA AND PERCEIVED UNFAIR TREATMENT

Figure 14.1 shows the prevalence of perceived stigma among current smokers and ex smokers. Most respondents agree that most people would not hire a smoker to take care of their children (81 percent) and that most nonsmokers would be reluctant to date someone who smokes (72 percent). Fewer agreed that most people believe that smoking is a sign of personal failure (21 percent) or that most people think less of a person who smokes (39 percent). The first two scale items measure an aspect of stigma that is somewhat different from the second two. The first two reflect the smoker's perception of social distancing by nonsmokers, while the latter two measures more explicitly capture respondents' perception of how other people view them. Because the perception of social distancing by others can be psychologically painful, albeit justified from the vantage point of nonsmokers, we believe the social distance items have reasonable face validity as measures of stigma—an assessment consistent with the α correlation score.

Fewer respondents reported instances of perceived unfair treatment. Thirteen percent said they were charged more for or were refused health insurance because of their smoking. Only 2 percent of respondents said they had been turned down for a job for which they were qualified, and 4 percent reported difficulty renting an apartment because of their smoking. Overall, 16 percent reported experiencing any of these three forms of unfair treatment.

ARE STIGMA AND DISCRIMINATION ASSOCIATED WITH BEING AN EX-SMOKER?

Respondents who perceive more stigma are less likely to report being a current smoker. In table 14.1 we show bivariate associations between age, gender, race/ethnicity, education, income, parental status, marital status, employment status, health status, number of life stressors experienced in the last 12 months, perceived stigma, and current smoking status. In bivariate analyses, only stigma is significantly associated with current smoking status. Respondents who perceive high levels of stigma are less likely to be current smokers than respondents who perceive low levels of stigma (OR=0.42, 95 percent CI [0.21, 0.82]). In a multivariate logistic regression model, respondents who perceive high levels of stigma as compared to those who perceive low levels of stigma remain significantly less likely to be current smokers (OR=0.47, 95 percent CI [0.23, 0.97]).

These results are consistent with the idea that perceived stigma makes people more likely to quit. However, these results are also open to other interpretations. For example, people might acknowledge more stigma once they quit, and stigma might not be the reason why they quit. Although we cannot test this possibility directly with a cross-sectional study, in another paper we examine if ex-smokers are less sympathetic to smokers using a survey item on the difficulty of quitting. When a smoker quits, he or she may feel that other smokers should also be able to quit and, thus, may have less sympathy for those who continue to smoke. We show that ex-smokers were indeed more likely than current smokers to agree that quitting is not difficult, but that including this measure in the analysis doesn't explain the higher levels of stigma reported by ex-smokers (Stuber, Galea, and Link 2008).

TABLE 14.1   Predictors of Being a Current Smoker ($N = 835$) as Compared to an Ex-Smoker Who Quit Recently ($N = 80$)

	TOTAL		BIVARIATE		MULTIVARIATE	
	N	%	OR	95% CI	OR	95% CI
Age						
18–34	273	33.52	Ref	Ref	Ref	Ref
35–54	429	45.10	1.01	(0.55, 1.85)	1.03	(0.55, 1.95)
55+	207	21.38	1.28	(0.63, 2.58)	2.45	(1.01, 6.94)
Female versus male	417	43.8	0.85	(0.50, 1.45)	1.01	(0.59, 1.71)
Race/ethnicity						
White	401	43.94	Ref	Ref	Ref	Ref
Black	250	27.04	1.41	(0.69, 2.88)	1.24	(0.60, 2.57)
Hispanic	193	23.38	0.64	(0.34, 1.19)	0.64	(0.33, 1.27)
Other	44	5.72	2.17	(0.49, 9.53)	1.78	(0.36, 8.81)
Education						
<High school	120	14.46	Ref	Ref	Ref	Ref
High school grad/GED	220	24.42	1.04	(0.40, 2.70)	0.88	(0.37, 2.11)
Some college or college grad	448	48.76	1.25	(0.50, 3.07)	1.25	(0.52, 3.03)
Graduate school	127	12.32	1.22	(0.43, 3.43)	1.33	(0.43, 4.10)
Income						
<$40,000	395	42.36	Ref	Ref	Ref	Ref
$40,000–80,000	271	29.70	1.10	(0.59, 2.07)	0.74	(0.35, 1.58)
$80,000+	159	18.06	0.85	(0.42, 1.72)	0.54	(0.22, 1.27)
Missing	90	9.87	0.84	(0.34, 2.10)	0.52	(0.19, 1.42)
Parent or primary caretaker	346	40.31	1.02	(0.60, 1.73)	0.90	(0.51, 1.60)
Marital status						
Married	293	38.02	Ref	Ref	Ref	Ref
Divorced, widowed, separated	268	24.26	0.79	(0.42, 1.52)	0.61	(0.31, 1.22)
Never married	354	37.72	1.11	(0.60, 2.05)	1.15	(0.58, 2.29)

TABLE 14.1 (*Continued*)

	TOTAL		BIVARIATE		MULTIVARIATE	
	N	%	OR	95% CI	OR	95% CI
Employment status						
Full-time	458	49.21	Ref	Ref	Ref	Ref
Part-time	92	11.07	0.50	(0.21, 1.20)	0.40	(0.17, 0.97)
Unemployed	115	13.40	1.02	(0.42, 2.52)	0.85	(0.32, 2.27)
Other	248	26.32	0.46	(0.26, 0.83)	0.36	(0.18, 0.70)
Health status fair or poor versus excellent, very good, or good	228	24.82	0.72	(0.39, 1.33)	0.78	(0.40, 1.52)
Life stressors last 12 months						
0	221	23.20	Ref	Ref	Ref	Ref
1	261	28.92	0.72	(0.37, 1.41)	0.74	(0.36, 1.55)
2	200	23.15	0.95	(0.44, 2.05)	1.06	(0.47, 2.39)
3+	221	24.72	1.56	(0.72, 3.38)	2.25	(0.85, 5.99)
Tobacco dependent	180	19.86	1.27	(0.68, 2.35)	1.20	(0.69, 2.49)
Stigma						
Low	215	23.46	Ref	Ref	Ref	Ref
Medium	278	31.72	0.83	(0.40, 1.72)	0.90	(0.42, 1.94)
High	308	32.79	0.42	(0.21, 0.82)	0.47	(0.23, 0.97)
Missing	114	12.03	0.58	(0.21, 1.63)	0.77	(0.27, 2.26)

Notes: OR, odds ratio; CI, confidence interval; Ref, reference category.
Source: New York Social Environment Study.

IS STIGMA ASSOCIATED WITH KEEPING ONE'S SMOKING STATUS A SECRET FROM A HEALTH CARE PROVIDER AND WITH SOCIAL WITHDRAWAL FROM NONSMOKING PEERS?

Among current smokers, we find positive associations between smoker-related stigma and both social withdrawal from nonsmoking peers (0.36, $p < 0.001$) and keeping one's smoking status a secret (0.18, $p < 0.001$). These correlations suggest that while stigma, social withdrawal, and secrecy are positively related, they are separate constructs. Thus, current smokers who perceive more smoker-related stigma are more likely to keep their smoking status a secret and to withdraw socially from nonsmoking peers.

DOES STIGMA CONTRIBUTE TO DISPARITIES IN THE SMOKING EPIDEMIC?

We now turn to the question of whether the perception of stigma varies by age, gender, race/ethnicity, or socioeconomic status. Table 14.2 shows there are significant associations between one's education and one's race and smoker-related stigma. Specifically, respondents with some college, a college education, or a graduate school education are more likely to perceive high levels of smoker-related stigma compared to respondents with less than a high school education ($p = 0.0002$). Table 14.2 also shows that whites are more likely to perceive high stigma than are blacks or Latinos ($p = 0.0002$). These results persist in multivariate analyses that control for income, age, gender, and current smoking status (see table 14.3). Although blacks and Latinos currently have lower smoking

TABLE 14.2 Differentiating Characteristics Between Current Smokers and Smokers Who Quit Since January 2002 Who Perceive High Versus Medium Versus Low Stigma

	TOTAL (N = 816)		LOW STIGMA (N = 222)		MEDIUM STIGMA (N = 280)		HIGH STIGMA (N = 314)		
	N	%	N	%	N	%	N	%	p-VALUE
Perceives one or more events of unfair treatment	134	16.95	30	14.21	42	14.10	62	21.64	0.05
Exposure to workplace smoke-free air law versus not	412	49.15	96	41.58	148	53.00	168	50.94	0.06
Exposure to smoke-free air law in neighborhood bars versus not	487	58.21	121	52.28	174	60.01	192	60.79	0.18
Education									0.0002
<High school	108	14.83	51	25.20	20	7.80	37	14.04	
High school grad/GED	188	24.41	58	26.72	61	22.32	69	24.74	
Some college or college grad	393	47.87	89	40.54	154	54.88	150	46.49	
Graduate school	119	12.89	21	7.53	42	15.00	56	14.73	

TABLE 14.2 *(Continued)*

	TOTAL (N = 816)		LOW STIGMA (N = 222)		MEDIUM STIGMA (N = 280)		HIGH STIGMA (N = 314)		p-VALUE
	N	%	N	%	N	%	N	%	
Income									0.20
<$40,000	345	41.15	104	47.76	104	34.87	136	42.25	
$40,000–80,000	249	30.70	64	27.55	93	33.74	92	30.07	
$80,000+	149	18.74	31	14.90	61	22.53	57	17.89	
Missing	73	9.46	22	9.79	22	8.85	29	9.80	
Race/ethnicity									0.0002
White	358	43.29	65	28.19	127	45.02	166	52.23	
Black	219	26.49	74	34.29	80	27.87	65	19.73	
Hispanic/Latino	180	24.54	61	29.68	54	22.72	65	22.64	
Other	40	5.69	14	7.84	12	4.39	14	5.40	
Current smoker	730	91.48	199	94.39	258	93.32	273	87.61	0.02
Age									0.11
18–34	262	35.39	65	32.52	86	33.89	111	38.89	
35–54	390	45.81	110	47.24	150	51.09	130	39.74	
55+	161	18.80	45	20.24	44	15.02	72	21.37	
Marital status									0.75
Married	260	38	69	39	96	38	95	36	
Divorced, separated, widowed	220	23	68	25	69	21	83	23	
Never married	331	40	81	36	114	42	136	41	
Female	366	43.37	94	39.50	130	45.77	142	43.86	0.44

Source: New York Social Environment Study.

TABLE 14.3 Polychotomous Regression Model Predicting High Compared to Low Stigma and Medium Compared to Low Stigma ($N = 816$)

	LOW STIGMA COMPARED TO HIGH STIGMA		LOW STIGMA COMPARED TO MEDIUM STIGMA	
	B	95% CI	B	95% CI
Perceives one or more events of unfair treatment	1.68	(0.46, 6.39)	1.14	(0.28, 4.67)
Education				
< High school	0.30	(0.13, 0.81)	0.19	(0.07, 0.52)
High school grad/GED	0.50	(0.22, 1.15)	0.49	(0.21, 1.12)
Some college or college grad	0.67	(0.33, 1.41)	0.72	(0.35, 1.50)
Graduate school	Ref	Ref	Ref	Ref
Race/ethnicity				
White	3.26	(1.23, 8.65)	2.87	(1.14, 7.25)
Black	1.13	(0.42, 3.09)	1.73	(0.69, 4.37)
Hispanic/Latino	1.38	(0.50, 3.79)	1.76	(0.68, 4.55)
Other	Ref	Ref	Ref	Ref
Smokers who quit since January 2002 as compared to current smokers	0.42	(0.02, 0.85)	0.83	(0.39, 1.76)

Notes: This final model also controls for age, gender, and income. B, regression coefficient; CI, confidence interval; Ref, reference category.
Source: New York Social Environment Study.

rates than whites, these differences in perceived stigma could mean that whites experience more pressure to quit, and might lead to a reversal in this pattern.

ARE TOBACCO CONTROL POLICIES ASSOCIATED WITH PERCEIVED STIGMA?

In this study we were unable to assess participants' exposure to the types of anti-tobacco interventions that might contribute to the formation of smoking as a stigmatized social status. However, we found some suggestive evidence that tobacco control policies may contribute to smoking-related stigma. In bivariate analyses, respondents who experienced one or more forms of unfair treatment were more likely to perceive smoking-related stigma ($p = 0.05$) (see table 14.2).

DISCUSSION

This study is one of the first to examine the prevalence of perceived stigma and its consequences among smokers. We find a high prevalence of perceived stigma in our study population, although experiences of unfair treatment are less common. We also find that perceived stigma is associated with being an ex-smoker. From one perspective, stigma may have a positive effect on public health by lowering smoking rates. But we also found that stigma is also associated with keeping one's smoking status a secret and with social withdrawal from nonsmoking peers. Stigma is also perceived less by persons of lower socioeconomic status and by certain minority groups, potentially contributing to tobacco-related disparities. Thus, we find evidence for stigma in the smoking context as a double-edged sword.

This research was motivated by concern that more vigorous anti-tobacco interventions, such as those proposed by the IOM, would lead to stigmatization of smokers and thereby to negative consequences for those who are unable or unwilling to stop smoking. Although there are sound theoretical reasons to believe that anti-tobacco interventions could promote stigmatization, this is an area that clearly needs more research. Our study was limited to a single jurisdiction; future work should examine the prevalence of stigma and discrimination across multiple jurisdictions to assess whether perceptions of stigma are associated with different types of anti-tobacco interventions. State and local variation in anti-tobacco interventions and the rapid pace of policy change offer many opportunities for such research.

This research could help us understand how tobacco control policies work. In some cases, as with tobacco excise taxes, the way policies work is relatively transparent. In others, such as smoking bans, it is less clear. Smoking bans might reduce smoking by generating stigma, but they might also work by making smoking less convenient. Media campaigns are another example. We do not understand whether media campaigns can change social norms about smoking without stigmatizing people who smoke. Understanding when and how anti-tobacco interventions lead to stigma can inform the design of policies to avoid the counterproductive aspects of stigma generation.

Future studies should also assess how stigma is associated with smoking behavior, including both cessation and initiation, and whether there are group differences in the influence of stigma. For instance, it is possible that stigma has a different effect on adolescents than it does on adults. Stigma may accentuate an oppositional identity associated with smoking and thus heighten its appeal to some adolescents.

In addition, it is far from clear how the stigmatization of smoking will affect disparities in tobacco use (Bayer 2008; Bell et al. 2010). The pronounced social class disparities in smoking prevalence are currently not well understood. Previous studies have shown that blue-collar workers experience a normative environment that is generally more supportive of smoking (Sorensen et al. 2002, 2004). It is possible that differences in perceived stigma are one reason for social class disparities in smoking prevalence.

Similarly, patterns of stigma may have implications for racial differences in smoking. Blacks and Latinos currently smoke less than whites. Tobacco use is one of the few chronic disease risk factors for which blacks and Latinos are at an advantage relative to whites. This pattern could change if anti-tobacco interventions affect some groups more strongly than others. As chapter 16 discusses, we know little about whether anti-tobacco interventions have differential effects by gender, socioeconomic status, or race and ethnicity. Our findings have implications for this question. Whites in our survey reported higher levels of stigma than blacks or Latinos. While we are unable to tie perceptions of stigma directly to changes in anti-tobacco interventions, if white smokers experience more stigma than black or Latino smokers, smoking rates could decline more steeply for whites than for other racial/ethnic groups.

It would also be worthwhile to consider perceptions of stigma among the seriously mentally ill population. As chapter 15 discusses, the quit rates for persons with serious mental illness are substantially lower than those for the general population. It may be that seriously mentally ill persons perceive less smoker-related stigma than non–mentally ill persons. The smoking prevalence in this population is higher; thus, the normative environment surrounding persons with a severe mental illness may be more supportive of smoking. Also, this population already contends with intense stigma related to their mental illness; smoker-related stigma may seem inconsequential by comparison. Thus, it is possible that stigma leads to disparities in the smoking epidemic in yet another way, affecting persons with a severe mental illness less than those without.

We hope this study promotes awareness and discussion within the tobacco control community about how anti-tobacco interventions may lead to stigmatization, and about the implications of stigma for smokers. On the one hand, smoking-related stigma may promote smoking cessation and thus avert disease and premature mortality. On the other hand, it may have unintended consequences for smokers who find quitting more difficult. This issue merits attention because the population of smokers has shifted over time: smokers are increasingly a group that is disproportionately disadvantaged in terms of socioeconomic status. Indeed, it is only because the social class composition of smokers has changed that stigmatization against smokers becomes possible. Decisions about alternative anti-tobacco interventions and media campaign strategy choices should weigh the potential negative consequences of stigma for people who continue to smoke.

15

THE UNMET NEEDS OF SMOKERS
WITH MENTAL ILLNESS OR ADDICTION

JILL M. WILLIAMS, CRISTINE DELNEVO, AND DOUGLAS M. ZIEDONIS

Mental illness is estimated to affect approximately 20 to 30 percent of the U.S. population (U.S. Department of Health and Human Services 1999). Tobacco use among individuals with either a mental illness or an alcohol or other drug use disorder is a significant health problem, with numerous studies showing higher rates of smoking and lower rates of smoking cessation in this population. Indeed, Lasser et al. (2000) estimated that these groups consume nearly half of all cigarettes in the United States.

The consequences of these elevated smoking rates are considerable. Smokers with mental illnesses incur significant tobacco-caused medical illnesses and lose up to 25 years of life expectancy (Brown, Inskip, and Barraclough 2000; Lichtermann et al. 2001; Miller, Paschall, and Svendsen 2006; Stroup, Gilmore, and Jarskog 2000). Mentally ill smokers may experience increased psychiatric symptoms and need higher medication doses compared to nonsmokers (Desai, Seabolt, and Jann 2001; Goff, Henderson, and Amico 1992; Ziedonis et al. 1994). For smokers with an alcohol problem, the health consequences of smoking are complicated by the synergistic effects of alcohol and tobacco, which raise the risk of developing pancreatitis and oral cancers; in fact, alcoholics are more likely to die from smoking than from alcohol-related diseases (Hurt et al. 1996; U.S. Department of Health and Human Services 1982).

Although public health interventions have led to lower smoking rates in the United States over the last 40 years, smokers with mental illness or addiction have benefited less from these efforts. At this time, little is being done nationally at the mental health or public health systems level to promote smoking cessation in this population. Moreover, we know little about smokers with mental illness or addiction: we lack critical information on their tobacco use patterns and the effects of tobacco control measures such as excise taxes, advertising, or clean indoor air laws on this population. If current trends continue, smokers with mental health or other substance use problems may become the majority of tobacco users in the United States. Some speculate that this has already contributed to plateaus in smoking rates that have been observed in the past 15 years despite aggressive tobacco control measures. Evidence-based interventions and enhanced surveillance of this population will be increasingly important to meet national goals for reduction of tobacco use as well as help this group overcome tobacco dependence.

The first part of this chapter reviews existing knowledge about smoking among individuals with mental illness or other addictions. In this context, we present findings from a nationally representative sample that confirm the high smoking prevalence among people with serious mental illness. The second part of this chapter considers the efficacy of tobacco control strategies in this population, with a focus on measures recommended by the IOM. This discussion considers why established tobacco control techniques may prove ineffective for smokers with mental illness or addiction comorbidity. We close with recommendations for future areas of study and policy development.

ASSOCIATIONS BETWEEN TOBACCO USE AND MENTAL ILLNESS

It is well established that smoking rates are higher among patients with psychiatric illnesses and substance use disorders than in the general population. A seminal study by Hughes et al. (1986) demonstrated higher smoking rates among psychiatric outpatients compared to population-based controls. Higher rates of smoking have also been noted among individuals with major depression (Glassman 1998; Kandel, Huang, and Davies 2001); bipolar disorder (Gonzalez-Pinto et al. 1998; Vanable et al. 2003); anxiety disorders (Breslau, Kilbey, and Andreski 1992; Covey et al. 1994; Patton et al. 1998), including panic disorder (McCabe et al. 2004) and posttraumatic stress disorder (Beckham 1999; Breslau, Davis, and Schultz 2003); schizophrenia (de Leon et al. 1995; de Leon and Diaz 2005; Ziedonis et al. 1994); attention deficit disorders (Barkley, DuPaul, and McMurray 1990; Kollins, McClernon, and Fuemmeler 2005; Upadhyaya et al. 2005); alcohol dependence (Covey et al. 1994; Hughes 1996); and drug dependence (Richter et al. 2001; Stark and Campbell 1993; Zickler 2000). However, we know little about the temporal and causal ordering of smoking behavior and mental illness. Some believe that the presence of mental illness leads to increased smoking, others that smoking predisposes one to certain types of mental illness, and still others that shared factors contribute to both (Breslau, Novak, and Kessler 2004).

Addiction to nicotine is also more common among smokers with mental illness. Measures of nicotine dependence such as the Fagerstrom Test for Nicotine Dependence (FTND) show elevated levels in smokers with schizophrenia (George et al. 2002; Williams, Ziedonis, and Foulds 2004), bipolar disorder (de Leon et al. 2002), and substance abuse (Hughes and Kalman 2006; Sullivan and Covey 2002). Studies of smokers with schizophrenia have also found increased levels of nicotine and its metabolites (Olincy, Young, and Freedman 1997; Williams et al. 2005), suggesting higher nicotine intake per cigarette and higher levels of dependence. Studies of individuals with major depression have found mixed results, with some showing higher levels of dependence (Lerman et al. 1996) and others reporting no relationship of nicotine dependence severity to presence or severity of major depression (Breslau and Johnson 2000; Dierker et al. 2002; Pomerleau et al. 1994). This research has practical significance because smokers with more severe nicotine dependence are less likely to be able to quit and have a greater need for pharmacotherapy to support cessation attempts.

Questions persist about how mental illness affects the ability to quit smoking. There are likely to be differences in cessation rates among individuals with different disorders as well as by illness severity or presence of a current episode of illness, but the evidence is limited. A cross-sectional analysis by Lasser et al. (2000), using data from the National Comorbidity Survey (NCS), found lower quit rates among smokers with current mental illness than among those without. Several studies have found that smokers with a history of depression had less success at smoking cessation (Anda et al. 1990; Covey et al. 1994; Glassman et al. 1988; Hall et al. 1998), but a 2003 meta-analysis of 15 studies showed no effect of history of major depression on either short-term (<3 months) or long-term (>6 months) abstinence rates (Hitsman et al. 2003).

A history of alcohol dependence is not associated with lower ability to quit smoking (Covey et al. 1994). A review of 16 smoking studies found that smokers with past alcohol problems (defined as no problem in the last year) could quit as easily as those with no such history (Hughes and Kalman 2006). Substance abusers in treatment for current problems showed similar success rates for quitting smoking in early substance recovery as when their tobacco cessation treatment was delayed for 6 months (Joseph et al. 2003).

Less is known about cessation rates in individuals with more serious forms of mental illnesses, persistent mental health symptoms, and/or current substance use. In schizophrenia, schizoaffective disorder, and bipolar disorder, which are more severe forms of mental illness often characterized by persistent mental symptoms, small clinical studies have found that quit rates are low (de Leon et al. 2002; Williams and Hughes 2003). Two population surveys found virtually no quitting in individuals with schizophrenia (Covey et al. 1994; Lasser et al. 2000), and clinical trials of combined counseling and medication indicate smoking cessation rates that are about half those of other smokers. Predictors of cessation failure in these seriously mentally ill smokers include greater deficits in cognitive function (Dolan et al. 2004) and lifetime drug abuse (de Leon et al. 2005). Cessation rates may also be low for individuals with ADHD and PTSD (Hapke et al. 2005; Humfleet et al. 2005).

Most studies relating mental illness to smoking rely on clinical samples; few studies use population-level data. Two important exceptions merit attention. First, using data from the NCS, implemented in 1991–1992, Lasser and colleagues (2000) showed that persons with past month mental health problems were twice as likely to smoke and consumed nearly half (44.3 percent) of all cigarettes sold in the United States. More recently, Grant et al. (2004) examined results from the 2001–2002 National Epidemiologic Survey on Alcohol and Related Conditions (NESARC) and found that individuals with a current psychiatric disorder (with and without nicotine dependence) made up 30.3 percent of the population but consumed 46.3 percent of all cigarettes smoked in the United States. It important to note that these two studies relied on surveys that were designed to examine the prevalence of psychiatric conditions in the United States and were not primarily concerned with tobacco indicators such as consumption or quitting behaviors.

Besides NCS and NESARC, few other population-based data sets collect both mental health and tobacco use measures, and most have limitations in the assessment of either the tobacco or mental health items. Anxiety, depressive, and substance use disorders are measured reasonably well in population studies, but individuals with more severe illnesses may not be accurately assessed. Thus, our knowledge is limited about the most vulnerable smokers with the more serious forms of mental illness since, to our knowledge, there are no population-based data sets that comprehensively assess both serious mental illness (that is diagnosis specific) and tobacco use. The National Survey on Drug Use and Health (NSDUH) and the National Health Interview Survey (NHIS) both include an assessment with established psychometric properties for detecting individuals with serious psychological distress (SPD). Measurement of SPD is a useful proxy measure for serious mental illnesses in the population, such as schizophrenia (Kessler et al. 1998; Poulin et al. 2005). The presence of SPD, albeit not a specific mental disorder, signifies a disabling disorder and the need for mental health care.

TOBACCO USE MEASURES IN INDIVIDUALS WITH SPD

To document smoking rates in individuals with serious illnesses who may be missed in certain population studies, we analyzed data from the 2002 National Survey on Drug Use and Health using the proxy measure of SPD (Hagman et al. 2008). Screening for SPD has been operationalized using the K6 scale. The K6 consists of six questions that ask respondents how frequently they experienced symptoms of psychological distress during the past year. Respondents with scores of 13 and higher based on a summary of the six items are considered to have SPD, although the measure can also be used linearly as an index of severity. Although the K6 is not diagnosis specific, the scale has been clinically validated and screens accurately for serious psychological distress (Kessler et al. 2002, 2003). Its brevity, strong psychometric properties, and ability to discriminate DSM-IV cases from noncases makes the K6 ideal for general population-based health surveys (Kessler et al. 2002).

Comparisons between those with and without SPD indicated that, on average, adults with SPD are younger, less educated, unemployed, and more likely to be female than adults without SPD (Hagman et al. 2008). In addition, those with SPD are less likely to be covered by any form of health insurance.

Ever use and current (past month) use of tobacco are higher for those with SPD than for those without, with cigarettes being the most common tobacco product utilized. Among those with SPD, 44.9 percent reported use in the past month, compared to 26.0 percent without SPD. Adults with SPD were also more likely to be daily smokers than those without SPD (30.2 percent vs. 16.7 percent; Hagman et al. 2008). Figure 15.1 depicts the relationship between SPD scores and the prevalence of past-month cigarette smoking. SPD symptom severity is associated with greater likelihood of being a current smoker. In addition, compared to current smokers without SPD, smokers with SPD were more likely to be nicotine dependent and exhibited greater smoking urgency (i.e., smoking within five minutes after waking).

Smoking cessation also differed significantly by SPD status. According to the 2002 NSDUH, 47 percent of U.S. adults who had ever smoked were former smokers at the time of the survey. The quit ratio for adults without SPD was 0.49, compared with 0.29 for those with SPD (Hagman et al. 2008).

These findings from a population-based sample confirm results of prior clinical studies showing evidence of higher ever and daily use of tobacco, higher likelihood of having nicotine dependence, and greater smoking urgency among persons with serious mental illness. We found a strong linear relationship between the severity of SPD and likelihood of being a current smoker. In addition, these data suggest that individuals with SPD are either less successful at cessation or more resistant to quitting.

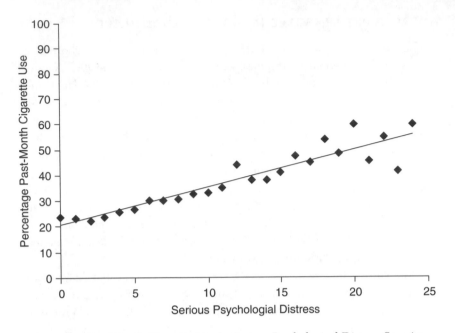

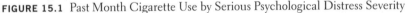

FIGURE 15.1 Past Month Cigarette Use by Serious Psychological Distress Severity

Source: National Survey on Drug Use and Health, http://oas.samhsa.gov/nhsda.htm.

NEUROBIOLOGICAL LINKS BETWEEN MENTAL ILLNESS AND SMOKING

Some researchers have speculated that individuals with mental illness are more likely to smoke because they are self-medicating with nicotine. Certain neuro-psychiatric disorders, including Alzheimer's disease, ADHD, and schizophrenia, are associated with abnormalities in the nicotinic cholinergic systems. Nicotine reduces the symptoms of ADHD (Conners et al. 1996; Levin et al. 2001; Potter and Newhouse 2004) and improves aspects of cognition in schizophrenia (Sacco, Bannon, and George 2004; Smith et al. 2002), suggesting that individuals with disorders of attention and cognition may benefit from smoking or taking nicotinic agonists.

Smoking may have other antidepressant effects beyond the effects of nicotine. Noninvasive brain positron emission tomography studies show that the brains of living smokers have 40 percent less of the enzyme monoamine oxidase B (MAO B) than those of nonsmokers or former smokers (Fowler et al. 1996). Researchers believe that a yet-unidentified component of cigarette smoke inhibits monoamine oxidase (MAO) in the brain, with an effect similar to that of a class of antidepressant medications, the MAO inhibitors.

Although the self-medication hypothesis is attractive and may help explain the higher smoking prevalence and lower quit rates among those with mental illness, its importance should not be exaggerated (Ziedonis et al. 2008); psychosocial risk factors and treatment system factors may also be important. Long-term studies are needed on the effect of smoking cessation on neuropsychological and other symptoms in this population. The effects of genetics, environment, and development are also important to consider for adolescent smokers who develop mental illness or other addictions later in life.

EFFECTS OF TOBACCO CONTROL STRATEGIES ON SMOKERS WITH MENTAL ILLNESS

Since 1965, the prevalence of adult smoking in the United States has declined by almost half (Giovino 2002; U.S. Department of Health and Human Services 2000). Tobacco control strategies that have been effective at reducing smoking initiation, prevalence, and consumption include increases in tobacco excise taxes, clean indoor air laws and workplace tobacco bans, state prevention and cessation initiatives, restriction of tobacco sales to minors, and anti-tobacco counter-marketing efforts (Bierer and Rigotti 1992; Centers for Disease Control and Prevention 1999; National Cancer Institute 2005a; Wakefield and Chaloupka 2000). The extent to which these strategies are effective in smokers with mental illness is largely unknown. Below we discuss each of the major areas of tobacco control strategies that are effective in the general population and discuss their impact on smokers with mental illness.

TAXES AND PRICE

Few studies have looked explicitly at the impact of increased tobacco prices and taxation on smokers with mental illness. Taxes or high tobacco prices reduce the consumption of tobacco in the general population (U.S. Department of Health and Human Services 2000). An analysis by Saffer and Dave (2002) provides the first economic analysis of the price elasticity of cigarettes among those with mental illness. They find that individuals with a history of mental illness are responsive to price, although the price elasticities may differ somewhat. Their model controlled statistically for factors such as poverty, stressful life events, and family history of addiction but did not include level of dependence, which can affect the price elasticity of tobacco use.

It should be noted, however, that price-related marketing efforts by the tobacco industry, including multipack discounts and coupons, may negate some of the effects of higher price. The use of discount/generic cigarettes increased nationally from 6 percent in 1988 to 26 percent in 2004 and is associated with lower household income, higher daily cigarette consumption, and lower cessation rates (Cummings et al. 1997a; Harris and Chan 1999; Maxwell 2004). Individuals with serious mental illness tend to smoke more generic or discount value brands than other smokers (Steinberg, Williams, and Ziedonis 2004; Williams et al. 2007). Tobacco industry documents clearly show that price-related marketing efforts became more prevalent in response to competitive pressures and reduce the impact of tax increases (Chaloupka et al. 2002).

Cigarettes are already a significant expense for many smokers with a serious mental illness. One study of a small sample of smokers with schizophrenia found they spent almost a third of their monthly disability income on cigarettes (Steinberg, Williams, and Ziedonis 2004). Studies of individuals with schizophrenia, a group with very high levels of dependence, have shown that smokers will go to great lengths to continue using tobacco, such as buying cigarettes instead of food and other basic necessities, buying bulk tobacco, or buying from Internet or Indian reservation sources in order to economize (Steinberg, Williams, and Ziedonis 2004; Williams et al. 2007). Smokers in the general population who buy cigarettes from lower-taxed sources, such as the Internet and American Indian reservations, tend to smoke heavily, have high levels of tobacco dependence, are less likely to make a quit attempt, and have lower cessation rates (Hrywna, Delnevo, and Staniewska 2004; Hyland et al. 2005).

CLEAN INDOOR AIR POLICIES

Clean indoor air policies are a powerful way to discourage smoking (Bauer 2005; Farrelly, Evans, and Sfekas 1999; U.S. Department of Health and Human Services 2006). Policies that restrict or ban smoking in public places have become more common over the last 30 years. Most of these have focused on the workplace, with the primary intent of reducing exposure to environmental tobacco smoke (ETS). The federal government requires employers to provide a work environment that is reasonably free of recognized hazards, and courts have ruled that this includes protection for nonsmoking employees from ETS (U.S. Department of Health and Human Services 2000). Thirty-eight states and the District of Columbia have local laws affecting municipalities that require smoke-free workplaces, restaurants, and/or bars. As of April 1, 2010, 32 states had enacted statewide smoke-free laws that protect workplaces and/or restaurants (American Nonsmokers' Rights Foundation 2010). For reducing exposure to ETS, smoking bans are more effective than smoking restrictions, which usually designate specific areas where smoking is allowed to continue (Hopkins et al. 2001).

The impact of clean indoor air laws has not been studied in smokers with mental illness. Many in this disadvantaged group are missed by workplace smoking bans because they are less likely to work. In addition, disparities exist in workplace smoking bans such that blue-collar and food/hospitality service employees (bartenders, restaurant servers, prep cooks) are less likely to be protected, as are workers who earn less than $50,000 annually or who have a high school education or less (Delnevo, Hrywna, and Lewis 2004; Gerlach et al. 1997). Because individuals with serious mental illness have lower levels of education and income and are more likely to work part-time, they are less likely to work in smoke-free workplaces. States with comprehensive smoking bans in public places are more likely to see an impact on smokers with mental illness because the venues covered include not only bars and restaurants but also recreational facilities, shopping malls, places of worship, and public buses.

For individuals with a mental illness or addiction, treatment settings are critical sites for intervention. In 1992, the Joint Commission on the Accreditation of Health Organizations (JCAHO) developed an accreditation standard that restricted smoking in hospitals and has led to efforts to provide smoke-free indoor environments. In the United States, hospitals are the only industry that has voluntarily implemented such a nationwide smoking ban. JCAHO standards have not been consistently implemented in psychiatric hospitals and inpatient substance abuse facilities, however. Most programs still provide an adjacent or outdoor smoking area, allowing patients and staff to continue to smoke. Hospitals with a psychiatric or substance abuse unit in the hospital have lower compliance than do other hospitals with the JCAHO tobacco control standards (Joseph et al. 1995; Longo et al. 1998).

In addition, other venues frequented by persons with a mental illness or addiction, including residential group homes, recovery-based treatment programs, and social clubs, often continue to permit smoking, exposing both clients and staff to ETS. Furthermore, functions may take place outside these venues, such as in motor vehicles, on outdoor campuses, on recreational outings, or at 12-step meetings. Living with a current smoker is responsible for at least 50 percent of an individual's total exposure to ETS, and policies banning smoking in mental health residences are needed.

Perhaps one of the biggest barriers is that smoking remains part of the culture in most mental health and residential facilities. Daily schedules, for instance, routinely include smoking breaks. Mental health professionals and family advocacy groups have not been vocal in demanding tobacco treatment services for smokers with mental illness. Indeed, these groups have continued to lobby for exemptions from smoke-free air provisions for hospitals and other mental health treatment facilities (Longo et al. 1998; Williams 2008).

The definition of smoke-free or tobacco-free facilities extends beyond requirements for clean indoor air and refers to environments that are entirely free of tobacco use. Studies of psychiatric and behavioral health inpatient units that become entirely smoke-free show that this change can occur without adverse effects on treatment (Haller, McNiel, and Binder 1996; Patten et al. 1995). Although many patients may resume smoking after discharge, it is still useful to reinforce healthy behaviors and drug-free environments in the treatment setting.

Only a few states require licensed residential addiction treatment programs to have tobacco-free grounds, but there is evidence of growing support for tobacco-free treatment centers. A survey of more than 200 U.S. state psychiatric hospitals indicates that almost half have already implemented some form of smoke-free policy, with many more planning to make changes in the following year (National Association of State Mental Health Program Directors 2006). In July 2006 the National Association of State Mental Health Program Directors released a policy statement supporting assertive steps to stop tobacco use in the public mental health system. New tobacco control policies aimed at treatment facilities may be an important step in reducing tobacco use among individuals with mental illness. To this end, educational efforts targeting clients, their families, and staff may help build support for smoke-free treatment facilities and for greater access to smoking cessation treatment.

CESSATION TREATMENT POLICIES

QUITLINES Smoking cessation techniques shown to be effective in the general population, such as telephone quitlines (Fiore et al. 2000; Zhu et al. 2002), have not been studied in a mentally ill population. This type of intervention may face practical barriers; for instance, many low-income individuals lack stable access to a telephone line. Boarding home residents often share a single pay telephone, making quitlines less accessible for them. In addition to simple logistical issues, there are concerns that tobacco counselors providing quitline services are not trained in assessing mental health and would be unable to manage complex clinical issues. Finally, cessation services are typically brief and rely on a highly motivated and organized client who is ready to quit.

The invisibility of mentally ill clients is evident from a new initiative for evaluating quitlines. In 2003 the North American Quitline Consortium (NAQC) developed what it called a minimal data set (MDS), a set of standard intake and follow-up questions administered to callers. The MDS facilitates performance monitoring and allows for the assessment of national trends and comparisons between states. Unfortunately, the MDS does not include questions about mental illness or addiction in smokers who call the quitline. In explaining why these questions were not included in the MDS, the NAQC noted that counselors are not trained to provide interventions to callers with those conditions. This response is consistent with anecdotal reports that many quitline tobacco counselors feel unprepared to assist smokers with mental illness and addiction comorbidity. However, it fails to move the field forward by not taking steps to address this inequity. The effectiveness of quitlines for smokers with mental illness or addiction cannot be evaluated until gaps in data collection are addressed.

INSURANCE COVERAGE FOR TREATMENT Although Medicaid was not designed as a mental health program, it is now a major source of financing for mental health services and care, especially for the seriously mentally ill. Estimates are that about 1 in 10 Medicaid dollars is spent on behavioral health services, and 1 in 7 Medicaid dollars is spent on tobacco-related illness, although the degree of overlap in these two groups is not known (Centers for Disease Control and Prevention 2005b; Mark et al. 2003).

Tobacco control organizations agree that Medicaid coverage for treatment of tobacco dependence should be increased dramatically. The number of state Medicaid programs providing some coverage for tobacco-dependence counseling or medication increased to 42 states and the District of Columbia by 2006 (National Cancer Institute 2010), but only one program offers all the treatments recommended by the 2000 U.S. Clinical Practice Guideline for Treating Tobacco (Fiore et al. 2000). Some programs do cover the prescription nicotine products such as Zyban (bupropion) and Chantix (varenicline). Medicaid coverage for the over-the-counter (OTC) products such as the nicotine patch or gum also varies by state. Patients on disability or other fixed income may not be able to afford OTC products, which cost an average of $35–$55 for each two-week supply. Thus, cost and insurance issues often dictate treatment choice for tobacco treatment medications. Options for these vulnerable smokers will remain limited until Medicaid coverage of tobacco dependence treatment is expanded.

PHYSICIAN INTERVENTIONS/ACCESS TO TOBACCO TREATMENT IN BEHAVIORAL HEALTH SETTINGS Mental health professionals assess or treat their patients' tobacco use only infrequently (Montoya et al. 2005; Peterson, Hryshko-Mullen, and Cortez 2003; Thorndike, Stafford, and Rigotti 2001). Despite recommendations made more than 10 years ago by the American Psychiatric Association (1996) that psychiatrists should treat tobacco in all patients they see for a mental health problem, most do not. Psychiatrists are estimated to treat tobacco use in about 9 percent of smoking patients (Montoya et al. 2005) and 12 percent of patient visits with smokers (Himelhoch and Daumit 2003). The probability of receiving smoking-cessation counseling from a psychiatrist was significantly higher for those older than 50 and for those with a medical diagnosis of obesity, hypertension, or diabetes mellitus (Himelhoch and Daumit 2003). Indeed, primary care physicians are more likely than psychiatrists to counsel smokers with mental illness (Thorndike, Stafford, and Rigotti 2001). Although psychiatry residents report considerable interest in this area, they appear unprepared to treat nicotine dependence (Prochaska, Fromont, and Hall 2005). In addition, public and private mental health and addiction services seldom provide tobacco dependence treatment.

The infrequency of receiving tobacco treatment from psychiatrists is a concern because smokers with serious mental illness have special needs. They may enter tobacco treatment with lower motivation levels, fewer quit experiences, and higher levels of nicotine dependence. Most brief tobacco dependence interventions, which can be effective in the general population, may lack the intensity or specialization needed to be effective for this population (Steinberg, Hall, and Rustin 2003). Studies of conventional cessation methods such as the nicotine patch, bupropion, and cognitive behavioral therapy have shown lower quit rates in mentally ill smokers (Evins et al. 2005; Williams and Ziedonis 2004; Ziedonis and George 1997), pointing to a need for more intensive treatments and perhaps a longer duration of treatment to allow for multiple quit attempts.

Further, it is well documented that individuals with serious mental illness do not receive adequate general medical care for a variety of reasons, including the chaotic and disorganized lifestyles often associated with mental illness, as well as the lack of health insurance. Additional factors sometimes include lack of the skills required to access health care and difficulty in communicating needs and following through with recommendations (Desai and Rosenheck 2005; Swartz et al. 2003). Stigma or misunderstanding by medical professionals toward individuals with serious mental illness makes matters worse.

Integrated care in mental health settings may be optimal for tobacco treatment in this population (Hall 2007). Mental health providers are in the best position to help psychiatric patients obtain prevention or educational services (Cournos, McKinnon, and Sullivan 2005; McKinnon, Cournos, and Herman 2002), and the model of integrated care has been successful in interventions for other co-occurring substance use disorders (Drake and Mueser 2001; Substance Abuse and Mental Health Services Administration 2002; Ziedonis 2004). The mental health setting is well suited to treatment of tobacco dependence, a chronic, relapsing condition that may require multiple attempts to achieve abstinence. Most clients in mental health settings resume stable functioning and remain in treatment for a period of years (Ziedonis 2004). If integrated care is indeed the most effective model, there is a need to integrate tobacco dependence treatment into curricula for the next generation of mental health trainees, including psychiatrists.

OTHER TOBACCO CONTROL STRATEGIES

Little is known about the effect on smokers with mental illness of other tobacco control measures, including bans on tobacco advertising, counteradvertising/ public health messages, and restrictions on youth access methods. We do not know, for example, if smokers with mental illness respond to media messages in the same way as other smokers, or even the degree to which they are reached by media campaigns. Tobacco industry documents, however, reveal evidence of targeting to psychologically vulnerable populations including the mentally ill (Apollonio and Malone 2005; Prochaska, Hall, and Bero 2008).

It is likely that tobacco control programs targeting smokers with mental illness may have to change norms around smoking because smoking is an accepted part of the mental health culture. Lawn (2004) describes the role of cigarettes as "the currency by which economic, social and political exchange took place" among hospitalized Australian psychiatric patients. Treatment settings commonly use cigarettes to reward appropriate behaviors. Although mental health advocacy groups have been effective in reducing the stigma associated with mental illness and working for parity of mental health treatment, they have not advocated for increased access to tobacco dependence treatment for smokers with mental illness. Virtually none of the Master Settlement Agreement funds were directed toward helping smokers with mental illness, and only a handful of states (New York, Colorado, Ohio) have spent any of their comprehensive tobacco control funds on mental health initiatives. There is evidence, though, that this is beginning to change. A prominent advocacy organization, the National Alliance on Mental Illness (NAMI), has recently reversed its position on tobacco. Previously NAMI encouraged all psychiatric hospitals and facilities to provide designated smoking areas. Now the organization has called on physicians and other health care providers to implement education and smoking cessation programs to help mental health consumers reduce and stop smoking (National Alliance on Mental Illness 2006).

THE "HARDENING" HYPOTHESIS

Despite the success of past tobacco control efforts, decreases in the prevalence of smoking have leveled off in the recent past. A prominent explanation for this plateau in smoking prevalence is that remaining smokers are "hardened" or relatively resistant to quitting (Warner and Burns 2003). This hypothesis posits that for biological or psychological reasons, the current population of smokers is more unwilling or unable to quit than the average smoker of previous eras. Alternatively, current smokers may have fewer resources with which to overcome their addiction or face greater barriers to behavior change. For these reasons, specific groups of smokers, such as the poor or individuals with mental disorders, may constitute a growing share of those who continue to smoke (Burns and Warner 2003).

To date, the evidence on this hypothesis is limited and inconclusive. Longitudinal data are scarce, and research is limited as well by the lack of data on nicotine dependence (Hughes 2001). Measures of cessation vary from study to study and range from measures of quit attempts to long-term abstinence rates. Last, as noted previously, the limited data on mental illness or other addiction and tobacco use makes it difficult to assess whether individuals with mental illness—who find it more difficult to quit—are becoming more prevalent among smokers.

It is important to emphasize that "hardening" is in part a function of tobacco control and public health policy. Given the emphasis in tobacco control on conventional measures aimed at the general population, combined with the very limited measures taken to promote smoking cessation in individuals with mental illness, it is likely that smoking rates will remain elevated in mentally ill populations. More vigorous tobacco treatment efforts targeted at mentally ill populations could counterbalance the greater difficulty faced by this population, preventing the emergence of a "hard-core" residual population of smokers.

CONCLUSION

Given their higher levels of dependence and reduced cessation, smokers with serious mental illness are likely to remain a sizable and perhaps growing share of smokers in the United States. Our analysis of the 2002 NSDUH supports prior studies of clinical samples demonstrating that individuals with serious psychological distress, a proxy measurement for serious mental illness, are more likely to be current and lifetime smokers and to have higher rates of nicotine dependence and lower cessation success than smokers without serious mental illness.

Significant gaps remain in our overall knowledge of smokers with mental illness, including major deficiencies in our understanding of how tobacco control strategies affect these smokers. Reducing tobacco dependence in this population is likely to require not only clinical interventions but also policy and other system-level changes. With the passage of a law in June 2009 granting the Food and Drug Administration (FDA) authority to regulate tobacco products, the FDA has been empowered to require changes in tobacco products such as the removal or reduction of harmful ingredients. A change in the product ingredients may impact the level of dependence within this population. More research is needed to better understand the scope of this problem and measure trends over time. Adding tobacco use measures to existing and ongoing psychiatric data sets may be an efficient way to increase our base of evidence. Future tobacco control efforts are likely to be impeded unless we can identify and implement effective strategies for smokers with mental illness or substance use disorder.

16

THE EFFECT OF TOBACCO CONTROL POLICIES ON INEQUITIES IN SMOKING PREVALENCE: SOCIAL CLASS, RACE/ETHNICITY, AND GENDER

EDITH D. BALBACH, CATHY HARTMAN, AND ELIZABETH M. BARBEAU

I f the United States adopted much stronger tobacco control policies, such as those proposed by the Institute of Medicine (IOM) and described in previous chapters, should we expect existing differences in smoking rates among subgroups of the general population to get smaller, get larger, or stay the same? In particular, how would differences in smoking prevalence by social class, race/ethnicity, and gender change with increases in tobacco excise taxes, clean indoor air/smoke-free worksites, access to cessation treatment, school-based education, stronger media campaigns, and restrictions on youth access to tobacco? To explore this "what if" question, we begin with a brief discussion of smoking patterns by social category. Then, drawing on existing research on each of these policies, we engage in evidence-based speculation about how stronger policies in each of these areas might affect disparities in smoking.

PATTERNS OF TOBACCO USE BY SUBGROUP

Smoking prevalence is inversely related to social class. Those who have less education and lower incomes, and who are employed in working-class occupations, are more likely to smoke than their more advantaged counterparts (Barbeau, Krieger, and Soobader 2004). For example, according to 2008 data, smoking rates among those with a General Educational Development diploma were 41.3 percent, compared to only 5.7 percent among those with a graduate degree. The poor—that is, those living below the federal poverty threshold—were more likely to smoke than those at or above the threshold (31.5 percent vs. 19.6 percent) (Centers for Disease Control and Prevention 2009a). This pattern has become more pronounced over the past several decades. Smoking rates have gone down among disadvantaged groups, but not as quickly as among the more advantaged.

Smoking prevalence also varies substantially by race and ethnicity. Among adults, in 2008, American Indians/Alaska Natives had the highest prevalence (32.4 percent), followed by non-Hispanic whites (22.0 percent), non-Hispanic blacks (21.3 percent), Hispanics (15.8 percent), and Asians (9.9) (Centers for Disease Control and Prevention 2009a). These prevalence rates have declined over the last several decades, but the racial/ethnic differences have changed little. In contrast, youth smoking rates differed little by race or ethnicity in the 1970s but declined more steeply for African American and Hispanic youth over the last three decades. Among twelfth-graders, a recent study found, the 30-day prevalence rate (proportion smoking at any time during the last month) was 28.2 percent for whites, 18.5 percent for Hispanics, and 10.1 percent for African Americans (Tauras 2007).

Cigarette smoking is and always has been more prevalent among men than women. However, a once-wide gender gap in smoking narrowed until the mid-1980s and has since remained fairly constant. In 2008, 18.3 percent of women reported smoking, compared to 23.1 percent of men (Centers for Disease Control and Prevention 2009a).

One caveat about these survey-based measures of smoking prevalence, particularly in the most recent surveys, is the growing percentage of households that only have wireless phones. Those living in wireless-only households are more likely to be younger, poorer, and either non-Hispanic black or Hispanic than those who live in households with landline phones. Because most surveys rely on calls to landlines, they may not be reaching the populations discussed in this chapter (Blumberg and Luke 2010).

DIFFERENTIAL EFFECTS OF TOBACCO CONTROL POLICIES

Before we review the evidence as to how tobacco control policy might affect different populations, we first note that this exercise may be unrealistically optimistic about the likelihood of adoption of the IOM recommendations. Public policies are rarely crafted by lawmakers or implemented by regulatory agencies solely on the basis of recommendations of experts in a particular field. If a modified version of the IOM recommendations were adopted by lawmakers, we must further consider at what governmental level this is likely to take place, because the level at which a policy might be implemented will in turn influence its effectiveness in reaching various population segments. Federal-level adoption would presumably reach all population groups equally, while policies implemented at the state or local level may not.

When it comes to tobacco control policies, the U.S. federal government has until recently had a poor policy record. It has passed only one national clean indoor air law (prohibition of smoking in U.S. commercial airplanes in 1989) (Pan et al. 2005), left tobacco excise taxes low (until a 2009 increase, the rate was only 39 cents and had not changed since a 5 cent increase in 2002), required compliance checks to ensure that tobacco retailers are not selling tobacco products to minors but has not adequately enforced this requirement (DiFranza and Dussault 2005), created a national smoking cessation quitline phone number (with transfer to state quitlines, where available) but failed to provide adequate funding for promoting it to the public, and has not sponsored any national media campaigns on smoking cessation for decades. Given this record, it is far from clear that tobacco control policies will be adopted at the federal level that will expose all population groups equally to strong tobacco control policies.

While the federal government has taken only limited steps to curb tobacco use, the states and many local communities have been more active. For example, 25 states and 654 communities have passed laws requiring smoke-free workplaces, and 30 states now have excise taxes of $1.00 or more (American Nonsmokers' Rights Foundation 2010; Campaign for Tobacco-Free Kids 2010). Likewise, communities have adopted their own school-based programs and youth access enforcement initiatives. Were it not for tobacco control advocates at the state and local levels, there would be nowhere near the declines in smoking prevalence we have observed over the past few decades. However, not every community adopts policies at the same rate. In Massachusetts, for example, prior to passage of a statewide ban on smoking in public places in 2005, bans on smoking in local communities were more prevalent in wealthy compared to poor communities (Deverell et al. 2006; Skeer et al. 2004). Poor residents were thus more likely to be exposed to secondhand smoke. Because smoking bans tend to drive down smoking rates, it was less likely that poor communities would experience any ban-associated declines in smoking prevalence.

Finally, even if policies are adopted by states or communities, implementation may vary widely. Consider school-based anti-smoking programs. Research suggests that for these programs to be effective, proper implementation is critical, entailing formal processes, adequate resources, school-based leadership, a supportive internal and external environment, and compatibility with schools' characteristics (Gingiss, Roberts-Gray, and Boerm 2006). Poorly resourced schools, likely to be located in low-income communities, will have the least capacity to implement programs, limiting chances for success. Thus, an important caveat to this chapter and its conclusions is that, based on recent history in tobacco control policymaking, we question whether tobacco control policies would be adopted as recommended by the IOM and, if adopted, implemented evenly across all segments of society in such a way as to confer equal public health benefits.

With these caveats about the policy process, we turn now to evidence regarding how smoking rates in various population subgroups might be affected by tobacco control policies (excise taxes, clean indoor air/smoke-free worksites, access to cessation treatment, school-based education, youth access, and media campaigns). The subgroups we consider are defined by social class, race/ethnicity, and gender. (Although we had originally intended to discuss sexual orientation as well, we found no studies of policy effects that differentiated by sexual orientation.) Differential impact might occur because of differences in exposure to a given policy intervention; for instance, smoke-free workplace regulations will affect the employed more than the unemployed. In addition, individuals with similar exposure to an intervention may respond differently. Explaining why responses might differ is beyond the scope of this chapter; our purpose here, instead, is to evaluate this evidence and, when possible, use it to project likely trends in disparities under a more vigorous tobacco control regime.

TOBACCO EXCISE TAXES

Research indicates that higher cigarette prices, which can be induced through taxation, result in both lower smoking rates and lower quantities of tobacco consumed by smokers among the general population (Hopkins et al. 2001; Liang et al. 2003), and that low-income groups may be more price sensitive. The most common measure of the effect of increases in tobacco excise taxes is the price elasticity of demand, or the percentage change in consumption that results from a 1 percent change in price (Hopkins et al. 2001). Most studies find that price elasticity is greatest in low-income populations (Centers for Disease Control and Prevention 1998; Farrelly and Bray 1998; Meier and Licari 1997; Wilson et al. 2004), meaning that low-income adult smokers are more likely than higher-income smokers to quit or cut back on tobacco consumption as a result of price increases. Likewise, higher tobacco taxes have been found to discourage lower-income youth from starting to smoke (Centers for Disease Control and Prevention 1998). Considering the effect of taxes in relation to smokers' education level, one study found that less-educated tobacco users were the most responsive to increased cigarette prices (Meier and Licari 1997). In a review of the impact of public policies on youth smoking in the 1990s, Gruber (2000) found that socioeconomically disadvantaged youth, including blacks and those with less-educated parents, were more responsive to increases in cigarette prices than white teens and those with more-educated parents.

Tobacco taxes have been an important policy lever for tobacco control activists, and so one might legitimately wonder why the social class gap in smoking is growing rather than diminishing. One reason for this apparent paradox is that many smokers quit for reasons other than the price of cigarettes; in fact, concern about health is the most often reported motivation for cessation attempts (Hyland et al. 2004). In addition, tobacco taxes at the federal level (those that affect all smokers) may be too low to offset other factors that tend to raise prevalence in disproportionately low-income smokers. The average excise tax on cigarettes in the United States is well below that of most other industrialized nations (U.S. Department of Health and Human Services 2000).

The regressivity of tobacco taxes has received limited attention in the public health and tobacco control literature but deserves special mention in a chapter dealing with social disparities. The regressive tax argument is that tobacco use is highest among low-income groups; thus, tax increases fall disproportionately on these groups, creating financial hardship among smokers who do not or cannot quit (Townsend 1996; Wilson et al. 2004). Others counter that taxes are actually progressive public health policy because they reduce smoking rates among those with low incomes and less education, reducing class disparities in tobacco use and health (Emery et al. 2001; Gruber and Köszegi 2004). Policymakers must decide whether the financial hardship that taxes impose on smokers is an acceptable cost in order to reduce smoking rates and class disparities in smoking.

There is some evidence that as cigarette prices increase, racial/ethnic minority populations are more likely than whites to smoke less and to quit smoking altogether (Centers for Disease Control and Prevention 1998; Hu et al. 1995). After controlling for income and education in National Health Interview Survey data collected from 1976 through 1993, Hispanic and non-Hispanic black smokers across all age groups were more likely than white smokers to reduce or quit smoking in response to increased cigarette prices (Centers for Disease Control and Prevention 1998). Two studies have found that young black and Hispanic smokers aged 18–24 are substantially more responsive to cigarette price increases than young white men (Centers for Disease Control and Prevention 1998; Chaloupka and Pacula 1999). Thus, higher excise taxes may widen the gap in smoking rates between whites on the one hand and black and Hispanic populations on the other. One study did show that smokers who purchased cigarettes on Indian reservations, where presumably Indians themselves were likely to purchase cigarettes, were half as likely to attempt to quit. We know very little about the influence of policies on Native Americans, the ethnic group with the highest smoking rates. However, people buying cigarettes sold on Indian reservations do not pay state excise taxes; thus, state tax policies are likely to have less influence on Native Americans than on other ethnic groups (Hyland et al. 2005).

Evidence about price sensitivity by gender is mixed. One might expect women smokers to be more likely to respond to increased cigarette prices because of gender differences in income. However, a number of studies, although not all, have found evidence that men's smoking behavior is more influenced by price than is women's smoking (Chaloupka and Warner 1999).

CLEAN INDOOR AIR/SMOKE-FREE WORKSITES

In addition to protecting the public from secondhand smoke exposure, clean indoor air laws also influence smokers' behavior. In a review of studies that tracked employee smoking behaviors before and after implementation of smoke-free worksite policies, Fichtenberg and Glantz (2002a) reported that such policies reduce both smoking prevalence and the number of cigarettes smoked per day among workers.

Based on the evidence to date, it is unclear whether clean indoor air or smoke-free worksite policies impact smoking behavior differentially by class, race/ethnicity, or gender. A few studies have reported differences in the effects of these policies on smoking (Shavers et al. 2006), but others do not (Dinno and Glantz 2009; Levy, Mumford, and Compton 2006; Thomas et al. 2008). However, there are differences by social category in current exposure to these policies and thus in the likely effect of policy change. Workers in lower-status occupations and with less education are far less likely to be employed in worksites that have implemented smoke-free policies (Bauer 2005; Gerlach et al. 1997), but gender and race/ethnic differences in access to workplace smoking bans may vary by place or occupational sector (Moore et al. 2006; Plescia et al. 2005; Shavers et al. 2006). Thus, if a national, comprehensive smoke-free law were passed, it could reduce the social class gap in smoking prevalence by ensuring that workers in lower-status occupations have the same access to smoke-free workplaces. To the extent that racial/ethnic minorities and women are overrepresented in lower-status jobs, which are less likely to offer smoke-free worksite policies, minority and female workers would also benefit more from a comprehensive national clean air policy. However, because employment rates are lower among racial/ethnic minorities and among women, the proportion of these subgroups exposed to smoke-free policies at the workplace will be lower. The effect of a national clean air law on race/ethnic and gender disparities in smoking is uncertain.

ACCESS TO TOBACCO CESSATION TREATMENTS

Proven tobacco cessation treatments include individual, group, and telephone counseling and pharmacotherapy (e.g., nicotine replacement therapies or medication such as bupropion) (Fiore et al. 2000). Tobacco control policies that promote use of smoking cessation treatments and services include (1) efforts to have health insurers cover the costs of treatments and (2) promotion of free and confidential counseling via telephone quitlines. When insurers cover tobacco treatments, users receive treatment at lower cost, which is expected to increase utilization of treatment and lead to more successful quit attempts. State-managed telephone quitlines may also increase utilization by reducing barriers such as inconvenience, time, and travel. Both types of policies should lower barriers to smoking cessation for socioeconomically disadvantaged groups. But does improving access to fully covered treatments through insurance programs reduce smoking rates?

Three large, well-designed research studies indicate the answer is "yes" (Curry et al. 1998; Kaper et al. 2005b; Schauffler et al. 2001). Despite this convincing body of evidence on the effectiveness of these treatments, which have become recommended government practice for treating tobacco dependence, access to and use of these therapies remains low for all population groups (Friend and Levy 2001). While 70 percent of smokers report wanting to quit, and about 40 percent make a serious quit attempt each year, only about 20 percent report using an effective treatment (Barbeau, Krieger, and Soobader 2004; Cokkinides et al. 2005). Lowering barriers and promoting use of treatments is thus a critical public health challenge. Over time, more health maintenance organizations have begun to pay for cessation treatments, creating greater access to cessation treatments for the insured (McPhillips-Tangum et al. 2002).

For low-income smokers, many of whom lack private insurance, Medicaid is a key source of health care coverage. In 2007, almost 57 million low-income persons in the United States received their health coverage through the federal-state Medicaid program (http://www.ssa.gov/policy/docs/statcomps/supplement/2009/8e.html#table8.e2). Medicaid recipients have approximately 53 percent greater smoking prevalence than the overall U.S. population but are less likely to receive tobacco cessation counseling due to lack of access to and cost of effective treatment (Schauffler, Mordavsky, and Orleans 2001). One study found that use of the NRT patch increased by 57 percent among Medicaid recipients when full financial coverage was provided, even after accounting for other sociodemographic characteristics (Cummings et al. 1997b). State Medicaid health plans are beginning to pay for government-recommended tobacco treatments. By 2006, 42 states and the District of Columbia required coverage for at least one recommended treatment, although benefits varied substantially across states and a few states covered tobacco dependence treatments only for pregnant women (National Cancer Institute 2010). In addition, awareness of Medicaid coverage for smoking cessation treatment is low (McMenamin, Halpin, and Bellows 2006; Murphy et al. 2003). Because smoking rates are high among Medicaid recipients and their access to coverage of tobacco treatments is low, this low-income group is disproportionately burdened by lack of insurance coverage for effective treatments.

Union health and welfare funds provide health insurance to 10 million union-ized workers, largely in blue-collar occupations, and their dependents. When a smoking cessation program involving telephone counseling and pharmaco-therapy was offered free of charge to a population of unionized blue-collar workers through their health and welfare fund, 13.4 percent of insured smokers enrolled in the program within two years (Ringen et al. 2002). This rate is much higher than the 1–2 percent rate typical for state-based quitlines. Very few health and welfare funds carry this type of coverage for their union members, however (Barbeau et al. 2001).

Socioeconomically disadvantaged smokers are less likely than more advan-taged smokers to have any kind of health insurance, including private, union, or public health insurance. According to the National Health Interview Survey, in 2004 29 percent of poor and near-poor adults lacked health insurance, com-pared to just 9 percent of nonpoor persons (Centers for Disease Control and Prevention 2004a). If they are insured through Medicaid or their union, they are less likely to have access to paid smoking cessation treatments.

In contrast, telephone-based quitlines provide more equal access to smoking cessation services. In 2004, the U.S. Department of Health and Human Services announced plans for a national network of smoking cessation quitlines to pro-vide all smokers in the United States access to the support and tools they need to quit (1-800-QUIT NOW) (North American Quitline Consortium; U.S. Depart-ment of Health and Human Services 2004b). A national toll-free telephone number serves as a single access point to the national network of state-managed quitlines. The program includes funding to expand existing quitlines, establish new quitlines in states that did not have them, and provide interim services to individuals in states that currently lack quitlines. By 2006, all 50 states had pub-licly funded quitlines (Keller et al. 2010). Telephone quitlines offer a variety of services including counseling, web-based and mailed self-help resources, refer-rals to group cessation programs and community resources, and provision of nico-tine replacement therapies. These services are available to callers regardless of their geographic location, race/ethnicity, or socioeconomic status, and Spanish as well as English language services are generally available (Keller et al. 2010). Telephone quitlines are effective in helping smokers quit (Ossip-Klein and Mc-Intosh 2003; Stead and Lancaster 2001; Zhu et al. 2002) but not many people call them. On the low end, 1.1 percent to 1.7 percent of adult smokers were esti-mated to have called a quitline in North America over the span of one year; and in one HMO, only 2.4 percent of smokers used their quitline (Glasgow et al. 1993; Ossip-Klein and McIntosh 2003). The low rate of use might be attributable to limited funds for advertising and staffing the quitlines (Zhu et al. 2000).

An emphasis on smoking cessation treatments in tobacco control policy could widen class disparities in smoking. Although telephone-based quitlines ostensibly create broad access to counseling services, what little data exist on their use among subpopulations indicate that they are most likely to be used by those in higher social classes. Reports from California's quitline, established in 1992, indicates that female, better-educated, and white smokers are more likely to call the quitline. Use of the quitline by various groups appears to be tied to promotion practices (Zhu et al. 2000). Similarly, policies requiring health insurance plans to provide cessation services will benefit those with health insurance. Therefore, expansion of these policies could widen class-based inequities in smoking prevalence.

Similarly, insurance-based coverage of cessation treatments is not equally beneficial to all racial/ethnic groups because these groups do not have equal access to health insurance. Racial/ethnic minorities are overrepresented in low-income groups and, as a result, are less likely to have health insurance. In 2004, about 33.0 percent of Hispanics and 17.7 percent of blacks lacked health insurance, compared with 16.5 percent of whites. If insurance companies increase coverage of smoking cessation treatments, therefore, smoking rates among whites are likely to fall more than smoking rates among blacks or Latinos. It remains to be seen what implications the Patient Protection and Affordable Care Act of 2010 will have for equity of access for support of smoking cessation.

If women are more likely than men to call telephone quitlines (Zhu et al. 2000), reliance on this policy might increase the gender gap in smoking prevalence. In addition, women are less likely to be uninsured than men (15.2 percent vs. 18.1 percent for adults under age 65) (Adams, Heyman, and Vickerie 2009), which would also indicate that improved access to treatment through insurance plans would have a greater impact on them, thus increasing the gender gap.

Compared with insurance-based coverage, increased use of telephone-based quitlines could benefit different segments of the population more equally, at least for those who have access to telephone service. However, the effectiveness of quitlines depends largely on their promotion. Research shows that promotion efforts can be effective in increasing use of quitlines among underserved populations. One important study, using a strong design, tested the effectiveness of a media campaign to increase use of the National Cancer Information Service (a telephone-based quitline) among African Americans and reported that use of the service was higher among residents in the intervention versus control communities (Boyd et al. 1998).

SCHOOL-BASED SMOKING PREVENTION PROGRAMS

Tobacco education programs in schools are appealing for two important reasons. First, if we can prevent smoking initiation in the teenage years, adult smoking prevalence is likely to drop; few people begin smoking after age 19. Second, most teenagers are in school for some or all of their teenage years, making them an easy target to reach. School-based programs have only modest effects on smoking rates (Backinger et al. 2003). An expert panel was convened in 1987 by the National Cancer Institute (NCI) to assess the evidence on school-based programming and to recommend what might be the essential elements of such programs (Glynn 1989). The panel found that the programs to date had shown some positive effects but that those effects had been both modest and limited in scope.

These programs do not reach all youth equally. The NCI panel concluded that school-based programs had been less effective in reaching high-risk youth, including youth from low socioeconomic status or racial/ethnic minority backgrounds as well as school dropouts. One study of Canadian youth tracked dropouts who had been exposed to a tobacco prevention curriculum in middle school but then left school, and found that 68 percent of them had begun smoking, compared with 28 percent of those still in school at grade 12 (Flay et al. 1989).

The difficulty in reaching dropouts with school-based prevention programs might even begin while dropouts are still in school. Research using the National Longitudinal Study of Adolescent Health conducted in 1995–1996, which surveyed students from 132 middle, junior, and high schools, found that trouble in school predicted both smoking initiation and progression to regular smoking for both boys and girls (Van Den Bree, Whitmer, and Pickworth 2004). It is not surprising that those who struggle in other classes may also not be successfully absorbing lessons from health classes. This problem is not limited to the United States. An Australian study also found that those with low levels of involvement in school activities and a low interest in having a healthy school were most likely to smoke (Schofield, Lynagh, and Mishra 2003). Similarly, an English study found that smokers were twice as likely to be absent from school as nonsmokers (Aveyard et al. 1999).

Schools are attractive sites for interventions because they represent an easy channel for reaching youth. But youth of low socioeconomic status, who are at greatest risk of smoking, may be among the least attentive students, and schools may well not be an appropriate venue for reaching them. There is a similar problem with trying to reach young adults (people aged 18–25). The easiest way to find a large population of this age group is at college, but college students are relatively unlikely to smoke (Barbeau, Leavy-Sperounis, and Balbach 2004). School-based tobacco education programs, therefore, may widen class-based differences in smoking rates.

School-based programs may be differentially available to different racial-ethnic groups because dropout rates are higher among Hispanics and blacks than among whites. While 7 percent of white students drop out of high school,

17 percent of blacks and 25 percent of Hispanics drop out (U.S. Department of Education 2006), creating uneven exposure to school-based tobacco control education. Because blacks and Hispanics have lower smoking rates than whites, school-based education may close the race-ethnicity smoking gap among these groups. However, because boys are more likely than girls to drop out of school, school-based programs could widen the gender gap in smoking.

RESTRICTING YOUTH ACCESS

Because most smokers begin smoking as teenagers, youth access programs have been developed to try to disrupt the supply of cigarettes to underage smokers. The assumption of these programs is that if a teenager or adolescent cannot buy cigarettes, he or she will be less likely to smoke. Tobacco control advocates also hope to establish a strong norm against teen tobacco use by implementing, monitoring, and publicizing such programs. Elements of a youth access program can include laws setting age minima for buying tobacco products, licensing tobacco retailers, signage requirements, penalties for selling tobacco products, penalties for buying cigarettes, bans on self-service displays, limits on vending machine placement, and enforcement and monitoring plans. To assess compliance, some communities have audit programs in which youth attempt to buy cigarettes from retailers (Brownson et al. 1995; Liang et al. 2003). The Synar Amendment, passed in 1993, required that all states have laws that prohibit cigarette sales to minors, establish youth access programs, and monitor compliance with the law. Failure to comply puts states at risk of losing up to nearly half of their federal funding in the area of substance abuse (Gilpin, Lee, and Pierce 2004b).

Controversy has marked youth access restrictions since their inception. One key area of controversy is whether these restrictions might actually encourage youth to smoke by making smoking seem exciting, rebellious, and adult (Unger et al. 1999). In addition, because many beginning smokers and more than half of all underage smokers do not buy their own cigarettes but rely on peers or family as sources (Harrison, Fulkerson, and Park 2000), it is unclear that youth access programs focused on sales can really block underage smokers from getting cigarettes.

Both of these concerns arise in considering class disparities in smoking. Because low-socioeconomic-status adults have higher smoking rates, youth from these families will continue to have social access to cigarettes even if youth access laws restrict their purchase of cigarettes. Thus, youth access programs may have a smaller impact on low-socioeconomic-status youth than on others. In addition, if youth in this population perceive themselves as "rebels" or "outside the mainstream," youth access programs might make smoking more appealing as a mark of rebellion against authority. For both of these reasons, youth access policies could increase class disparities in smoking rates.

While research indicates that youth access laws may reduce cigarette sales and thereby smoking prevalence (Forster et al. 1998; Jason et al. 1999), most such studies have been conducted in predominantly white communities, leaving us little basis for predictions about how this policy might affect racial-ethnic differences in smoking. Moreover, it has been difficult to understand how race or ethnicity affects access to cigarettes because many studies fail to control statistically for social class or neighborhood characteristics (Harrison, Fulkerson, and Park 2000). A 1999 study found that merchants were 2.5 times more likely to sell cigarettes to African American and Latino youth than to white youth, replicating the results of a similar study conducted in 1993–1995, which also found differences in sales rates by race/ethnicity (Landrine et al. 2000). On the other hand, a large-scale national survey found that youth of color reported lower perceived availability of cigarettes than white youth (Johnston, O'Malley, and Terry-McElrath 2004). The effect of tougher youth access laws on race/ethnic disparities in smoking is difficult to anticipate based on existing evidence.

Research indicates that women are more likely to be able to buy cigarettes despite youth access restrictions (Clark et al. 2000; DiFranza, Savageau, and Aisquith 1996). Another study found that women are more than twice as likely as men to rely on social sources for cigarettes, a method of bypassing youth access laws (Harrison, Fulkerson, and Park 2000). On the other hand, a recent systematic review concluded that youth access programs that involved enforcement and education might be more effective for girls than for boys (Thomas et al. 2008). The effect of youth access restrictions on the gender gap in smoking is thus difficult to anticipate.

MEDIA CAMPAIGNS

In general, there are very few studies that compare the effectiveness of media campaigns across population subgroups. A few studies consider differential effects among youth. For instance, the American Legacy Foundation's "Truth" campaign has been found to be more effective with African Americans than with other racial/ethnic groups. Anti-industry beliefs were associated with lower smoking prevalence, thus indicating that "truth"-type campaigns may be particularly effective with this population (Hersey et al. 2005). However, other research finds little difference by social category in the association between exposure to counterindustry media campaigns and smoking attitudes or behavior (Sly et al. 2001). It is unclear how generalizable these studies are to the adult population. Among adults, there is mixed evidence that the effects of media campaigns on smoking behavior differ by social category (Bala, Strzeszynski, and Cahill 2008; Levy, Mumford, and Compton 2006). The efficacy of mass media anti-smoking campaigns is likely to depend on the fit between message and market segment (Dietz et al. 2008). Overall, the evidence base is too thin even for speculation about differential impacts of media campaigns by social category.

SUMMARY AND CONCLUSIONS

Smoking rates vary by social category. The gender gap in smoking between men and women has narrowed, though men continue to be more likely than women to smoke. Black-white smoking differences have fluctuated, with whites now slightly more likely to be smokers than blacks; Native Americans have the highest prevalence of smoking. Once a habit of the most affluent in society (Kluger 1996), smoking is now increasingly concentrated among the socioeconomically disadvantaged, and the inverse relationship between smoking and socioeconomic status has been steadily increasing.

Because these differentials in smoking contribute to health disparities, it is critical to understand how more vigorous tobacco control measures might affect them. We reviewed evidence about the six policy instruments in the IOM scenario in order to examine how these policies were likely to affect disparities in smoking. The evidence regarding differential impacts of tobacco control policies remains very limited; our conclusions are provisional and often based as much on presumed differences in exposure to the policies as on differences in their effects. Nonetheless, this preliminary evaluation provides a place to start and will, we hope, spur further research. Indeed, signs of increasing attention to this question include recently published research articles or reviews (Dinno and Glantz 2009; Thomas et al. 2008) as well as special theme issues in the *Journal of Epidemiology and Community Health* (September 2006 supplement on "Tobacco Control Policy and Low Socioeconomic Status Women and Girls"), *Addiction* (October 2007 special issue on "Conceptual and Methodological Issues for Research on Tobacco-Related Health Disparities"), and the *American Journal of Preventive Medicine* (August 2009 supplement on "Tobacco Policy and Its Unintended Consequences Among Low-Income Women"). Some of this research was spurred by the Tobacco Research Network on Disparities (TReND), a transdisciplinary research network organized by the NCI and the American Legacy Foundation (Clayton 2006).

Of the six policies, two of them are likely to reduce class disparities, reducing smoking rates more among those of lower socioeconomic status: excise tax increases and national clean air policies. On the other hand, while expanding insurance coverage of smoking cessation treatments will help smokers who have health insurance, it will do nothing for disadvantaged populations who lack public and private health care coverage. (The new health care reform law is likely to temper this inequality, but it is too soon to understand its impact.) In addition, school-based smoking prevention programs will miss dropouts, and youth access restrictions are likely to have less impact on youth of lower socio-economic status, who can more readily get access to cigarettes through their social networks. Because black and Latino populations have higher jobless and dropout rates and lower insurance coverage, they are less likely than whites to be reached by some IOM policy measures, but they may be more price-sensitive and thus more likely to respond to changes in the excise tax; the net effect is uncertain. Finally, gender disparities may be reduced under the IOM policy measures if, as many studies find, males are more price sensitive than females; in addition, to the extent that men have higher employment rates than women, men are more likely to be affected by clean air regulations that ban or restrict smoking in the workplace. The data on the potential effects of youth access programs are mixed.

There were some social categories for which we found essentially no evidence at all. Native Americans have the highest smoking rates of any racial/ethnic sub-group in the United States, while Asian Americans have the lowest; we know very little about how tobacco control policies affect either of these ethnic groups. In addition, although smoking rates tend to be relatively high among gay men and lesbian and bisexual women, we know little about how tobacco control policies affect these populations (Ryan et al. 2001; Tang et al. 2004).

We should also caution that the tobacco industry could adapt to new policy scenarios by targeting promotion efforts to specific groups, thereby changing smoking disparities in ways that are difficult to predict a priori. We know, for instance, that the industry has executed specific marketing efforts to attract low-income (Barbeau, Leavy-Sperounis, and Balbach 2004), African American (Balbach, Gasior, and Barbeau 2003), immigrant (Acevedo-Garcia et al. 2004), and lesbian/gay/bisexual groups (Smith, Offen, and Malone 2005). Although we cannot predict what changes the industry might undertake under different policy scenarios and how these in turn would affect different population groups, it is nonetheless important to situate tobacco control policies in a larger, dynamic policy context.

In recent years, several tobacco control (and other public health) agencies and foundations have begun to designate some groups as "special" or "priority populations," that is, those deserving of special attention in terms of programs and resources. These typically include relatively disadvantaged or marginalized populations such as women, people of color, youth, lesbians and gays, and the poor (Barbeau, Krieger, and Soobader 2004; Krieger 2004). Smoking rates and the risk of tobacco-related disease, however, do not align well with this conventional health disparities framework. Complementing this framework, it may be worthwhile to consider institutional location both in identifying disparities and in planning interventions. Some institutional locations are relatively tolerant of smoking; examples include the military, prisons, some homeless shelters, and institutions that serve people with a mental illness. Other institutional locations, such as schools and civilian workplaces, are more likely to prohibit smoking and may also provide smoking prevention or cessation services. These contrasts in institutional policies may deepen the divide in smoking rates between advantaged and disadvantaged populations.

For those concerned with how tobacco control policies might affect disparities in smoking prevalence, a fundamental and value-laden question remains: ought we as a society give priority to policies that confer the most benefit to the population overall, regardless of the implications for disparities in smoking? Is it, for example, justifiable to expend public resources on school-based smoking cessation education when we know the youth most at risk of smoking have already dropped out? Or should we prioritize policies that target particular groups with elevated smoking rates, even if they represent a relatively small proportion of the population (Adler and Newman 2002)? For example, this approach might lead us to pinpoint resources to vocational or trade schools and job training programs for high school dropouts.

There is no consensus within the public health or tobacco control advocacy communities on this question, and we don't attempt to answer it here. Instead, we suggest that readers consider the potential for inequity as we discuss how various policy levers work in reducing smoking prevalence across social category. By choosing some policies and not others, tobacco control advocates may widen some inequities and mitigate or eliminate others. More research is needed to understand the extent of these trade-offs.

PART 4

EPILOGUE

17

AFTER TOBACCO

PETER BEARMAN, KATHRYN M. NECKERMAN, AND LESLIE WRIGHT

There is no question that reducing smoking would improve health and reduce mortality among smokers and others exposed to tobacco smoke. People who smoke face risks of disease that are considerably higher for certain types of cancer as well as heart disease, stroke, and respiratory disease. Maternal smoking also increases the risk of low birth weight, preterm delivery, and sudden infant death syndrome. These well-documented effects of smoking on health have motivated more than four decades of tobacco control policy.

Although policymakers understand the gains from tobacco control, they have not understood its costs. Americans smoke several hundred billion cigarettes each year, and those cigarettes represent income for farmers, factory workers, retailers, and governments, among others. There is concern that a steep decline in smoking could be disruptive or costly in many ways, or that stronger tobacco control policies could have undesirable side effects. Given this uncertainty about the magnitude of these economic and social consequences, even modest tobacco control measures—a small tax increase, for instance, or a smoking ban in restaurants—can become embroiled in controversy. Yet it is clear that without much more vigorous measures, smoking will remain the largest single preventable cause of illness and premature mortality. Thus, it is critical to understand what would happen if Americans stopped smoking.

This chapter highlights key findings from the preceding chapters and discusses their implications for future research and policy.

KEY FINDINGS

ECONOMIC IMPACTS ON TOBACCO PRODUCERS

A drop in smoking rates obviously has implications for the producers of tobacco leaf and cigarettes and for the southeastern communities where tobacco production is concentrated. Tobacco gives farmers a much higher return per acre than other crops and has long sustained rural families through the uncertainties of farm life. Cigarette manufacturing pays higher wages than blue-collar workers are likely to earn elsewhere. It is not that surprising that many elected officials from tobacco-producing states have been stalwart supporters of the industry.

There is no question that farmers and cigarette production workers would face some losses if smoking rates fell substantially. Under the high-impact scenario, if cigarette consumption fell by three-quarters, Sumner and Alston (chapter 3) estimate, growers' revenue from tobacco sales would be a third lower in 2025. The projected decline in revenue is not greater because tobacco farmers produce for the international market as well as the domestic one; international trade in tobacco and cigarettes is likely to protect farmers from the full impact of declining U.S. consumption. Under the same high-impact scenario, Espinosa and Evans (chapter 4) project some 4,300 fewer cigarette manufacturing production workers would be employed in 2025 than would be the case with no change in tobacco control policy. Although some displaced workers would find other jobs, their expected earnings would be 24 percent lower than what they would have earned making cigarettes.

The impact of tobacco control is less severe than it would have been only a few decades ago because the tobacco-producing sector is smaller than it was. Between 1982 and 2002 the number of tobacco farmers fell by two-thirds, and the number of cigarette factory workers fell by half. Over the same period, as chapter 5 reports, the percentage of counties defined as economically dependent on tobacco dropped from 23.6 to only 4.2 percent. The decline in smoking is only one reason for this change. Because of technological advances, tobacco leaf and cigarettes can now be produced more efficiently—with less labor—than ever before. In addition, U.S. manufacturers are using more imported tobacco leaf in their cigarettes, and growing competition from abroad has reduced exports of tobacco leaf and products. For all these reasons, by 2002 tobacco farming and manufacturing had already downsized significantly, and the impact of a further decline in smoking is correspondingly reduced.

ECONOMIC IMPACTS IN OTHER SECTORS

In the Southeast, concern about the impact of tobacco control has focused on tobacco farmers and manufacturers, but elsewhere the hospitality and retail sectors have attracted more attention, with restaurant, bar, and convenience store owners fearing a loss of business. Other sectors that could be affected include nonprofit organizations and state and local governments.

In general, we find that the economic costs of tobacco control policy for these sectors are very limited and in some cases may be offset by gains. Among retailers, Ribisl and colleagues (chapter 6) report, stores that specialize in tobacco products would inevitably be hit hard by a substantial drop in smoking rates. Convenience stores, where cigarettes represent an average of 12.4 percent of sales, face a much smaller impact. Other types of retailers would be little affected. In fact, some might benefit as discretionary income previously spent on tobacco is now spent on other consumer goods. Overall, the effect on the retail sector is expected to be minimal: retail employment is projected to be less than 1 percent lower in 2025 under the high-impact scenario than in the status quo.

The impact of smoking bans on the hospitality industry is one of the most widely studied questions in tobacco research. As Hyland and colleagues (chapter 7) discuss, most independently funded research finds that clean air laws and other anti-smoking measures have no negative impact on restaurants and bars. A national smoking ban is even less likely to show a negative impact than current research might suggest because many existing studies examine local-level smoking bans, which allow smokers to cross city or county boundaries to find venues where they can smoke. Under a nationwide clean air law, there would be no incentive for this kind of boundary crossing. Moreover, these studies do not measure a potential benefit for the industry: employees will be healthier. There is little indication that tougher smoking bans would lead to a loss of business in the hospitality industry, but if there were a negative impact, it would likely diminish over time as smoking rates dropped among consumers.

The large cigarette companies such as Philip Morris (now Altria) and R. J. Reynolds (now Reynolds American) have made extensive philanthropic contributions to education, the arts, disaster relief, and other causes as well as to hometown organizations. Because corporate contributions are closely tied to corporate profits, a decline in the scale or profitability of the tobacco industry is likely to lead to a decline in philanthropy. However, as Rooney and Frederick (chapter 8) point out, because corporate philanthropy is such a small share of the budgets of nonprofit organizations, a decline in donations from only one industry would have a negligible effect on nonprofit organizations, although the impact in Winston-Salem or Richmond, where the two largest cigarette manufacturers are headquartered, could be more significant. Even there, however, the industry comprises a falling share of an increasingly diversified local economy, and the impact of a decline in tobacco would be much smaller than it would have been several decades ago.

States and localities have raised tobacco excise taxes sharply over the last decade for both public health and fiscal reasons. The tobacco control scenarios discussed here have mixed implications for state revenue: the increase in tax rates would raise revenues while the decline in smoking rates would decrease revenues. As Chernick (chapter 9) discusses, the net impact of tobacco control policy on state budgets depends on how much smoking rates fall. States fare better under the IOM scenario than the high-impact scenario because smoking rates would remain higher. In addition, the fiscal impact depends on whether the tax is imposed (and retained) by the federal government or by state governments. In 2005, the per-capita tobacco tax revenue in the average state was $65; in 2010, under the IOM scenario, that figure was projected to be $115 if the tax were imposed by the states and $35 if the tax were imposed by the federal government. The impact on total tax revenues would be small, however, because tobacco taxes are a small fraction of total state revenue. The estimated change in per-capita state tax revenues between 2005 and 2025 would range from an increase of 0.5 percent (IOM scenario, state tax) to a decline of 2.5 percent (high-impact scenario, federal tax). The impact is even smaller when considered in the context of all (tax and nontax) sources of state revenue.

HEALTH AND LONGEVITY

Tobacco control policy has implications for health and mortality, but some of the benefit of reducing smoking takes a long time to appear. Although there is an immediate boost to health from smoking cessation, former smokers continue to have elevated rates of disease and mortality for years after they quit. In addition, many tobacco control measures, including those modeled here, aim to prevent smoking among young people. Because smoking-related illness typically does not appear until middle age, the health benefits of preventing smoking among teenagers do not become evident for many years.

For both of these reasons, tobacco control policies have a relatively small near-term effect on outcomes related to health and longevity. Compared with the status quo scenario, Apelberg and Samet (chapter 10) estimate that the IOM scenario would reduce the number of premature deaths occurring between 2006 and 2025 by about 450,000, or 1 percent; the reduction in mortality would be about 1.1 million (3 percent) under the high-impact scenario and 2.8 million under the 100 percent cessation scenario. Almost 40 percent of this decline in mortality reflects a reduction in deaths from lung cancer, 8 percent from other cancers, and 30 percent from cardiovascular disease.

The studies of medical care expenditures and Social Security find parallel results. Levy and Newhouse (chapter 11) report that, compared with the status quo scenario, medical care expenditures between 2006 and 2025 would be 0.43 percent lower under the IOM scenario and 0.88 percent lower under the high-impact scenario. A decline in smoking would have the largest effect on Medicaid spending because smoking rates are higher in low-income populations, but the savings are still quite modest. Hurd and colleagues (chapter 12) find that a decline in smoking would increase payments for old age benefits due to rising longevity but would also decrease disability payments through improving health. In addition, because healthier workers tend to earn more and retire later, a decline in smoking rates would increase Social Security tax receipts. The net effect is small: in 2024, net Social Security outlays would be 0.1 percent lower under the IOM scenario and 2.7 percent higher under the 100 percent cessation scenario. In today's policy context, this modest and gradual effect of tobacco control policy on health is a double-edged sword. Some might hope that a decline in smoking could solve the crisis of rising health care costs, but that hope is unrealistic. Some might fear that tobacco control will create a new fiscal crisis in Social Security; that fear, too, is unlikely to be realized.

LAW AND SOCIETY

As discussed above, tobacco control policy could have unintended consequences that temper its benefits for health. The classic historical referent is the Prohibition era, when a ban on the sale of alcohol spurred a rise in organized crime. The final chapters in this book explore the implications of tobacco control for enforcement costs, stigmatization of smokers, mentally ill populations, and health disparities. Taken together, these chapters highlight the ways in which policy design matters. What we might consider the social costs of tobacco control depend critically on how policy objectives are achieved.

While enforcement of tobacco control regulations involves expenses for tax collection and for inspections in restaurants, stores, and other businesses, perhaps the most prominent concern is that higher excise tax rates will lead to more tax evasion—illegal activities such as smuggling—as well as tax avoidance through cross-border shopping. As Chaloupka and colleagues (chapter 13) write, however, simple legal and regulatory measures such as improved tax stamps and licensing of those involved in cigarette distribution can reduce the risk of tax evasion. In addition, states have efficient ways to curtail tax evasion through Internet sales, and the federal government could support these efforts by enforcing existing laws. Reducing the large differences in state tax rates would also remove much of the incentive for smuggling.

A second concern about tobacco control policies is that they might stigma-tize those who continue to smoke. Stigma could undermine health by causing stress; it could also lead smokers to isolate themselves or to conceal their smok-ing status. Research by Stuber and colleagues (chapter 14) finds that some smokers do perceive stigma, and that those who do are more likely to have quit; however, they are also more likely to keep their smoking a secret and to with-draw socially from nonsmokers. Although we don't know whether tobacco con-trol policies cause stigmatization, some policy measures—such as media cam-paigns with negative portrayals of smoking—seem more likely than others to do so; future research should examine both the causes and consequences of the stigmatization of smokers.

Anti-smoking policies are sometimes believed to be more burdensome for people with mental illness or multiple addictions. These vulnerable populations smoke more, and there is some evidence that quitting may be more difficult; people may self-medicate by smoking to relieve both their symptoms and the side effects of their medications. As Williams and colleagues (chapter 15) write, smokers with mental illness have lower quit rates in part because tobacco control policies are not designed to address the particular challenges faced by this popu-lation. Some residential and clinic settings tolerate smoking, and not all health care providers make smoking cessation a priority for patients with mental illness. With appropriate support, however, these patients can quit and enjoy significant health benefits from doing so.

Finally, there is concern that tobacco control policy could widen socio-economic or racial/ethnic disparities in health. This might occur if tobacco control measures have a greater impact on people who hold more privileged positions in society. As Balbach and colleagues (chapter 16) write, so far we know little about whether tobacco control measures affect some social groups more than others. However, there are certainly differences in exposure to policies meant to reduce smoking. For instance, smoking prevention programs aimed at teenagers are of-ten based in schools; as a result, students are exposed to these programs while school dropouts are not. Among adults, people in higher-status occupations are more likely than people in lower-status occupations to be in workplaces that ban smoking, while the jobless are not exposed at all to workplace smoking bans. Here as well, policy design matters. Disparities in smoking rates could be re-duced by policies that are applied more universally, such as clean air laws that cover all public places. In considering the implications of tobacco control, it will be important to attend to marginalized populations, such as the incarcerated or homeless, who occupy institutions where smoking is tolerated or who fall en-tirely outside the reach of mainstream institutions.

IMPLICATIONS FOR FUTURE RESEARCH

Predicting the future is a complex undertaking. Any project of this kind has limitations—questions left unexamined or shortcomings of existing data and methods—and ours is no exception. For the present, readers should simply keep these caveats in mind. For the future, these limitations represent an agenda for study that we hope other researchers will engage.

To begin, we made some simplifying assumptions about the policy process that are unlikely to be borne out in reality. Policy change seldom occurs in the quick and orderly fashion that the SimSmoke model assumes. As Balbach and colleagues write, as long as many anti-smoking regulations and programs are legislated, funded, and implemented at the state and local levels, their reach is likely to be uneven because of differences across communities in political support and budgetary resources. Disparities may result: for instance, lower-income communities may have more limited funding to support cessation programs or enforcement of clean air laws.

In addition, we did not consider the possibility that recently enacted tobacco policy measures might be rolled back or that the impact of tobacco control measures might be offset by more vigorous marketing and price offsets by the industry. Neither is out of the question. In fact, incremental rollbacks occur often, when states fail to adjust their tobacco tax rates for inflation, or when they reduce funding for enforcement of youth access or tobacco cessation programs in response to budgetary or political pressure. In addition, it is well known that the major tobacco companies have increased their marketing and discounts significantly since the Master Settlement Agreement restricted advertising for tobacco products.

We should also keep in mind that the SimSmoke projections that were developed by Levy and Mumford (chapter 2) and that drive most chapters in this volume are based on the experience of the last 10 to 20 years. Key parameters of that experience may have changed or could change in the future. For instance, some observers believe that as tobacco control policies have been strengthened, the smokers who are the least addicted or the most motivated to stop have quit first, leaving a population of smokers who are more heavily addicted or more resistant to quitting. As smoking rates decline, this "hardening hypothesis" suggests, the remaining smokers are less likely to be responsive to an increase in excise taxes or other policy measures (Warner and Burns 2003). If this is true, the SimSmoke model may overstate the smoking decline likely to occur in the future in response to the IOM policy measures.

Moreover, the current generation of simulation models—including SimSmoke, the most widely used of these models—are not able to account for the ways that social influences might affect the predicted decline in smoking. Like many activities, smoking is patterned by social networks. A recent study finds that when one friend, co-worker, or relative quits, others are likely to follow (Christakis and Fowler 2008). Yet research on tobacco control policy treats people as individuals, isolated from the social networks that shape their behavior. We do not understand the implications of social networks for the efficacy of anti-smoking policies. It may be that social networks would amplify these policies and accelerate the decline in smoking rates. On the other hand, if smoking becomes more concentrated among socially isolated individuals, or if smokers and nonsmokers become more isolated from each other, patterns of social influence might reduce quit rates. Indeed, Christakis and Fowler found that over time smokers became more peripheral and the number of social ties between smokers and nonsmokers declined.

Among the questions we did not consider are the potential benefits of reducing smoking for quality of life as well as the health benefits of reducing exposure to secondhand smoke. In addition, although the risk of some tobacco-related disease is higher for some racial/ethnic groups than for others (Haiman et al. 2006), the analyses of mortality, medical care expenditures, and Social Security do not take race or ethnicity into account. For race and ethnicity, as for social class or poverty status, data limitations made it difficult to account for such factors. And as previous chapters discuss, there are contingencies that could alter projections about the effects of tobacco control. For instance, the global trade in tobacco affects the demand for U.S. tobacco leaf and cigarettes and could offset the effects of domestic tobacco control policy on farmers and factory workers. Advances in medical treatment for smoking-related diseases could alter our conclusions about the effects of tobacco control on health and longevity and thus on medical care expenditures and on Social Security. Changes in health care policy would likely affect estimates of the costs of smoking-related illness.

In addition, although we considered the economic costs of tobacco control, we did not directly examine some kinds of economic benefits. For instance, reducing smoking may improve employee health and productivity (Halpern et al. 2001) or increase household wealth (Zagorsky 2004). People who stop smoking will have more discretionary income they can spend on other goods and services, increasing demand in other sectors of the economy; in fact, Kenneth Warner and colleagues concluded a decade ago that eliminating smoking could create 130,000 jobs nationwide (Jha and Chaloupka 1999; Warner et al. 1996). The analysis by Ribisl and colleagues explores this possibility by examining the effects of a decline in smoking on stores selling wine, beer, or liquor, but the implications may extend beyond the retail sector, for instance to manufacturing or services. Although researchers have begun to examine this question (Busch et al. 2005), we know too little about the trade-offs consumers make to anticipate where such benefits might appear.

Overall, this volume errs on the side of caution, presenting what are likely to be "worst case" estimates of the consequences of tobacco control policy. We have focused on the negative consequences of tobacco control, giving less attention to the benefits for health and quality of life or to possible economic benefits of reducing smoking. In addition, it is unlikely that tobacco control policies and smoking patterns will change as quickly and consistently as the SimSmoke model assumes; the impact of change in policy is likely to be more gradual and uneven. As better data and more sophisticated simulation models become available, we may find that our estimates have been too pessimistic and that tobacco control measures are less disruptive and less costly than the results in this volume imply.

IMPLICATIONS FOR PUBLIC POLICY

The research reported here should reassure those concerned about the impact of stronger anti-smoking efforts. Even a steep decline in smoking is likely to have minimal effects on large sectors of the economy including the retail and hospitality industries, nonprofit organizations, and state governments, and on medical care expenditures and Social Security. This is because tobacco accounts for a small share of retail sales, taxes paid, and donations given; because the costs of a drop in smoking are sometimes offset by benefits, as when income that had been spent on cigarettes is spent on other consumer items; and because the effects of tobacco control on health—and hence on medical care and Social Security—unfold very gradually over time. In these domains of the economy, there is little reason for public action to mitigate the economic consequences of reducing smoking. Perhaps the best guidance for policymakers is to minimize the differences across jurisdictions in tax rates and regulations. Reducing the variation in excise tax rates would limit the incentives for tax evasion and avoidance, easing enforcement. Similarly, eliminating the variation in clean air laws would remove the incentive for consumers to cross city or county lines to patronize restaurants or bars where they can smoke.

However, a small number of stakeholders could suffer significant economic losses from a decline in smoking. In 2002, these included the owners and employees of roughly 57,000 farms growing tobacco, about 16,600 cigarette manufacturing employees, and the owners and employees of almost 6,200 stores specializing in tobacco products. In addition, in 2002, 29 southeastern counties were classified as "tobacco dependent," meaning that more than 5 percent of the earnings generated in the county were related to tobacco production. Not all of these stakeholders and communities would lose their livelihood even if smoking rates in the United States fell to zero. Most farms sell other products in addition to tobacco, and some farmers and manufacturing workers would continue to produce for the global trade in tobacco leaf and cigarettes. Yet many farmers, workers, and communities are not well positioned to find alternatives to tobacco production or distribution. If policymakers want to mitigate the economic consequences of tobacco control, these stakeholders and communities are relatively straightforward to identify for assistance. In fact, many such programs are already in place, including the payments associated with the quota buyout and the MSA-funded farm diversification and economic development funds.

It is straightforward to identify the proprietors, employees, and communities facing economic losses because of a decline in tobacco production. It is more challenging to devise policies that address the needs of tobacco consumers. As we see in the final chapters in this volume, the most significant risk we may face from a more vigorous tobacco control policy is a widening of disparities in health and health behavior. Anti-smoking policies have worked well for the more advantaged members of our society, who have the knowledge to understand how smoking damages their health and the health care access and social resources to support quitting. These policies do not work as well for people who are disadvantaged or marginalized—for those who lack health insurance, who are unemployed or unstably housed, or who live their lives outside of mainstream institutions. To advance public health objectives without stigmatizing and isolating the minority who continue to smoke, tobacco control policies must be crafted with careful attention to the economic and social contexts of vulnerable populations.

More research will provide more precise and up-to-date estimates of the consequences of tobacco control, but it is unlikely to alter the basic picture. The economic costs and social disruptions we might expect even with a dramatic plunge in smoking rates are relatively modest. For the most part these consequences can be addressed either through careful policy design or through programs to assist those involved directly in tobacco production and distribution. Set against a toll of some 433,000 deaths a year attributed to smoking, these consequences seem a small price to pay.

ACKNOWLEDGMENTS AND LIST OF CONTRIBUTORS

The editors gratefully acknowledge the financial support of the American Legacy Foundation through a grant to Columbia University (CU02493001, Principal Investigator: Peter Bearman). This grant provided support for project administration and editorial work carried out at Columbia University and funded small grants to the authors to support preparation of all but one of the chapters. (Funding for chapter 14 is acknowledged below.) The contents of the chapters are solely the responsibility of the authors and editors and do not necessarily represent the official views of the American Legacy Foundation. At Columbia University's Institute for Social and Economic Research and Policy (ISERP), Nancy Davenport and Joyce Robbins assisted with background research for this project; Fletcher Haulley coordinated the authors' conferences; and Carmen Morillo, Ariel Schwartz, and Paulette Yousefzadeh helped prepare the manuscript for publication. The editors also appreciate the assistance of referees who reviewed the chapters and chapter proposals. At the Columbia University Press, the editors would like to thank Lauren Dockett for her enthusiastic support of the project and Brad Hebel, Meredith Howard, and Derek Warker for managing communications. In addition, we thank John Donohue and Westchester Book Group for their meticulous copyediting.

CONTRIBUTORS

Chapters 1 and 17: Peter Bearman is the Jonathan Cole Professor of the Social Sciences at Columbia University. Kathryn M. Neckerman is Research Associate in the Department of Medicine (Section of Hospital Medicine), University of Chicago. At the time this project was conducted, Leslie Wright was Assistant Director of the Institute for Social and Economic Research and Policy at Columbia University.

Chapter 2: David T. Levy is Professor of Economics at the University of Baltimore. At the time this research was completed, Elizabeth Mumford was Associate Research Scientist at Pacific Institute for Research and Evaluation.

Chapter 3: Daniel A. Sumner is Director of the University of California Agricultural Issues Center and the Frank H. Buck Jr. Professor in the Department of Agricultural and Resource Economics at the University of California, Davis. Julian M. Alston is Director of the Robert Mondavi Institute Center for Wine Economics and a Professor in the Department of Agricultural and Resource Economics of the University of California, Davis. The authors thank the editors and reviewers for suggestions and Sébastien Pouliot, Antoine Champetier de Ribes, and Haley Boriss for research assistance.

Chapter 4: Javier Espinosa is Assistant Professor of Economics at the Rochester Institute of Technology. William N. Evans is the Keough-Hesburgh Professor of Economics at the University of Notre Dame.

Chapter 5: Kathryn M. Neckerman is Research Associate in the Department of Medicine (Section of Hospital Medicine), University of Chicago. Christopher C. Weiss is Director of the Quantitative Methods in the Social Sciences Program at Columbia University. The authors thank Michael Benigno, Silvett Garcia, Heidi Gorham, Audra Query, and Kelly Rader for assistance in compiling the tobacco dependence measures; Samuel Field and James Kim for advice on the analysis; and James W. Quinn for making the maps included in the chapter.

Chapter 6: Kurt M. Ribisl is Associate Professor at the Gillings School of Global Public Health at the University of North Carolina at Chapel Hill. William N. Evans is the Keough-Hesburgh Professor of Economics at the University of Notre Dame. Ellen C. Feighery is Associate Director of International Research at the Campaign for Tobacco-Free Kids.

Chapter 7: Andrew Hyland is an Associate Member in the Department of Health Behavior at Roswell Park Cancer Institute, Buffalo, New York. Mark Travers is an HRI Scientist in the Department of Health Behavior at Roswell Park Cancer Institute. Brian Fix is a Senior Research Specialist in the Department of Health Behavior at Roswell Park Cancer Institute. Special thanks are extended to Anita Lal at the Cancer Council Victoria in Melbourne, Australia, who assisted with the coding of the studies that examined the economic impact of smoke-free laws on the hospitality industry.

Chapter 8: Patrick M. Rooney is Executive Director of the Center on Philanthropy at Indiana University. At the time this research was conducted, Heidi K. Frederick was Assistant Director of Research at the Center on Philanthropy at Indiana University. The authors would like to thank the editors and referees for many useful comments on the penultimate draft. They also thank Diana Agidi for the statistical analyses and Christine Weisenbach for editorial assistance. Any remaining errors or omissions remain their sole responsibility.

Chapter 9: Howard Chernick is Professor of Economics at Hunter College and the Graduate Center, City University of New York. The author would like to thank Phillip Cook, Phillip DeCicca, David Merriman, and Joel Slemrod for helpful comments, and Paul Sturm for superlative research assistance. He would also like to thank Kathryn Neckerman, both for excellent substantive comments and for substantial editorial assistance.

Chapter 10: Benjamin J. Apelberg is an Assistant Scientist at the Johns Hopkins Bloomberg School of Public Health. Jonathan M. Samet is Professor and Flora L. Thornton Chair for the Department of Preventive Medicine at the Keck School of Medicine of USC at the University of Southern California. The authors acknowledge Georgiana Onicescu for her assistance in the statistical programming for the analysis presented here.

Chapter 11: Douglas E. Levy is Assistant Professor of Medicine at Harvard Medical School and the Mongan Institute for Health Policy at Massachusetts General Hospital. Joseph P. Newhouse is the John D. MacArthur Professor of Health Policy and Management at Harvard University. Dr. Levy acknowledges the generous support of the Agency for Healthcare Research and Quality (T32-HS000020).

Chapter 12: Michael Hurd is Director of the Center for the Study of Aging and Senior Principal Researcher at the RAND Corporation. Yuhui Zheng is a Postdoctoral Research Fellow at the Harvard Center for Population and Development Studies. Federico Girosi is a Senior Policy Researcher at the RAND Corporation. Dana Goldman is Professor and the Norman Topping Chair in Medicine and Public Policy at the University of Southern California.

Chapter 13: Frank J. Chaloupka is Distinguished Professor of Economics at the University of Illinois at Chicago. Philip J. Cook is ITT/Terry Sanford Professor of Public Policy and Professor of Economics and Sociology at the Sanford School of Public Policy, Duke University. Richard M. Peck and John A. Tauras are both Associate Professor of Economics at the University of Illinois at Chicago.

Chapter 14: Jennifer Stuber is Assistant Professor in the School of Social Work at the University of Washington. Sandro Galea is the Gelman Professor and

Chair of the Department of Epidemiology at Columbia University's Mailman School of Public Health. Bruce Link is Professor of Epidemiology and Professor of Sociomedical Sciences at Columbia University's Mailman School of Public Health. Funding for the survey supplement was provided by the Robert Wood Johnson Foundation Health and Society Scholars program at Columbia University.

Chapter 15: Jill M. Williams is Associate Professor of Psychiatry and Director of the Division of Addiction Psychiatry at the University of Medicine and Dentistry of New Jersey–Robert Wood Johnson Medical School. Cristine Delnevo is Associate Professor and Director of the Center for Tobacco Surveillance and Evaluation Research at the University of Medicine and Dentistry of the New Jersey School of Public Health. Douglas M. Ziedonis is Professor and Chair of the Department of Psychiatry at the University of Massachusetts Medical School and UMass Memorial Medical Center.

Chapter 16: Edith D. Balbach is Senior Lecturer in the undergraduate Community Health Program at Tufts University. Cathy Hartman is Vice President for Product Management at Healthrageous, Inc. Elizabeth M. Barbeau is Chief Science Officer at Healthrageous, Inc.

REFERENCES

Abidoye, O., M. K. Ferguson, and R. Salgia. 2007. "Lung Carcinoma in African Americans." *Nature Clinical Practice Oncology* 4: 118–29.

Abrams, S. M., M. C. Mahoney, A. Hyland, K. M. Cummings, W. Davis, and L. Song. 2006. "Early Evidence on the Effectiveness of Clean Indoor Air Legislation in New York State." *American Journal of Public Health* 96: 296–98.

Acevedo-Garcia, D., E. Barbeau, J. A. Bishop, J. Pan, and K. M. Emmons. 2004. "Undoing an Epidemiologic Paradox: The Tobacco Industry's Targeting of US Immigrants." *American Journal of Public Health* 94: 2188–93.

Adams, E. K., G. Solanki, and L. S. Miller. 1997. "Medical-Care Expenditures Attributable to Cigarette Smoking During Pregnancy—United States, 1995." *MMWR—Morbidity & Mortality Weekly Report* 46: 1048–50.

Adams, P. F., and C. A. Schoenborn. 2006. "Health Behaviors of Adults: United States, 2004–05." Hyattsville, MD: National Center for Health Statistics.

Adams, P., K. Heyman, and J. Vickerie. 2009. "Summary Health Statistics for the U.S. Population: National Health Interview Survey, 2008." Hyattsville, MD: National Center for Health Statistics.

Adams, S., and C. D. Cotti. 2007. "The Effect of Smoking Bans on Bars and Restaurants: An Analysis of Changes in Employment." *The B.E. Journal of Economic Analysis & Policy* 7: Article 12.

Adler, N. E., and K. Newman. 2002. "Socioeconomic Disparities in Health: Pathways and Policies." *Health Affairs* 21: 60–76.

Ahmad, S. 2005. "Increasing Excise Taxes on Cigarettes in California: A Dynamic Simulation of Health and Economic Impacts." *Preventive Medicine* 41: 276–83.

Ahmad, S., and G. A. Franz. 2008. "Raising Taxes to Reduce Smoking Prevalence in the US: A Simulation of the Anticipated Health and Economic Impacts." *Public Health* 122: 3–10.

Alamar, B., and S. A. Glantz. 2006a. "Author's Response to M. R. Pakko." *Tobacco Control* 15: 69.

Alamar, B., and S. A. Glantz. 2006b. "Effect of Increased Social Unacceptability of Cigarette Smoking on Reduction in Cigarette Consumption." *American Journal of Public Health* 96: 1359–63.

Alberg, A. J., M. V. Brock, and J. M. Samet. 2005. "Epidemiology of Lung Cancer: Looking to the Future." *Journal of Clinical Oncology* 23: 3175–85.

Altman, D. G., V. Rosenquist, J. S. McBride, B. Bailey, and D. Austin. 2000. "Churches, Tobacco Farmers, and Community Sustainability: Insights from the Tobacco South." *Journal of Community Psychology* 28: 151–68.

American Association for Public Opinion Research. 2003. "Standard Definitions: Final Dispositions of Case Codes and Outcome Rates for Surveys." Deerfield, IL: American Association for Public Opinion Research.

American Lung Association. 2006. "State Legislated Actions on Tobacco Issues (SLATI)." 17th ed. http://lungusa.org.

American Nonsmokers' Rights Foundation. 2010. "Overview List—How Many Smokefree Laws?" April 1. http://www.no-smoke.org/goingsmokefree.php?id=519.

American Psychiatric Association. 1996. "Practice Guideline for the Treatment of Patients with Nicotine Dependence. American Psychiatric Association." *American Journal of Psychiatry* 153: 1–31.

An, L. C., B. A. Schillo, A. M. Kavanaugh, R. B. Lachter, M. G. Luxenberg, A. H. Wendling, and A. M. Joseph. 2006. "Increased Reach and Effectiveness of a Statewide Tobacco Quitline After the Addition of Access to Free Nicotine Replacement Therapy." *Tobacco Control* 15: 286–93.

Anda, R. F., D. F. Williamson, L. G. Escobedo, E. E. Mast, G. A. Giovino, and P. L. Remington. 1990. "Depression and the Dynamics of Smoking: A National Perspective." *Journal of the American Medical Association* 264: 1541–45.

Anonymous. 1995. "Self-Serving Surveys: The 30 Percent Myth." *Consumer Reports* (March): 142–47.

Apollonio, D. E., and R. E. Malone. 2005. "Marketing to the Marginalised: Tobacco Industry Targeting of the Homeless and Mentally Ill." *Tobacco Control* 14: 409–15.

Armitage, P., and R. Doll. 1957. "A Two-Stage Theory of Carcinogenesis in Relation to the Age Distribution of Human Cancer." *British Journal of Cancer* 11: 161–69.

Armour, B. S., and M. M. Pitts. 2006. "Smoking: Taxing Health and Social Security." Working Paper 2006–12. Atlanta: Federal Reserve Bank of Atlanta.

Aveyard, P., K. Cheng, J. Almond, E. Sherratt, R. Lancashire, and T. Lawrence. 1999. "Cluster Randomised Controlled Trial of Expert System Based on the Transtheoretical ('Stages of Change') Model for Smoking Prevention." *British Medical Journal* 319: 948–53.

Babcock, B. A., and W. E. Foster. 1991. "Measuring the Potential Contribution of Plant Breeding to Crop Yields: Flue-Cured Tobacco, 1954–87." *American Journal of Agricultural Economics* 73: 850–59.

Backinger, C., P. Fagan, E. Matthews, and R. Grana. 2003. "Adolescent and Young Adult Tobacco Prevention and Cessation: Current Status and Future Directions." *Tobacco Control* 46: 46–53.

Bain, C., D. Feskanich, F. E. Speizer, M. Thun, E. Hertzmark, B. A. Rosner, and G. A. Colditz. 2004. "Lung Cancer Rates in Men and Women with Comparable Histories of Smoking." *Journal of the National Cancer Institute* 96: 826–34.

Bala, M., L. Strzeszynski, and K. Cahill. 2008. "Mass Media Interventions for Smoking Cessation in Adults." *Cochrane Database of Systematic Reviews* no. 1: CD004704.

Balbach, E. D., R. J. Gasior, and E. M. Barbeau. 2003. "R.J. Reynolds' Targeting of African Americans: 1988–2000." *American Journal of Public Health* 93: 822–27.

Baltagi, B. H., and D. Levin. 1986. "Estimating Dynamic Demand for Cigarettes Using Panel Data: The Effects of Bootlegging, Taxation and Advertising Reconsidered." *Review of Economics and Statistics* 68: 148–55.

Banthin, C. 2004. "Cheap Smokes: State and Federal Responses to Tobacco Tax Evasion Over the Internet." *Health Matrix* 14: 325–56.

Barbeau, E., N. Krieger, and M. Soobader. 2004. "Working Class Matters: Socioeconomic Disadvantage, Race/Ethnicity, Gender and Smoking in the National Health Interview Survey, 2000." *American Journal of Public Health* 94: 269–78.

Barbeau, E., A. Leavy-Sperounis, and E. Balbach. 2004. "Smoking, Social Class, and Gender: What Can Public Health Learn from the Tobacco Industry About Disparities in Smoking?" *Tobacco Control* 13: 115–20.

Barbeau, E., Y. Li, G. Sorensen, K. Conlan, R. Youngstrom, and K. Emmons. 2001. "Coverage of Smoking Cessation Treatment by Union Health and Welfare Funds." *American Journal of Public Health* 91: 1412–15.

Barkley, R. A., G. J. DuPaul, and M. B. McMurray. 1990. "Comprehensive Evaluation of Attention Deficit Disorder with and Without Hyperactivity as Defined by Research Criteria." *Journal of Consulting and Cinical Psychology* 58: 775–89.

Bartlett, J. C., L. S. Miller, D. P. Rice, and W. B. Max. 1994. "Medical-Care Expenditures Attributable to Cigarette Smoking—United States, 1993." *MMWR—Morbidity & Mortality Weekly Report* 43: 469–72.

Bauer, J. E. 2005. "A Longitudinal Assessment of the Impact of Smoke-Free Worksite Policies on Tobacco Use." *American Journal of Public Health* 95: 1024–29.

Bayer, R. 2008. "Stigma and the Ethics of Public Health: Not Can We But Should We." *Social Science and Medicine* 67: 463–72.

Bayer, R., and J. Stuber. 2006. "Tobacco Control, Stigma, and Public Health: Rethinking the Relations." *American Journal of Public Health* 96: 47–50.

Becker, G. S., M. Grossman, and K. M. Murphy. 1994. "An Empirical Analysis of Cigarette Addiction." *American Economic Review* 84: 396–418.

Beckham, J. C. 1999. "Smoking and Anxiety in Combat Veterans with Chronic Posttraumatic Stress Disorder: A Review." *Journal of Psychoactive Drugs* 31: 103–10.

Beghin, J., and F. Hu. 1995. "Declining U.S. Tobacco Exports to Australia: A Derived Demand Approach to Competitiveness." *American Journal of Agricultural Economics* 77: 260–67.

Bell, K., A. Salmon, M. Bowers, J. Bell, and L. McCullough. 2010. "Smoking, Stigma and Tobacco 'Denormalization': Further Reflections on the Use of Stigma as a Public Health Tool. A Commentary on Social Science & Medicine's Stigma, Prejudice, Discrimination and Health Special Issue (67: 3)." *Social Science & Medicine* 70: 795–99.

Bernard, A. B., J. B. Jensen, and P. K. Schott. 2005. "Assessing the Impact of Trade Liberalization on Import-Competing Industries in the Appalachian Region." Washington, DC: Appalachian Regional Commission.

Bernat, D. H., E. G. Klein, L. E. A. Fabian, and J. L. Forster. 2009. "Young Adult Support for Clean Indoor Air Laws in Restaurants and Bars." *Journal of Adolescent Health* 45: 102–4.

Bierer, M. F., and N. A. Rigotti. 1992. "Public Policy for the Control of Tobacco-Related Disease." *Medical Clinics of North America* 76: 515–39.

Black, D. A., T. McKinnish, and S. G. Sanders. 2003. "Does the Availability of High-Wage Jobs for Low-Skilled Men Affect Welfare Expenditures? Evidence from Shocks to the Coal and Steel Industries." *Journal of Public Economics* 87: 1919–40.

Blanchflower, D. G., A. J. Oswald, and P. Sanfey. 1996. "Wages, Profits, and Rent-Sharing." *The Quarterly Journal of Economics* 111: 227–51.

Bloom, P. N. 2001. "Role of Slotting Fees and Trade Promotions in Shaping How Tobacco Is Marketed in Retail Stores." *Tobacco Control* 10: 340–44.

Blumberg, S., and J. Luke. 2010. "Wireless Substitution: Early Release of Estimates from the National Health Interview Survey, July–December 2008." Hyattsville, MD: National Center for Health Statistics.

Bondy, S. J., B. Zhang, N. Kreiger, P. Selby, N. Benowitz, H. Travis, A. Florescu, N. R. Greenspan, and R. Ferrence. 2009. "Impact of an Indoor Smoking Ban on Bar Workers' Exposure to Secondhand Smoke." *Journal of Occupational and Environmental Medicine* 51: 612–19.

Borland, R., N. Owen, D. Hill, and S. Chapman. 1990. "Changes in Acceptance of Workplace Smoking Bans Following Their Implementation: A Prospective Study." *Preventive Medicine* 19: 314–22.

Boyd, N. R., C. Sutton, C. T. Orleans, M. W. McClatchey, R. Bingler, L. Fleisher, D. Heller, S. Baum, C. Graves, and J. Ward. 1998. " 'Quit Today'—a Targeted Communications Campaign to Increase Use of the Cancer Information Services as a Quit Smoking Resource Among African American Smokers." *Preventive Medicine* 27: S50–S60.

Brandt, A. M. 1990. "The Cigarette, Risk and American Culture." *Daedalus* 119: 155–76.

Brandt, A. M. 1998. "Blow Some Smoke My Way: Passive Smoking, Risk and American Culture." In *Ashes to Ashes: The History of Smoking and Health*, ed. S. Lock, L. Reynolds, and E. Tansey, pp. 164–91. Amsterdam, The Netherlands: Rodopi BV.

Brandt, A. M. 2007. *The Cigarette Century: The Rise, Fall, and Deadly Persistence of the Product That Defined America*. New York: Basic Books.

Breslau, N., G. C. Davis, and L. R. Schultz. 2003. "Posttraumatic Stress Disorder and the Incidence of Nicotine, Alcohol, and Other Drug Disorders in Persons Who Have Experienced Trauma." *Archives of General Psychiatry* 60: 289–94.

Breslau, N., and E. O. Johnson. 2000. "Predicting Smoking Cessation and Major Depression in Nicotine-Dependent Smokers." *American Journal of Public Health* 90: 1122–27.

Breslau, N., M. M. Kilbey, and P. Andreski. 1992. "Nicotine Withdrawal Symptoms and Psychiatric Disorders: Findings from an Epidemiologic Study of Young Adults." *American Journal of Psychiatry* 149: 464–69.

Breslau, N., S. P. Novak, and R. C. Kessler. 2004. "Psychiatric Disorders and Stages of Smoking." *Biological Psychiatry* 55: 69–76.

Brown, A. B. 1995. "Cigarette Taxes and Smoking Restrictions: Impacts and Policy Implications." *American Journal of Agricultural Economics* 77: 946–51.

Brown, A. B., R. R. Rucker, and W. N. Thurman. 2007. "The End of the Federal Tobacco Program: Economic Impacts of the Deregulation of U.S. Tobacco Production." *Review of Agricultural Economics* 29: 635–55.

Brown, C., and J. Medoff. 1989. "The Employer Size–Wage Effect." *Journal of Political Economy* 105: 1027–59.

Brown, M., W. Chin, and P. Rooney. n.d. "Estimating Corporate Charitable Giving for *Giving USA*." Indianapolis, IN: Center on Philanthropy at Indiana University.

Brown, S., H. Inskip, and B. Barraclough. 2000. "Causes of the Excess Mortality of Schizophrenia." *British Journal of Psychiatry* 177: 212–17.

Brownson, R. C., D. M. Koffman, T. E. Novotny, R. G. Hughes, and M. P. Eriksen. 1995. "Environmental and Policy Interventions to Control Tobacco Use and Prevent Cardiovascular Disease." *Health Education Quarterly* 22: 478–98.

Bulow, J., and P. Klemperer. 1999. "The Tobacco Deal." In *Brookings Papers on Economic Activity: Microeconomics: 1998*, ed. Clifford Winston, Martin N. Baily, and Peter C. Reiss, pp. 323–94. Washington, DC: Brookings Institution Press.

Buntin, M. B., and A. M. Zaslavsky. 2004. "Too Much Ado About Two-Part Models and Transformation? Comparing Methods of Modeling Medicare Expenditures." *Journal of Health Economics* 23: 525–42.

Burns, D. M., and K. E. Warner. 2003. "Smokers Who Have Not Quit: Is Cessation More Difficult and Should We Change Our Strategies?" In *Smoking and Control*, monograph no. 15, pp. 1–31. Bethesda, MD: National Cancer Institute.

Burton, S., L. Clark, G. Elliott, and F. Siciliano. 2005. "The Impact of Retail Distribution on Tobacco Consumption: Research Agenda." Paper presented at ANZMAC Conference, Fremantle, Western Australia, December 5–7.

Busch, S. H., M. Jofre-Bonet, T. A. Falba, and J. L. Sindelar. 2005. "Burning a Hole in the Budget: Tobacco Spending and Its Crowd-Out of Other Goods." *Applied Health Economics and Health Policy* 3: 263–72.

Byrnes, N. 2005. "Smarter Corporate Giving." *BusinessWeek*, November 28.

California Environmental Protection Agency. 2005. "Proposed Identification of Environmental Tobacco Smoke as a Toxic Air Contaminant. Part B: Health Effects." Sacramento: State of California.

Campaign for Tobacco-Free Kids. 2010. "State Cigarette Excise Tax Rates & Rankings." http://www.tobaccofreekids.org/research/factsheets/pdf/0097.pdf.

Capehart, T. 2004. "Trends in Tobacco Farming." Washington, DC: Economic Research Service, U.S. Department of Agriculture.

Capehart, T. 2005a. *Tobacco Situation and Outlook Yearbook*. Washington, DC: Economic Research Service, U.S. Department of Agriculture.

Capehart, T. 2005b. "Long-Lived Tobacco Program to End." *Amber Waves* 3: 2–3.

Capehart, T. 2006. "U.S. Tobacco Sector Regroups." *Amber Waves* 4: 2.

Card, D. 1997. "Deregulation and Labor Earnings in the Airline Industry." In *Regulatory Reform and Labor Markets*, ed. J. Peoples, pp. 183–230. Norwell, MA: Kluwer Academic Press.

Carroll, R. J., and C. J. Carroll. 1988. *Transformation and Weighting in Regression*. Boca Raton, FL: CRC Press.

Centers for Disease Control. 1990. "Progress in Chronic Disease Prevention State Laws Restricting Minors' Access to Tobacco." *MMWR—Morbidity & Mortality Weekly Report* 39: 349–52.

Centers for Disease Control. 1991. "State Tobacco Prevention and Control Activities: Results of the 1989–1990 Association of State and Territorial Health Officials (ASTHO) Survey Final Report." *MMWR—Morbidity & Mortality Weekly Report* 40, no. RR-11: 1–40.

Centers for Disease Control and Prevention. 1998. "Response to Increases in Cigarette Process by Race/Ethnicity, Income, and Age Groups—United States, 1976–1993." *MMWR—Morbidity & Mortality Weekly Report* 47: 605–9.

Centers for Disease Control and Prevention. 1999. "Best Practices for Comprehensive Tobacco Control Programs." Atlanta: U.S. Department of Health and Human Services, Centers for Disease Control and Prevention, National Center for Chronic Disease Prevention and Health Promotion, Office on Smoking and Health.

Centers for Disease Control and Prevention. 2002. "Annual Smoking-Attributable Mortality, Years of Potential Life Lost, and Economic Costs—United States, 1995–1999." *MMWR—Morbidity & Mortality Weekly Report* 51: 300–303.

Centers for Disease Control and Prevention. 2004a. "Health Insurance Coverage: Estimates from the NHIS, 2004." http://www.cdc.gov/nchs/data/nhis/earlyrelease/insur200506.pdf.

Centers for Disease Control and Prevention. 2004b. "State Medicaid Coverage for Tobacco-Dependence Treatments—United States, 1994–2002." *MMWR—Morbidity & Mortality Weekly Report* 53: 54–57.

Centers for Disease Control and Prevention. 2005a. "Annual Smoking-Attributable Mortality, Years of Potential Life Lost, and Productivity Losses—United States, 1997–2001." *MMWR—Morbidity & Mortality Weekly Report* 54: 625–28.

Centers for Disease Control and Prevention. 2005b. "Preventing Chronic Diseases: Investing Wisely in Health-Preventing Tobacco Use" (fact sheet). Washington, DC: U.S. Department of Health and Human Services.

Centers for Disease Control and Prevention. 2006. "Youth Tobacco Surveillance—United States, 2001–2002." *MMWR—Morbidity & Mortality Weekly Report* 55: 1–60.

Centers for Disease Control and Prevention. 2008. "Smoking-Attributable Mortality, Years of Potential Life Lost, and Productivity Losses—United States, 2000–2004." *MMWR— Morbidity & Mortality Weekly Report* 57: 1226–28.

Centers for Disease Control and Prevention. 2009a. "Cigarette Smoking Among Adults and Trends in Smoking Cessation—United States, 2008." *MMWR—Morbidity & Mortality Weekly Report* 58: 1227–32.

Centers for Disease Control and Prevention. 2009b. "Federal and State Cigarette Excise Taxes—United States, 1995–2009." *MMWR—Morbidity & Mortality Weekly Report* 58: 524–27.

Centers for Medicaid and Medicare Services. 2006. "National Health Expenditures Data by Age, Age Tables." http://www.cms.gov/Nationalhealthexpenddata/04_Nationalhealthac countsagephc.asp.

Chaloupka, F. J. 1991. "Rational Addictive Behavior and Cigarette Smoking." *Journal of Political Economy* 99: 722–44.

Chaloupka, F. J., K. M. Cummings, C. P. Morley, and J. K. Horan. 2002. "Tax, Price and Cigarette Smoking: Evidence from the Tobacco Documents and Implications for Tobacco Company Marketing Strategies." *Tobacco Control* 11, Suppl. 1: I62–I72.

Chaloupka, F. J., and R. Pacula. 1999. "Sex and Race Differences in Young People's Responsiveness to Price and Tobacco Control Policies." *Tobacco Control* 8, no. 4: 373–77.

Chaloupka, F. J., and K. E. Warner. 1999. "The Economics of Smoking." In *The Handbook of Health Economics*, ed. J. P. Newhouse and A. J. Cuyler, pp. 1539–627. New York: North-Holland, Elsevier Science B.V.

Chandra, S., and F. J. Chaloupka. 2003. "Seasonality in Cigarette Sales: Patterns and Implications for Tobacco Control." *Tobacco Control* 12: 105–7.

Chernick, H., and A. Reschovsky. 1990. "The Taxation of the Poor." *The Journal of Human Resources* 25: 712–35.

Christakis, N. A., and J. H. Fowler. 2008. "The Collective Dynamics of Smoking in a Large Social Network." *New England Journal of Medicine* 358: 2249–58.

Christoff, C. 2006. "State Busts Nearly 9,000 Who Dodged Cigarette Tax." *Detroit Free Press*, February 28.

Ciliberto, F., and N. V. Kuminoff. 2010. "Public Policy and Market Competition: How the Master Settlement Agreement Changed the Cigarette Industry." *The B.E. Journal of Economic Analysis & Policy* 10: Article 63.

Clark, P. I., S. L. Natanblut, C. L. Schmitt, C. Wolters, and R. Iachan. 2000. "Factors Associated with Tobacco Sales to Minors: Lessons Learned from the FDA Compliance Checks." *Journal of the American Medical Association* 284: 729–34.

Clayton, R. R. 2006. "The Tobacco Research Network on Disparities (Trend)." *Journal of Epidemiology and Community Health* 60: ii3–ii4.

Coats, R. M. 1995. "A Note on Estimating Cross-Border Effects of State Cigarette Taxes." *National Tax Journal* 48: 573–84.

Cohen, J. 2005. "Internet Cigarette Diversion." Conference presentation, Federation of Tax Administrators Tobacco Tax Section Conference, Big Sky, MT, September 12.

Cokkinides, V. E., E. Ward, A. Jemal, and M. J. Thun. 2005. "Under-Use of Smoking-Cessation Treatments." *American Journal of Preventive Medicine* 28: 119–22.

Conners, C. K., E. D. Levin, E. Sparrow, S. C. Hinton, D. Erhardt, W. H. Meck, J. E. Rose, and J. March. 1996. "Nicotine and Attention in Adult Attention Deficit Hyperactivity Disorder (ADHD)." *Psychopharmacology Bulletin* 32: 67–73.

Convenience Store News. 2006. "California Leads the Way in Fighting Tobacco Tax Evasion." http://www.csnews.com/csn/search/article_display.jsp?schema=&vnu_content_id=1001772077.

Cork, K., and C. Forman. 2008. "Legal and Political Obstacles to Smoke-Free Regulation in Minnesota Regions." *American Journal of Preventive Medicine* 35: S508–S518.

Cournos, F., K. McKinnon, and G. Sullivan. 2005. "Schizophrenia and Comorbid Human Immunodeficiency Virus or Hepatitis C Virus." *Journal of Clinical Psychiatry* 66, Suppl. 6: 27–33.

Covey, L. S., D. C. Hughes, A. H. Glassman, D. G. Blazer, and L. K. George. 1994. "Ever-Smoking, Quitting, and Psychiatric Disorders: Evidence from the Durham, North Carolina, Epidemiologic Catchment Area." *Tobacco Control* 3: 222–27.

Cowling, D. W., and P. Bond. 2005. "Smokefree Laws and Bar Revenues in California—the Last Call." *Health Economics* 14: 1273–81.

Cummings, K. M., B. Fix, P. Celestino, S. Carlin-Menter, R. O'Connor, and A. Hyland. 2006a. "Reach, Efficacy, and Cost-Effectiveness of Free Nicotine Medication Giveaway Programs." *Journal of Public Health Management and Practice* 12: 37–43.

Cummings, K. M., A. Hyland, B. Fix, U. Bauer, P. Celestino, S. Carlin-Menter, N. Miller, and T. R. Frieden. 2006b. "Free Nicotine Patch Giveaway Program 12-Month Follow-up of Participants." *American Journal of Preventive Medicine* 31: 181–84.

Cummings, K. M., A. Hyland, E. Lewit, and D. Shopland. 1997a. "Use of Discount Cigarettes by Smokers in 20 Communities in the United States, 1988–1993." *Tobacco Control* 6, Suppl. 2: S25–S30.

Cummings, K. M., A. Hyland, J. K. Ockene, N. Hymowitz, and M. Manley. 1997b. "Use of the Nicotine Skin Patch by Smokers in 20 Communities in the United States, 1992–1993." *Tobacco Control* 6: S63–S70.

Curry, S. J., L. C. Grothaus, T. McAfee, and C. Pabiniak. 1998. "Use and Cost Effectiveness of Smoking-Cessation Services Under Four Insurance Plans in a Health Maintenance Organization." *New England Journal of Medicine* 339: 673–79.

Cutler, D. M., A. M. Epstein, R. G. Frank, R. Hartman, C. R. King, J. P. Newhouse, M. Rosenthal, and E. R. Vigdor. 2000. "How Good a Deal Was the Tobacco Settlement? Assessing Payments to Massachusetts." *Journal of Risk and Uncertainty* 21: 235–61.

Cutler, D. M., J. Gruber, R. S. Hartman, M. B. Landrum, J. P. Newhouse, and M. B. Rosenthal. 2002. "The Economic Impacts of the Tobacco Settlement." *Journal of Policy Analysis and Management* 21: 1–19.

Danaei, G., E. L. Ding, D. Mozaffarian, B. Taylor, J. R. Rehm, C. J. L. Murray, and M. Ezzati. 2009. "The Preventable Causes of Death in the United States: Comparative Risk Assessment of Dietary, Lifestyle, and Metabolic Risk Factors." *PLoS Medicine* 6: e1000058.

de Leon, J., G. Abraham, C. Nair, C. Verghese, A. McGrory, and E. McCann. 1995. "Nicotine Addiction in Chronic Schizophrenic Inpatients." *Biological Psychiatry* 37: 640.

de Leon, J., E. Becona, M. Gurpegui, A. Gonzalez-Pinto, and F. J. Diaz. 2002. "The Association Between High Nicotine Dependence and Severe Mental Illness May Be Consistent Across Countries." *Journal of Clinical Psychiatry* 63: 812–16.

de Leon, J., and F. J. Diaz. 2005. "A Meta-Analysis of Worldwide Studies Demonstrates an Association Between Schizophrenia and Tobacco Smoking Behaviors." *Schizophrenia Research* 76: 135–57.

de Leon, J., M. T. Susce, F. J. Diaz, D. M. Rendon, and D. M. Velasquez. 2005. "Variables Associated with Alcohol, Drug, and Daily Smoking Cessation in Patients with Severe Mental Illnesses." *Journal of Clinical Psychiatry* 66: 1447–55.

Delnevo, C. D., M. Hrywna, and M. J. Lewis. 2004. "Predictors of Smoke-Free Workplaces by Employee Characteristics: Who Is Left Unprotected?" *American Journal of Industrial Medicine* 46: 196–202.

Desai, H. D., J. Seabolt, and M. W. Jann. 2001. "Smoking in Patients Receiving Psychotropic Medications: A Pharmacokinetic Perspective." *CNS Drugs* 15: 469–94.

Desai, M. M., and R. A. Rosenheck. 2005. "Unmet Need for Medical Care Among Homeless Adults with Serious Mental Illness." *General Hospital Psychiatry* 27: 418–25.

Deverell, M., C. Randolph, A. Albers, W. Hamilton, and M. Siegel. 2006. "Diffusion of Local Restaurant Smoking Regulations in Massachusetts: Identifying Disparities in Health Protection for Population Subgroups." *Journal of Public Health Management and Practice* 12: 262–69.

Dierker, L. C., S. Avenevoli, M. Stolar, and K. R. Merikangas. 2002. "Smoking and Depression: An Examination of Mechanisms of Comorbidity." *American Journal of Psychiatry* 159: 947–53.

Dietz, N. A., J. Delva, M. E. Woolley, and L. Russello. 2008. "The Reach of a Youth-Oriented Anti-Tobacco Media Campaign on Adult Smokers." *Drug and Alcohol Dependence* 93: 180–84.

DiFranza, J. R. 2001. "State and Federal Compliance with the Synar Amendment: Federal Fiscal Year 1998." *Archives of Pediatric and Adolescent Medicine* 155: 572–78.

DiFranza, J. R. 2005. "Best Practices for Enforcing State Laws Prohibiting the Sale of Tobacco to Minors." *Journal of Public Health Management and Practice* 11: 559–65.

DiFranza, J. R., and M. Coleman. 2001. "Sources of Tobacco for Youths in Communities with Strong Enforcement of Youth Access Laws." *Tobacco Control* 10: 323–28.

DiFranza, J. R., and G. F. Dussault. 2005. "The Federal Initiative to Halt the Sale of Tobacco to Children—the Synar Amendment, 1992–2000: Lessons Learned." *Tobacco Control* 14: 93–98.

DiFranza, J. R., and J. J. Librett. 1999. "State and Federal Revenues from Tobacco Consumed by Minors." *American Journal of Public Health* 89: 1106–8.

DiFranza, J. R., R. M. Peck, T. E. Radecki, and J. A. Savageau. 2001. "What Is the Potential Cost-Effectiveness of Enforcing a Prohibition on the Sale of Tobacco to Minors?" *Preventive Medicine* 32: 168–74.

DiFranza, J. R., J. A. Savageau, and B. F. Aisquith. 1996. "Youth Access to Tobacco: The Effects of Age, Gender, Vending Machine Locks, and 'It's the Law' Programs." *American Journal of Public Health* 86: 221–24.

DiFranza, J. R., J. A. Savageau, and J. Bouchard. 2001. "Is the Measured Compliance Check Protocol a Valid Measure of Tobacco to Underage Smokers?" *Tobacco Control* 10: 227–32.

Dinno, A., and S. A. Glantz. 2009. "Tobacco Control Policies Are Egalitarian: A Vulnerabilities Perspective on Clean Indoor Air Laws, Cigarette Prices, and Tobacco Use Disparities." *Social Science & Medicine* 68: 1439–47.

Dohlman, E., L. Foreman, and M. Da Pra. 2009. The Post-Buyout Experience: Peanut and Tobacco Sectors Adapt to Policy Reform. Washington, DC: U.S. Department of Agriculture.

Dolan, S. L., K. A. Sacco, A. Termine, A. A. Seyal, M. M. Dudas, J. C. Vessicchio, B. E. Wexler, and T. P. George. 2004. "Neuropsychological Deficits Are Associated with Smoking Cessation Treatment Failure in Patients with Schizophrenia." *Schizophrenia Research* 70: 263–75.

Doll, R. 1971. "The Age Distribution of Cancer: Implications for Models of Carcinogenesis." *Journal of the Royal Statistical Society* A134: 133–66.

Doll, R., R. Peto, J. Boreham, and I. Sutherland. 2004. "Mortality in Relation to Smoking: 50 Years' Observations on Male British Doctors." *British Medical Journal* 328: 1519.

Drake, R. E., and K. T. Mueser. 2001. "Managing Comorbid Schizophrenia and Substance Abuse." *Current Psychiatry Reports* 3: 418–22.

Duan, N., W. G. Manning, C. N. Morris, and J. P. Newhouse. 1983. "A Comparison of Alternative Models for the Demand for Medical Care." *Journal of Business & Economic Statistics* 1: 115–26.

Economic Research Service. 2006. "Baseline Forecasts February 2006." Washington, DC: U.S. Department of Agriculture.

Eisner, M. D., A. K. Smith, and P. D. Blanc. 1998. "Bartenders' Respiratory Health After Establishment of Smoke-Free Bars and Taverns." *Journal of the American Medical Association* 280: 1909–14.

Emery, S., C. F. Ake, A. M. Navarro, and R. M. Kaplan. 2001. "Simulated Effect of Tobacco Tax Variation on Latino Health in California." *American Journal of Preventive Medicine* 21: 278–83.

Evans, W. N., J. S. Ringel, and D. Stech. 1999. "Tobacco Taxes and Public Policy to Discourage Smoking." In *Tax Policy and the Economy*, ed. J. Poterba, pp. 1–56. Cambridge, MA: MIT Press.

Evins, A. E., C. Cather, T. Deckersbach, O. Freudenreich, M. A. Culhane, C. M. Olm-Shipman, D. C. Henderson, D. A. Schoenfeld, D. C. Goff, and N. A. Rigotti. 2005. "A Double-Blind Placebo-Controlled Trial of Bupropion Sustained-Release for Smoking Cessation in Schizophrenia." *Journal of Clinical Psychopharmacology* 25: 218–25.

Farber, H. S. 2001. "Job Loss in the United States, 1981–1999." Working Paper 453. Princeton, NJ: Princeton University, Industrial Relations Section.

Farber, H. S. 2005. "What Do We Know About Job Loss in the United States? Evidence from the Displaced Workers Survey, 1981–2004." *Economic Perspectives, Federal Reserve Bank of Chicago* 29, no. 2: 13–28.

Farrelly, M. C., and J. W. Bray. 1998. "Office on Smoking and Health. Response to Increases in Cigarette Prices by Race/Ethnicity, Income and Age Groups—United States, 1976–1993." *MMWR—Morbidity & Mortality Weekly Report* 47: 605–9.

Farrelly, M. C., K. C. Davis, M. L. Haviland, P. Messeri, and C. G. Healton. 2005a. "Evidence of a Dose-Response Relationship Between 'Truth' Antismoking Ads and Youth Smoking Prevalence." *American Journal of Public Health* 95: 425–31.

Farrelly, M. C., W. N. Evans, and A. E. Sfekas. 1999. "The Impact of Workplace Smoking Bans: Results from a National Survey." *Tobacco Control* 8: 272–77.

Farrelly, M. C., C. T. Nimsch, and J. James. 2003. "State Cigarette Excise Taxes: Implications for Revenue and Tax Evasion." Research Triangle Park, NC: RTI International.

Farrelly, M. C., J. M. Nonnemaker, R. Chou, A. Hyland, K. K. Peterson, and U. E. Bauer. 2005b. "Changes in Hospitality Workers' Exposure to Secondhand Smoke Following the Implementation of New York's Smoke-Free Law." *Tobacco Control* 14: 236–41.

Farrelly, M. C., T. F. Pechacek, and F. J. Chaloupka. 2003. "The Impact of Tobacco Control Program Expenditures on Aggregate Cigarette Sales: 1981–2000." *Journal of Health Economics* 22: 843–59.

Federal Trade Commission. 2007. "Federal Trade Commission Cigarette Report for 2004 and 2005." Washington, DC: Federal Trade Commission.

Federal Trade Commission. 2009. "Federal Trade Commission Cigarette Report for 2006." Washington, DC: Federal Trade Commission.

Feighery, E. C., K. M. Ribisl, D. D. Achabal, and T. Tyebjee. 1999. "Retail Trade Incentives: How Tobacco Industry Practices Compare with Those of Other Industries." *American Journal of Public Health* 89: 1564–66.

Feighery, E. C., K. M. Ribisl, P. I. Clark, and H. H. Haladjian. 2003. "How the Tobacco Companies Ensure Prime Placement of Their Advertising and Products in Stores: Interviews with Retailers About Tobacco Company Incentive Programs." *Tobacco Control* 12: 184–88.

Feighery, E. C., K. M. Ribisl, N. C. Schleicher, and P. I. Clark. 2004. "Retailer Participation in Cigarette Company Incentive Programs Is Related to Increased Levels of Cigarette Advertising and Cheaper Cigarette Prices in Stores." *Preventive Medicine* 38: 876–84.

Fichtenberg, C. M., and S. A. Glantz. 2002a. "Effect of Smoke-Free Workplaces on Smoking Behaviour: Systematic Review." *British Medical Journal* 325: 188.

Fichtenberg, C. M., and S. A. Glantz. 2002b. "Youth Access Interventions Do Not Affect Youth Smoking." *Pediatrics* 109: 1088–92.

Filozof, C., M. C. Fernandez Pinilla, and A. Fernandez-Cruz. 2004. "Smoking Cessation and Weight Gain." *Obesity Reviews* 5: 95–103.

Fiore, M. C., W. Bailey, S. J. Cohen, S. F. Dorfman, M. G. Goldstein, E. R. Gritz, R. B. Heyman, C. R. Jaén, T. E. Kottke, H. A. Lando, R. E. Mecklenburg, P. D. Mullen, L. M. Nett, L. Robinson, M. L. Stitzer, A. C. Tommasello, L. Villejo, and M. E. Wewers. 2000. "Treating Tobacco Use and Dependence." Rockville, MD: U.S. Department of Health and Human Services, Public Health Service.

Fisher, B. E. 1999. "Turning Over a New Leaf: Tobacco." *Environmental Health Perspectives* 107: A206–A209.

Fisher, J. C. 1958. "Multiple-Mutation Theory of Carcinogenesis." *Nature* 181: 651–52.

Flay, B., D. Koepke, S. Thomson, S. Santi, J. Best, and K. Brown. 1989. "Six-Year Follow-up of the First Waterloo School Smoking Prevention Trial." *American Journal of Public Health* 79: 1371–76.

Fong, G. T., A. Hyland, R. Borland, D. Hammond, G. Hastings, A. McNeill, S. Anderson, K. M. Cummings, S. Allwright, M. Mulcahy, F. Howell, L. Clancy, M. E. Thompson, G. Connolly, and P. Driezen. 2006. "Reductions in Tobacco Smoke Pollution and Increases in Support for Smoke-Free Public Places Following the Implementation of Comprehensive Smoke-Free Workplace Legislation in the Republic of Ireland: Findings from the ITC Ireland/UK Survey." *Tobacco Control* 15: iii51–iii58.

Forrester Research, Inc. 2001. "Online Tobacco Sales Grow, States Lose." Cambridge, MA: Forrester Research.

Forster, J., D. M. Murray, M. Wolfson, T. M. Blaine, A. C. Wagenaar, and D. J. Hennrikus. 1998. "The Effects of Community Policies to Reduce Youth Access to Tobacco." *American Journal of Public Health* 88: 1193–98.

Fowler, J. S., N. D. Volkow, G. J. Wang, N. Pappas, J. Logan, C. Shea, D. Alexoff, R. R. MacGregor, D. J. Schlyer, I. Zezulkova, and A. P. Wolf. 1996. "Brain Monoamine Oxidase A Inhibition in Cigarette Smokers." *National Academy of Sciences of the United States of America* 93: 14065–69.

Frieden, T. R., F. Mostashari, B. D. Kerker, N. Miller, A. Hajat, and M. Frankel. 2005. "Adult Tobacco Use Levels After Intensive Tobacco Control Measures: New York City, 2002–2003." *American Journal of Public Health* 95: 1016–23.

Friend, K., and D. T. Levy. 2001. "Smoking Treatment Interventions and Policies to Promote Their Use: A Critical Review." *Nicotine & Tobacco Research* 3: 299–310.

Friend, K., and D. T. Levy. 2002. "Reductions in Smoking Prevalence and Cigarette Consumption Associated with Mass-Media Campaigns." *Health Education Research* 17: 85–98.

Friis, R. H., and A. M. Safer. 2005. "Analysis of Responses of Long Beach, California Residents to the Smoke-Free Bars Law." *Public Health* 119: 1116–21.

Gale, H. F., Jr. 1999. "Tobacco Communities Facing Change." *Rural Development Perspectives* 14: 36–43.

Gale, H. F., Jr., L. F. Foreman, and T. C. J. Capehart. 2000. "Tobacco and the Economy: Farms, Jobs, and Communities." Washington DC: Economic Research Service, U.S. Department of Agriculture.

Galea, S., D. Vlahov, H. Resnick, J. Ahern, E. Susser, J. Gold, M. Bucuvalas, and D. Kilpatrick. 2003. "Trends in Probable Posttraumatic Stress Disorder in New York City After the September 11 Terrorist Attacks." *American Journal of Epidemiology* 158: 514–24.

Gallet, C. A., and J. A. List. 2003. "Cigarette Demand: A Meta-Analysis of Elasticities." *Health Economics* 12: 821–35.

Gandini, S., E. Botteri, S. Iodice, M. Boniol, A. B. Lowenfels, P. Maisonneuve, and P. Boyle. 2008. "Tobacco Smoking and Cancer: A Meta-Analysis." *International Journal of Cancer* 122: 155–64.

Garfinkel, L. 1985. "Selection, Follow-up, and Analysis in the American Cancer Society Prospective Studies." *National Cancer Institute Monograph* 67: 49–52.

Garrett, T. A., and M. R. Pakko. 2009. "No Ifs, Ands or Butts: Illinois Casinos Lost Revenue After Smoking Banned." *The Regional Economist* (July): 14–15.

George, T. P., J. C. Vessicchio, A. Termine, T. A. Bregartner, A. Feingold, B. J. Rounsaville, and T. R. Kosten. 2002. "A Placebo Controlled Trial of Bupropion for Smoking Cessation in Schizophrenia." *Biological Psychiatry* 52: 53–61.

Gerlach, K. K., D. R. Shopland, A. M. Hartman, J. T. Gibson, and T. F. Pechacek. 1997. "Workplace Smoking Policies in the United States: Results from a National Survey of More Than 100,000 Workers." *Tobacco Control* 6: 199–206.

Gilpin, E. A., S. L. Emery, A. J. Farkas, J. M. Distefan, M. M. White, and J. P. Pierce. 2001. "The California Tobacco Control Program: A Decade of Progress, 1989–1999." La Jolla: University of California, San Diego.

Gilpin, E. A., S. L. Emery, A. J. Farkas, J. M. Distefan, M. M. White, and J. P. Pierce. 2003. "Tobacco Control Successes in California: A Focus on the Young People, Results from the California Tobacco Control Surveys, 1990–2002." La Jolla: University of California, San Diego.

Gilpin, E. A., L. Lee, and J. P. Pierce. 2004a. "Changes in Population Attitudes About Where Smoking Should Not Be Allowed: California Versus the Rest of the USA." *Tobacco Control* 13: 38–44.

Gilpin, E. A., L. Lee, and J. P. Pierce. 2004b. "Does Adolescent Perception of Difficulty in Getting Cigarettes Deter Experimentation?" *Preventive Medicine* 38: 485–91.

Gilpin, E. A., J. P. Pierce, and A. J. Farkas. 1997. "Duration of Smoking Abstinence and Success in Quitting." *Journal of the National Cancer Institute* 89: 572–76.

Gingiss, P. M., C. Roberts-Gray, and M. Boerm. 2006. "Bridget-It: A System for Predicting Implementation Fidelity for School-Based Tobacco Prevention Programs." *Prevention Science* 7: 197–207.

Giovino, G. A. 2002. "Epidemiology of Tobacco Use in the United States." *Oncogene* 21: 7326–40.

Glasgow, R. E., H. Lando, J. Hollis, S. G. McRae, and P. A. La Chance. 1993. "A Stop-Smoking Telephone Helpline That Nobody Called." *American Journal of Public Health* 83: 252–53.

Glassman, A. H. 1998. "Psychiatry and Cigarettes." *Archives of General Psychiatry* 55: 692–93.

Glassman, A. H., F. Stetner, B. T. Walsh, P. S. Raizman, J. L. Fleiss, T. B. Cooper, and L. S. Covey. 1988. "Heavy Smokers, Smoking Cessation, and Clonidine: Results of a Double-Blind, Randomized Trial." *Journal of the American Medical Association* 259: 2863–66.

Glynn, T. 1989. "Essential Elements of School-Based Smoking Prevention Programs." *Journal of School Health* 59: 181–88.

Goff, D. C., D. C. Henderson, and B. S. Amico. 1992. "Cigarette Smoking in Schizophrenia: Relationship to Psychopathology and Medication Side Effects." *American Journal of Psychiatry* 149: 1189–94.

Goldman, D. P., B. Shang, J. Bhattacharya, A. M. Garber, M. Hurd, G. F. Joyce, D. N. Lakdawalla, C. Panis, and P. G. Shekelle. 2005. "Consequences of Health Trends and Medical Innovation for the Future Elderly." *Health Affairs* 24: W5R5–W5R17.

Goldman, D., P. Shekelle, J. Bhattacharya, M. Hurd, G. Joyce, D. Lakdawalla, D. Matsui, S. Newberry, C. Panis, and B. Shang. 2004. "Health Status and Medical Treatment of the Future Elderly: Final Report." Santa Monica, CA: RAND Corporation.

Gonzalez-Pinto, A., M. Gutierrez, J. Ezcurra, F. Aizpuru, F. Mosquera, P. Lopez, and J. de Leon. 1998. "Tobacco Smoking and Bipolar Disorder." *Journal of Clinical Psychiatry* 59: 225–28.

Goolsbee, A., M. Lovenheim, and J. Slemrod. 2010. "Playing with Fire: Cigarettes, Taxes and Competition from the Internet." *American Economic Journal: Economic Policy* 2: 131–54.

Gottlob, B. J. 2003. "The Fiscal and Economic Impacts of Increasing the Tobacco Tax in New Hampshire." Dover, NH: PolEcon Research.

Graff, S. K. 2006. "State Taxation of Online Tobacco Sales: Circumventing the Archaic Bright Line Penned by Quill." *Florida Law Review* 58: 375–424.

Grant, B. F., D. S. Hasin, S. P. Chou, F. S. Stinson, and D. A. Dawson. 2004. "Nicotine Dependence and Psychiatric Disorders in the United States: Results from the National Epidemiologic Survey on Alcohol and Related Conditions." *Archives of General Psychiatry* 61: 1107–15.

Gruber, J. 2000. "Youth Smoking in the US: Prices and Policies." NBER Working Paper 7506. Cambridge, MA: National Bureau of Economic Research.

Gruber, J., and B. Köszegi. 2001. "Is Addiction 'Rational'? Theory and Evidence." *The Quarterly Journal of Economics* 116: 1261–303.

Gruber, J., and B. Köszegi. 2004. "Tax Incidence When Individuals Are Time-Inconsistent: The Case of Cigarette Excise Taxes." *Journal of Public Economics* 88: 1959–87.

Gruber, J., A. Sen, and M. Stabile. 2003. "Estimating Price Elasticities When There Is Smuggling: The Sensitivity of Smoking to Price in Canada." *Journal of Health Economics* 22: 821–42.

Hagman, B. T., C. D. Delnevo, M. Hrywna, and J. M. Williams. 2008. "Tobacco Use Among Those with Serious Psychological Distress: Results from the National Survey of Drug Use and Health, 2002." *Addictive Behaviors* 33: 582–92.

Haiman, C. A., D. O. Stram, L. R. Wilkens, M. C. Pike, L. N. Kolonel, B. E. Henderson, and L. Le Marchand. 2006. "Ethnic and Racial Differences in the Smoking-Related Risk of Lung Cancer." *New England Journal of Medicine* 354: 333–42.

Hall, S. M. 2007. "Nicotine Interventions with Comorbid Populations." *American Journal of Preventive Medicine* 33: S406–S413.

Hall, S. M., V. I. Reus, R. F. Munoz, K. L. Sees, G. Humfleet, D. T. Hartz, S. Frederick, and E. Triffleman. 1998. "Nortriptyline and Cognitive Behavioral Therapy in the Treatment of Cigarette Smoking." *Archives of General Psychiatry* 55: 683–90.

Haller, E., D. E. McNiel, and R. L. Binder. 1996. "Impact of a Smoking Ban on a Locked Psychiatric Unit." *Journal of Clinical Psychiatry* 57: 329–32.

Halper, E. 2005. "State's Tobacco Revenue Surges." *Los Angeles Times*, December 27.

Halpern, M. T., R. Shikiar, A. M. Rentz, and Z. M. Khan. 2001. "Impact of Smoking Status on Workplace Absenteeism and Productivity." *Tobacco Control* 10: 233–38.

Hamilton, H. 2003. "Sustainable Agriculture for Midsized Farms." *Choices: The Magazine of Food, Farm & Resource Issues* (August): 39–40.

Hapke, U., A. Schumann, H. J. Rumpf, U. John, U. Konerding, and C. Meyer. 2005. "Association of Smoking and Nicotine Dependence with Trauma and Posttraumatic Stress Disorder in a General Population Sample." *Journal of Nervous and Mental Disease* 193: 843–46.

Harris, J. 1994. "A Working Model for Predicting the Consumption and Revenue Impacts of Large Increases in the U.S. Federal Cigarette Tax Rate." NBER Working Paper 4803. Cambridge, MA: National Bureau of Economic Research.

Harris, J. E., and S. W. Chan. 1999. "The Continuum-of-Addiction: Cigarette Smoking in Relation to Price Among Americans Aged 15–29." *Health Economics* 8: 81–86.

Harrison, P. A., J. A. Fulkerson, and E. Park. 2000. "The Relative Importance of Social Versus Commercial Sources in Youth Access to Tobacco, Alcohol, and Other Drugs." *Preventive Medicine* 31: 39–48.

Hedrick, J. L. 1971. "The Economic Costs of Cigarette Smoking." *HSMHA Health Report* 86: 179–82.

Henschke, C. I., and O. S. Miettinen. 2004. "Women's Susceptibility to Tobacco Carcinogens." *Lung Cancer* 43: 1–5.

Herek, G. M. 1999. "Aids and Stigma." *American Behavioral Scientist* 42: 1106–16.

Hersey, J., J. Niederdeppe, W. Evans, J. Nonnemaker, S. Blahut, D. Holden, P. Messeri, and M. L. Haviland. 2005. "The Theory of 'Truth': How Counterindustry Media Campaigns Affect Smoking Behavior Among Teens." *Health Psychology* 24: 22–31.

Himelhoch, S., and G. Daumit. 2003. "To Whom Do Psychiatrists Offer Smoking-Cessation Counseling?" *American Journal of Psychiatry* 160: 2228–30.

Hirschhorn, N. 2004. "Corporate Social Responsibility and the Tobacco Industry: Hope or Hype?" *Tobacco Control* 13: 447–53.

Hitsman, B., B. Borrelli, D. E. McChargue, B. Spring, and R. Niaura. 2003. "History of Depression and Smoking Cessation Outcome: A Meta-Analysis." *Journal of Consulting and Clinical Psychology* 71: 657–63.

Hodgson, T. A. 1992. "Cigarette Smoking and Lifetime Medical Expenditures." *Milbank Quarterly* 70: 81–125.

Hollmann, F. W., T. J. Mulder, and J. E. Kallan. 2000. "Methodology and Assumptions for the Population Projections of the United States: 1999 to 2100." Population Division Working Paper 38. Washington, DC: Department of Commerce, U.S. Bureau of the Census.

Homer, J. B., and G. B. Hirsch. 2006. "System Dynamics Modeling for Public Health: Background and Opportunities." *American Journal of Public Health* 96: 452–58.

Hopkins, D. P., P. A. Briss, C. J. Ricard, C. G. Husten, V. G. Carande-Kulis, J. E. Fielding, M. O. Alao, J. W. McKenna, D. J. Sharp, J. R. Harris, T. A. Woollery, and K. W. Harris. 2001. "Reviews of Evidence Regarding Interventions to Reduce Tobacco Use and Exposure to Environmental Tobacco Smoke." *American Journal of Preventive Medicine* 20: 16–66.

Hopkins, D. P., S. Razi, K. D. Leeks, G. Priya Kalra, S. K. Chattopadhyay, and R. E. Soler. 2010. "Smokefree Policies to Reduce Tobacco Use: A Systematic Review." *American Journal of Preventive Medicine* 38: S275–S289.

Hrywna, M., C. D. Delnevo, and D. Stanicwska. 2004. "Prevalence and Correlates of Internet Cigarette Purchasing Among Adult Smokers in New Jersey." *Tobacco Control* 13: 296–300.

Hu, T. W., Q. F. Ren, T. E. Keeler, and J. Bartlett. 1995. "The Demand for Cigarettes in California and Behavioural Risk Factors." *Health Economics* 4: 7–14.

Hughes, J. R. 1996. "Treating Smokers with Current or Past Alcohol Dependence." *American Journal of Health Behavior* 20: 286–90.

Hughes, J. R. 2000. "Reduced Smoking: An Introduction and Review of the Evidence." *Addiction* 95: S3–S7.

Hughes, J. R. 2001. "Distinguishing Nicotine Dependence from Smoking: Why It Matters to Tobacco Control and Psychiatry." *Archives of General Psychiatry* 58: 817–18.

Hughes, J. R., D. K. Hatsukami, J. E. Mitchell, and L. A. Dahlgren. 1986. "Prevalence of Smoking Among Psychiatric Outpatients." *American Journal of Psychiatry* 143: 993–97.

Hughes, J. R., and D. Kalman. 2006. "Do Smokers with Alcohol Problems Have More Difficulty Quitting?" *Drug and Alcohol Dependence* 82: 91–102.

Humfleet, G. L., J. J. Prochaska, M. Mengis, J. Cullen, R. Munoz, V. Reus, and S. M. Hall. 2005. "Preliminary Evidence of the Association Between the History of Childhood Attention-Deficit/Hyperactivity Disorder and Smoking Treatment Failure." *Nicotine & Tobacco Research* 7: 453–60.

Hurt, R. D., K. P. Offord, I. T. Croghan, L. Gomez-Dahl, T. E. Kottke, R. M. Morse, and L. J. R. Melton. 1996. "Mortality Following Inpatient Addictions Treatment: Role of Tobacco Use in a Community-Based Cohort." *Journal of the American Medical Association* 275: 1097–103.

Hyatt, J. 1998. "Philip Morris Launches $100m Anti-Hunger Drive." PNNOnline, March 10, pnnonline.org.

Hyland, A., K. M. Cummings, and M. P. Wilson. 1999. "Compliance with the New York City Smoke-Free Air Act." *Journal of Public Health Management and Practice* 5: 43–52.

Hyland, A., C. Higbee, Q. Li, J. E. Bauer, G. A. Giovino, T. Alford, and K. M. Cummings. 2005. "Access to Low-Taxed Cigarettes Deters Smoking Cessation Attempts." *American Journal of Public Health* 95: 994–95.

Hyland, A., F. L. Laux, C. Higbee, G. Hastings, H. Ross, F. J. Chaloupka, G. T. Fong, and K. M. Cummings. 2006. "Cigarette Purchase Patterns in Four Countries and the Relationship with Cessation: Findings from the International Tobacco Control (ITC) Four Country Survey." *Tobacco Control* 15, Suppl. 3: iii59–iii64.

Hyland, A., Q. Li, J. E. Bauer, G. A. Giovino, C. Steger, and K. M. Cummings. 2004. "Predictors of Cessation in a Cohort of Current and Former Smokers Followed Over 13 Years." *Nicotine & Tobacco Research* 6: S363–S369.

Hymowitz, N., K. M. Cummings, A. Hyland, W. R. Lynn, T. F. Pechacek, and T. D. Hartwell. 1997. "Predictors of Smoking Cessation in a Cohort of Adult Smokers Followed for Five Years." *Tobacco Control* 6, Suppl. 2: S57–S62.

Hymowitz, N., M. Sexton, J. Ockene, and G. Grandits. 1991. "Baseline Factors Associated with Smoking Cessation and Relapse: MRFIT Research Group." *Preventive Medicine* 20: 590–601.

Indiana University Center on Philanthropy. 2005. "Giving USA 2005." Indianapolis, IN: Center on Philanthropy at Indiana University.

Institute of Medicine. 2007. "Ending the Tobacco Problem: A Blueprint for the Nation." Washington, DC: National Academies Press.

Institute of Medicine. 2009. "Secondhand Smoke Exposure and Cardiovascular Effects: Making Sense of the Evidence." Washington, DC: National Academies Press.

Jacobson, L. S., R. G. Lalonde, and D. G. Sullivan. 1993. "Earning Losses of Displaced Workers." *American Economic Review* 83: 685–709.

Jacobson, P. D., and J. Wasserman. 1997. "Tobacco Control Laws: Implementation and Enforcement." Santa Monica, CA: RAND Corporation.

Jacobson, P. D., and J. Wasserman. 1999. "The Implementation and Enforcement of Tobacco Control Laws: Policy Implications for Activists and the Industry." *Journal of Health Politics, Policy and Law* 24: 567–98.

Jaramillo, E. 1999. "Tuberculosis and Stigma: Predictors of Prejudice Against People with Tuberculosis." *Journal of Health Psychology* 4: 71–79.

Jason, L., M. Berk, D. L. Schnopp-Wyatt, and B. Talbot. 1999. "Effects of Enforcement of Youth Access Laws on Smoking Prevalence." *American Journal of Community Psychology* 27: 143–60.

Jemal, A., W. D. Travis, R. E. Tarone, L. Travis, and S. S. Devesa. 2003. "Lung Cancer Rates Convergence in Young Men and Women in the United States: Analysis by Birth Cohort and Histologic Type." *International Journal of Cancer* 105: 101–7.

Jha, P., and F. J. Chaloupka. 1999. "Curbing the Epidemic: Governments and the Economics of Tobacco Control." Washington, DC: The World Bank.

Jha, P., and F. Chaloupka, eds. 2000. *Tobacco Control in Developing Countries*. New York: Oxford University Press.

Johnston, L., P. M. O'Malley, and Y. M. Terry-McElrath. 2004. "Methods, Locations, and Ease of Cigarette Access for American Youth, 1997–2002." *American Journal of Preventive Medicine* 27: 267–76.

Jones, A. S., W. D. Austin, R. H. Beach, and D. G. Altman. 2007. "Funding of North Carolina Tobacco Control Programs Through the Master Settlement Agreement." *American Journal of Public Health* 97: 36–44.

Joossens, L., F. J. Chaloupka, D. Merriman, and A. Yurekli. 2000. "Issues in the Smuggling of Tobacco Products." In *Tobacco Control in Developing Countries*, ed. P. Jha and F. Chaloupka, pp. 393–406. Oxford: Oxford University Press.

Joseph, A. M., J. M. Knapp, K. L. Nichol, and P. L. Pirie. 1995. "Determinants of Compliance with a National Smoke-Free Hospital Standard." *Journal of the American Medical Association* 274: 491–94.

Joseph, A. M., D. B. Nelson, S. M. Nugent, and M. L. Willenbring. 2003. "Timing of Alcohol and Smoking Cessation (TASC): Smoking Among Substance Use Patients Screened and Enrolled in a Clinical Trial." *Journal of Addictive Diseases* 22: 87–107.

Junor, W., D. Collins, and H. Lapsley. 2004. "The Macroeconomic and Distributional Effects of Reduced Smoking Prevalence in New South Wales." Sydney, Australia: The Cancer Council New South Wales.

Kandel, D. B., F. Y. Huang, and M. Davies. 2001. "Comorbidity Between Patterns of Substance Use Dependence and Psychiatric Syndromes." *Drug and Alcohol Dependence* 64: 233–41.

Kaper, J., E. J. Wagena, J. L. Severens, and C. P. Van Schayck. 2005a. "Healthcare Financing Systems for Increasing the Use of Tobacco Dependence Treatment." *Cochrane Database of Systematic Reviews* no. 2: CD004305.

Kaper, J., E. J. Wagena, M. C. Willemsen, and C. P. van Schayck. 2005b. "Reimbursement for Smoking Cessation Treatment May Double the Abstinence Rate: Results of a Randomized Trial." *Addiction* 100: 1012–20.

Keeler, T. E., T.-W. Hu, P. G. Barnett, W. G. Manning, and H.-Y. Sung. 1996. "Do Cigarette Producers Price-Discriminate by State? An Empirical Analysis of Local Cigarette Pricing and Taxation." *Journal of Health Economics* 15: 499–512.

Keller, P., A. Feltracco, L. Bailey, Z. Li, J. Niederdeppe, T. Baker, and M. Fiore. 2010. "Changes in Tobacco Quitlines in the United States, 2005–2006." *Preventing Chronic Disease* 7(2), http://www.cdc.gov/pcd/issues/2010/mar/09_0095.htm.

Kenyon, D. 1994. "Hogs, Jobs, and the Environment." *Virginia's Rural Economic Analysis Program: Horizons* 6(5). Blacksburg: Virginia Polytechnic Institute and State University.

Kessler, R. C., G. Andrews, L. J. Colpe, E. Hiripi, D. K. Mroczek, S. L. Normand, E. E. Walters, and A. M. Zaslavsky. 2002. "Short Screening Scales to Monitor Population Prevalences and Trends in Non-Specific Psychological Distress." *Psychological Medicine* 32: 959–76.

Kessler, R. C., P. R. Barker, L. J. Colpe, J. F. Epstein, J. C. Gfroerer, E. Hiripi, M. J. Howes, S. L. Normand, R. W. Manderscheid, E. E. Walters, and A. M. Zaslavsky. 2003. "Screening for Serious Mental Illness in the General Population." *Archives of General Psychiatry* 60: 184–89.

Kessler, R. C., and T. B. Ustun. 2004. "The World Mental Health Survey (WMH) Initiative Version of the World Health Organization (WHO) Composite International Diagnostic Interview (CIDI)." *International Journal of Methods in Psychiatric Research* 13: 93–121.

Kessler, R. C., H. Wittchen, J. M. Abelson, K. Mcgonagle, N. Schwarz, K. S. Kendler, B. Knäuper, and S. Zhao. 1998. "Methodological Studies of the Composite International Diagnostic Interview (CIDI) in the US National Comorbidity Survey (NCS)." *International Journal of Methods in Psychiatric Research* 7: 33–55.

Khuder, S. A. 2001. "Effect of Cigarette Smoking on Major Histological Types of Lung Cancer: A Meta-Analysis." *Lung Cancer* 31: 139–48.

Kletzer, L. G. 1989. "Returns to Seniority After Permanent Job Loss." *American Economic Review* 79: 536–43.

Kluger, R. 1996. *Ashes to Ashes: America's Hundred-Year Cigarette War, the Public Health, and the Unabashed Triumph of Philip Morris.* New York: Alfred A. Knopf.

Kollins, S. H., F. J. McClernon, and B. F. Fuemmeler. 2005. "Association Between Smoking and Attention-Deficit/Hyperactivity Disorder Symptoms in a Population-Based Sample of Young Adults." *Archives of General Psychiatry* 62: 1142–47.

Kostandini, G., B. F. Mills, and G. W. Norton. 2006. "The Potential Impact of Tobacco Biopharming: The Case of Human Serum Albumin." *American Journal of Agricultural Economics* 88: 671–79.

Kreuzer, M., P. Boffetta, E. Whitley, W. Ahrens, V. Gaborieau, J. Heinrich, K. H. Jockel, L. Kreienbrock, S. Mallone, F. Merletti, F. Roesch, P. Zambon, and L. Simonato. 2000. "Gender Differences in Lung Cancer Risk by Smoking: A Multicentre Case-Control Study in Germany and Italy." *British Journal of Cancer* 82: 227–33.

Krieger, N. 2004. "Defining and Investigating Social Disparities in Cancer: Critical Issues." *Cancer Causes & Control* 16: 5–14.

Kristein, M. M. 1977. "Economic Issues in Prevention." *Preventive Medicine* 6: 252–64.

Lancaster, T., and L. Stead. 2004. "Physician Advice for Smoking Cessation." *Cochrane Database of Systematic Reviews* no. 2: CD000165.

Landrine, H., and E. A. Klonoff. 2003. "Validity of Assessments of Youth Access to Tobacco: The Familiarity Effect." *American Journal of Public Health* 93: 1883–86.

Landrine, H., E. A. Klonoff, R. Campbell, and A. Reina-Patton. 2000. "Sociocultural Variables in Youth Access to Tobacco: Replication 5 Years Later." *Preventive Medicine* 30: 433–37.

Lasser, K., J. W. Boyd, S. Woolhandler, D. U. Himmelstein, D. McCormick, and D. H. Bor. 2000. "Smoking and Mental Illness: A Population-Based Prevalence Study." *Journal of the American Medical Association* 284: 2606–10.

Lawn, S. J. 2004. "Systemic Barriers to Quitting Smoking Among Institutionalised Public Mental Health Service Populations: A Comparison of Two Australian Sites." *International Journal of Social Psychiatry* 50: 204–15.

Lee, J. P., R. S. Moore, and S. E. Martin. 2003. "Unobtrusive Observations on Smoking in Urban California Bars." *Journal of Drug Issues* (Fall): 983–1000.

Lee, K., E. J. Hahn, C. Riker, S. Head, and P. Seithers. 2007. "Immediate Impact of Smoke-Free Laws on Indoor Air Quality." *Southern Medical Journal* 100: 885–89.

Leistikow, B. N., D. C. Martin, and C. E. Milano. 2000. "Estimates of Smoking-Attributable Deaths at Ages 15–54, Motherless or Fatherless Youths, and Resulting Social Security Costs in the United States in 1994." *Preventive Medicine* 30: 353–60.

Lerman, C., J. Audrain, C. T. Orleans, R. Boyd, K. Gold, D. Main, and N. Caporaso. 1996. "Investigation of Mechanisms Linking Depressed Mood to Nicotine Dependence." *Addictive Behaviors* 21: 9–19.

Levin, E. D., C. K. Conners, D. Silva, W. Canu, and J. March. 2001. "Effects of Chronic Nicotine and Methylphenidate in Adults with Attention Deficit/Hyperactivity Disorder." *Experimental and Clinical Psychopharmacology* 9: 83–90.

Levin, M. L. 1953. "The Occurrence of Lung Cancer in Man." *Acta Unio Internationalis Contra Cancrum* 9: 531–41.

Levinson, A. H., S. Henderrshott, and T. E. Byers. 2002. "The ID Effect on Youth Access to Cigarettes." *Tobacco Control* 11: 296–99.

Levy, D. T., S. Bales, and L. Nikolayev. 2006. "The Role of Public Policies in Reducing Smoking and Deaths Caused by Smoking in Vietnam: Results from the Vietnam Tobacco Policy Simulation Model." *Social Science & Medicine* 62: 1819–30.

Levy, D. T., F. J. Chaloupka, and J. G. Gitchell. 2004. "The Effects of Tobacco Control Policies on Smoking Rates: A Tobacco Control Scorecard." *Journal of Public Health Management and Practice* 10: 338–51.

Levy, D. T., F. J. Chaloupka, J. Gitchell, D. Mendez, and K. E. Warner. 2002. "The Use of Simulation Models for the Surveillance, Justification and Understanding of Tobacco Control Policies." *Health Care Management Science* 5: 113–20.

Levy, D. T., K. M. Cummings, and A. Hyland. 2000a. "A Simulation of the Effects of Youth Initiation Policies on Overall Cigarette Use." *American Journal of Public Health* 90: 1311–14.

Levy, D. T., K. M. Cummings, and A. Hyland. 2000b. "Increasing Taxes as a Strategy to Reduce Cigarette Use and Deaths: Results of a Simulation Model." *Preventive Medicine* 31: 279–86.

Levy, D. T., and K. B. Friend. 2000. "A Simulation Model of Tobacco Youth Access Policies." *Journal of Health Politics, Policy and Law* 25: 1023–50.

Levy, D. T., and K. Friend. 2001. "A Computer Simulation Model of Mass Media Interventions Directed at Tobacco Use." *Preventive Medicine* 32: 284–94.

Levy, D. T., and K. Friend. 2002a. "Examining the Effects of Tobacco Treatment Policies on Smoking Rates and Smoking Related Deaths Using the SimSmoke Computer Simulation Model." *Tobacco Control* 11: 47–54.

Levy, D. T., and K. Friend. 2002b. "A Simulation Model of Policies Directed at Treating Tobacco Use and Dependence." *Medical Decision Making* 22: 6–17.

Levy, D. T., K. Friend, H. Holder, and M. Carmona. 2001. "Effect of Policies Directed at Youth Access to Smoking: Results from the SimSmoke Computer Simulation Model." *Tobacco Control* 10: 108–16.

Levy, D. T., K. Friend, and E. Polishchuk. 2001. "Effect of Clean Indoor Air Laws on Smokers: The Clean Air Module of the SimSmoke Computer Simulation Model." *Tobacco Control* 10: 345–51.

Levy, D., and E. Mumford. 2007. "Examining Trends in Quantity Smoked." *Nicotine & Tobacco Research* 9: 1287–96.

Levy, D. T., E. A. Mumford, and C. Compton. 2006. "Tobacco Control Policies and Smoking in a Population of Low Education Women, 1992–2002." *Journal of Epidemiology and Community Health* 60: ii20–ii26.

Levy, D. T., E. Mumford, and B. Pesin. 2003. "Tobacco Control Policies, and Reductions in Smoking Rates and Smoking-Related Deaths: Results from the SimSmoke Model." *Expert Review of Pharmacoeconomics and Outcomes Research* 3: 457–68.

Levy, D. T., N. Nikolayev, and E. A. Mumford. 2004. "The Role of Public Policies in Reducing Smoking Prevalence and Deaths Caused by Smoking in California: Results from the California Tobacco Policy Simulation Model." Calverton, MD: Pacific Institute.

Levy, D. T., N. Nikolayev, and E. A. Mumford. 2005a. "Recent Trends in Smoking and the Role of Public Policies: Results from the SimSmoke Tobacco Control Policy Simulation Model." *Addiction* 10: 1526–37.

Levy, D. T., N. Nikolayev, and E. A. Mumford. 2005b. "The Healthy People 2010 Smoking Prevalence and Tobacco Control Objectives: Results from the SimSmoke Tobacco Control Policy Simulation Model." *Cancer Causes & Control* 16: 359–71.

Levy, D., H. Ross, L. Powell, J. Bauer, and H. Lee. 2007. "The Role of Public Policies in Reducing Smoking Prevalence and Deaths Caused by Smoking in Arizona: Results from the Arizona Tobacco Policy Simulation Model." *Journal of Public Health Management and Practice* 13: 59–67.

Levy, D. T., C. P. Wen, D. T. Y. Cheng, and M. Oblak. 2005. "Increasing Taxes to Reduce Smoking Prevalence and Smoking-Attributable Mortality in Taiwan: Results from a Tobacco Policy Simulation Model." *Tobacco Control* 14, Suppl. 1: i45–i50.

Lewit, E. M., D. Coate, and M. Grossman. 1981. "The Effects of Government Regulation on Teenage Smoking." *Journal of Law and Economics* 24: 545–69.

Liang, L., F. J. Chaloupka, M. Nichter, and R. Clayton. 2003. "Prices, Policies and Youth Smoking." *Addiction* 98: 105–22.

Lichtermann, D., J. Ekelund, E. Pukkala, A. Tanskanen, and J. Lonnqvist. 2001. "Incidence of Cancer Among Persons with Schizophrenia and Their Relatives." *Archives of General Psychiatry* 58: 573–78.

Lieu, J. E., and A. R. Feinstein. 2000. "Confirmations and Surprises in the Association of Tobacco Use with Sinusitis." *Archives of Otolaryngology—Head & Neck Surgery* 126: 940–46.

Lindsted, K. D., G. E. Fraser, M. Steinkohl, and W. L. Beeson. 1996. "Healthy Volunteer Effect in a Cohort Study: Temporal Resolution in the Adventist Health Study." *Journal of Clinical Epidemiology* 49: 783–90.

Link, B. G., and J. C. Phelan. 2001. "Conceptualizing Stigma." *Annual Review of Sociology* 27: 363–85.

Lippiatt, B. C. 1990. "Measuring Medical Cost and Life Expectancy Impacts of Changes in Cigarette Sales." *Preventive Medicine* 19: 515–32.

Longo, D. R., M. M. Feldman, R. L. Kruse, R. C. Brownson, G. F. Petroski, and J. E. Hewett. 1998. "Implementing Smoking Bans in American Hospitals: Results of a National Survey." *Tobacco Control* 7: 47–55.

Luce, B. R., and S. O. Schweitzer. 1978. "Smoking and Alcohol Abuse: A Comparison of Their Economic Consequences." *New England Journal of Medicine* 298: 569–71.

Malarcher, A. M., J. Schulman, L. A. Epstein, M. J. Thun, P. Mowery, B. Pierce, L. Escobedo, and G. A. Giovino. 2000. "Methodological Issues in Estimating Smoking-Attributable Mortality in the United States." *American Journal of Epidemiology* 152: 573–84.

Manning, W. G. 1998. "The Logged Dependent Variable, Heteroscedasticity, and the Retransformation Problem." *Journal of Health Economics* 17: 283–95.

Manning, W. G., E. B. Keeler, J. P. Newhouse, E. M. Sloss, and J. Wasserman. 1989. "The Taxes of Sin: Do Smokers and Drinkers Pay Their Way?" *Journal of the American Medical Association* 261: 1604–9.

Manning, W. G., and J. Mullahy. 2001. "Estimating Log Models: To Transform or Not to Transform?" *Journal of Health Economics* 20: 461–94.

Manser, R. L., L. B. Irving, C. Stone, G. Byrnes, M. Abramson, and D. Campbell. 2004. "Screening for Lung Cancer." *Cochrane Database of Systematic Reviews* no. 1: CD001991.

Marang-van de Mheen, P. J., G. D. Smith, C. L. Hart, and D. J. Hole. 2001. "Are Women More Sensitive to Smoking Than Men? Findings from the Renfrew and Paisley Study." *International Journal of Epidemiology* 30: 787–92.

Mark, T. L., J. A. Buck, J. D. Dilonardo, R. M. Coffey, and M. Chalk. 2003. "Medicaid Expenditures on Behavioral Health Care." *Psychiatric Services* 54: 188–94.

Markley, D. M., M. I. Luger, L. S. Stewart, and J. Perry. 2001. "Understanding the Dimensions of Tobacco Dependency at the Community Level in North Carolina." Chapel Hill: Office of Economic Development, University of North Carolina at Chapel Hill.

Martinson, B. C., P. J. O'Connor, N. P. Pronk, and S. J. Rolnick. 2003. "Smoking Cessation Attempts in Relation to Prior Health Care Charges: The Effect of Antecedent Smoking-Related Symptoms?" *American Journal of Health Promotion* 18: 125–32.

Massachusetts Tobacco Control Program. 2006. "One-Year Review of the Massachusetts Smoke-Free Workplace Law." Boston: Massachusetts Department of Public Health.

Max, W. 2001. "The Financial Impact of Smoking on Health-Related Costs: A Review of the Literature." *American Journal of Health Promotion* 15: 321–31.

Maxwell, J. C., Jr. 2004. "The Maxwell Report: Year End and Fourth Quarter 2003 Sales Estimates for the Cigarette Industry, February 2004." Richmond, VA: John C. Maxwell, Jr.

McCabe, R. E., S. M. Chudzik, M. M. Antony, L. Young, R. P. Swinson, and M. J. Zolvensky. 2004. "Smoking Behaviors Across Anxiety Disorders." *Journal of Anxiety Disorders* 18: 7–18.

McDonald, J. D., and D. A. Sumner. 2003. "The Influence of Commodity Programs on Acreage Response to Market Price: With an Illustration Concerning Rice Policy in the United States." *American Journal of Agricultural Economics* 85: 857–71.

McGowan, R., and J. Mahon. 2005. "Collaborating with the Enemy: Tobacco, Alcohol and the Public Good?" *Business in the Contemporary World* 7: 69–92.

McKinnon, K., F. Cournos, and R. Herman. 2002. "HIV Among People with Chronic Mental Illness." *Psychiatric Quarterly* 73: 17–31.

McMenamin, S. B., H. A. Halpin, and N. M. Bellows. 2006. "Knowledge of Medicaid Coverage and Effectiveness of Smoking Treatments." *American Journal of Preventive Medicine* 31: 369–74.

McPhillips-Tangum, C., A. Cahill, C. Bocchino, and C. M. Cutler. 2002. "Addressing Tobacco in Managed Care: Results of the 2000 Survey." *Preventive Medicine in Managed Care* 3: 85–94.

McWhorter, W. P., G. M. Boyd, and M. E. Mattson. 1990. "Predictors of Quitting Smoking: The NHANES I Followup Experience." *Journal of Clinical Epidemiology* 43: 1399–1405.

Meier, K., and M. Licari. 1997. "The Effect of Cigarette Taxes on Cigarette Consumption: 1955 Through 1994." *American Journal of Public Health* 87: 1126–30.

Mendez, D., and K. E. Warner. 2004. "Adult Cigarette Smoking Prevalence: Declining as Expected (Not as Desired)." *American Journal of Public Health* 94: 251–52.

Mendez, D., K. E. Warner, and P. N. Courant. 1998. "Has Smoking Cessation Ceased? Expected Trends in the Prevalence of Smoking in the United States." *American Journal of Epidemiology* 148: 249–58.

Merriman, D., A. Yurekli, and F. J. Chaloupka. 2000. "How Big Is the Worldwide Cigarette Smuggling Problem?" In *Tobacco Control in Developing Countries*, ed. P. Jha and F. Chaloupka, pp. 365–92. Oxford: Oxford University Press.

Metzger, K. B., F. Mostashari, and B. D. Kerker. 2005. "Use of Pharmacy Data to Evaluate Smoking Regulations' Impact on Sales of Nicotine Replacement Therapies in New York City." *American Journal of Public Health* 95: 1050–55.

Miles, R., and K. Cameron. 1982. *Coffin Nails and Corporate Strategies.* Englewood Cliffs, NJ: Prentice-Hall.

Miller, B. J., C. B. Paschall III, and D. P. Svendsen. 2006. "Mortality and Medical Comorbidity Among Patients with Serious Mental Illness." *Psychiatric Services* 57: 1482–87.

Miller, D. P., K. F. Villa, S. L. Hogue, and D. Sivapathasundaram. 2001. "Birth and First-Year Costs for Mothers and Infants Attributable to Maternal Smoking." *Nicotine & Tobacco Research* 3: 25–35.

Miller, L. S., X. Zhang, T. Novotny, D. P. Rice, and W. Max. 1998b. "State Estimates of Medicaid Expenditures Attributable to Cigarette Smoking, Fiscal Year 1993." *Public Health Reports* 113: 140–51.

Miller, L. S., X. Zhang, D. P. Rice, and W. Max. 1998a. "State Estimates of Total Medical Expenditures Attributable to Cigarette Smoking, 1993." *Public Health Reports* 113: 447–58.

Miller, N., T. R. Frieden, S. Y. Liu, T. D. Matte, F. Mostashari, D. R. Deitcher, K. M. Cummings, C. Chang, U. Bauer, and M. T. Bassett. 2005. "Effectiveness of a Large-Scale Distribution Programme of Free Nicotine Patches: A Prospective Evaluation." *The Lancet* 365: 1849–54.

Miller, V. P., C. Ernst, and F. Collin. 1999. "Smoking-Attributable Medical Care Costs in the USA." *Social Science & Medicine* 48: 375–91.

Miner, B. M. 2005. "New York State CIAA Enforcement and Waiver Activity July 2003–December 2004." Troy, NY: New York State Department of Health.

Montoya, I. D., D. M. Herbeck, D. S. Svikis, and H. A. Pincus. 2005. "Identification and Treatment of Patients with Nicotine Problems in Routine Clinical Psychiatry Practice." *American Journal on Addictions* 14: 441–54.

Moore, R. S., J. P. Lee, T. M. J. Antin, and S. E. Martin. 2006. "Tobacco Free Workplace Policies and Low Socioeconomic Status Female Bartenders in San Francisco." *Journal of Epidemiology and Community Health* 60: ii51–ii56.

Mullahy, J. 1998. "Much Ado About Two: Reconsidering Retransformation and the Two-Part Model in Health Econometrics." *Journal of Health Economics* 17: 247–81.

Murphy, J. M., D. Shelley, P. M. Repetto, K. M. Cummings, and M. C. Mahoney. 2003. "Impact of Economic Policies on Reducing Tobacco Use Among Medicaid Clients in New York." *Preventive Medicine* 37: 68–70.

Musich, S., S. D. Faruzzi, C. Lu, T. McDonald, D. Hirschland, and D. W. Edington. 2003. "Pattern of Medical Charges After Quitting Smoking Among Those with and Without Arthritis, Allergies, or Back Pain." *American Journal of Health Promotion* 18: 133–42.

National Alliance on Mental Illness. 2006. "National Alliance on Mental Illness (NAMI) Public Policy Platform." Arlington, VA: National Alliance on Mental Illness.

National Association of State Mental Health Program Directors. 2006. "Smoking Policies and Practices: Survey Results." Paper presented at Summer 2006 Commissioners Meeting, NASMHPD Research Institute, Kissimmee, FL, July 11.

National Cancer Institute. 2000. "State and Local Legislative Action to Reduce Tobacco Use." Bethesda MD: U.S. Department of Health and Human Services.

National Cancer Institute. 2005a. "ASSIST: Shaping the Future of Tobacco Prevention and Control." Bethesda, MD: U.S. Department of Health and Human Services.

National Cancer Institute. 2005b. "Cancer Trends Progress Report—2005 Update." Bethesda, MD: U.S. Department of Health and Human Services.

National Cancer Institute. 2010. "Cancer Trends Progress Report—2009/2010 Update." Bethesda, MD: U.S. Department of Health and Human Services.

National Center for Health Statistics. 2002. *2002 Natality Detail Files, National Vital Statistics Section, National Center for Health Statistics.* http://www.cdc.gov/nchs/products/elec _prods/subject/natality.htm.

National Research Council. 1986. *Environmental Tobacco Smoke: Measuring Exposures and Assessing Health Effects.* Washington, DC: National Research Council Committee on Passive Smoking.

National Restaurant Association. 2010. "Restaurant Industry Fact Sheet." http://www.restau rant.org/research/facts/.

National Workrights Institute. 1994. "Lifestyle Discrimination in the Workplace." Princeton, NJ: National Workrights Institute.

Nevitt, J., G. W. Norton, B. F. Mills, J. M. Ellen, M. Ellerbrock, D. Reaves, K. Tiller, and G. Bullen. 2003. "Participatory Assessment of Social and Economic Impacts of Biotechnology." Blacksburg: Department of Agricultural and Applied Economics, Virginia Polytechnic Institute and State University.

Nilsson, S., J. M. Carstensen, and G. Pershagen. 2001. "Mortality Among Male and Female Smokers in Sweden: A 33 Year Follow Up." *Journal of Epidemiology and Community Health* 55: 825–30.

Nordling, C. O. 1952. "A New Theory on the Cancer-Inducing Mechanism." *British Journal of Cancer* 1: 69–72.

Nordlund, L. A., J. M. Carstensen, and G. Pershagen. 1999. "Are Male and Female Smokers at Equal Risk of Smoking-Related Cancer: Evidence from a Swedish Prospective Study." *Scandinavian Journal of Public Health* 27: 56–62.

Office of Technology Assessment. 1985. "Smoking-Related Deaths and Financial Costs." Washington, DC: United States Congress.

Office of Tobacco Control. 2005. "Smoke-Free Workplaces in Ireland: A One-Year Review." County Kildare, Ireland: Office of Tobacco Control.

O'Hara, P., J. E. Connett, W. W. Lee, M. Nides, R. Murray, and R. Wise. 1998. "Early and Late Weight Gain Following Smoking Cessation in the Lung Health Study." *American Journal of Epidemiology* 148: 821–30.

Olincy, A., D. A. Young, and R. Freedman. 1997. "Increased Levels of Nicotine Metabolite Cotinine in Schizophrenic Smokers Compared to Other Smokers." *Biological Psychiatry* 42: 1–5.

O'Neil, M. 2002. *Nonprofit Nation.* San Francisco: Jossey-Bass.

Orme, M. E., S. L. Hogue, L. M. Kennedy, A. C. Paine, and C. Godfrey. 2001. "Development of the Health and Economic Consequences of Smoking Interactive Model." *Tobacco Control* 10: 55–61.

Orzechowski and Walker. Various years. "The Tax Burden on Tobacco." Arlington, VA: Orzechowski and Walker.

Ossip-Klein, D. J., and S. McIntosh. 2003. "Quitlines in North America: Evidence Base and Applications." *American Journal of the Medical Sciences* 326: 201–5.

Oster, G., G. A. Colditz, and N. L. Kelly. 1984. "The Economic Costs of Smoking and Benefits of Quitting for Individual Smokers." *Preventive Medicine* 13: 377–89.

Oster, G., T. E. Delea, and G. A. Colditz. 1988. "Maternal Smoking During Pregnancy and Expenditures on Neonatal Health Care." *American Journal of Preventive Medicine* 4: 216–19.

Pakko, M. 2006. "Smokefree Law Did Affect Revenue from Gaming in Delaware." *Tobacco Control* 15: 68–69.

Pan, J., E. M. Barbeau, C. Levenstein, and E. D. Balbach. 2005. "Organized Labor and Occupational Health." *American Journal of Public Health* 95: 398–404.

Parasher, G., and G. L. Eastwood. 2000. "Smoking and Peptic Ulcer in the *Helicobacter pylori* Era." *European Journal of Gastroenterology & Hepatology* 12: 843–53.

Patten, C. A., B. K. Bruce, R. D. Hurt, K. P. Offord, J. W. Richardson, L. R. Clemensen, and S. M. Persons. 1995. "Effects of a Smoke-Free Policy on an Inpatient Psychiatric Unit." *Tobacco Control* 4: 372–79.

Patton, G. C., J. B. Carlin, C. Coffey, R. Wolfe, M. Hibbert, and G. Bowes. 1998. "Depression, Anxiety, and Smoking Initiation: A Prospective Study Over 3 Years." *American Journal of Public Health* 88: 1518–22.

Peterson, A. L., A. S. Hryshko-Mullen, and Y. Cortez. 2003. "Assessment and Diagnosis of Nicotine Dependence in Mental Health Settings." *American Journal on Addictions* 12: 192–97.

Pierce, J. P., and E. A. Gilpin. 2002. "Impact of Over-the-Counter Sales on Effectiveness of Pharmaceutical Aids for Smoking Cessation." *Journal of the American Medical Association* 288: 1260–64.

Plescia, M., S. Malek, D. Shopland, C. Anderson, and D. Burns. 2005. "Protecting Workers from Secondhand Smoke in North Carolina." *North Carolina Medical Journal* 66: 186–91.

Pomerleau, C. S., S. M. Carton, M. L. Lutzke, K. A. Flessland, and O. F. Pomerleau. 1994. "Reliability of the Fagerström Tolerance Questionnaire and the Fagerström Test for Nicotine Dependence." *Addictive Behaviors* 19: 33–39.

Potter, A. S., and P. A. Newhouse. 2004. "Effects of Acute Nicotine Administration on Behavioral Inhibition in Adolescents with Attention-Deficit/Hyperactivity Disorder." *Psychopharmacology (Berlin)* 176: 182–94.

Poulin, C., O. Lemoine, L.-R. Poirier, and J. Lambert. 2005. "Validation Study of a Nonspecific Psychological Distress Scale." *Social Psychiatry and Psychiatric Epidemiology* 40: 1019–24.

Prochaska, J. J., S. C. Fromont, and S. M. Hall. 2005. "How Prepared Are Psychiatry Residents for Treating Nicotine Dependence?" *Academic Psychiatry* 29: 256–61.

Prochaska, J. J., S. M. Hall, and L. A. Bero. 2008. "Tobacco Use Among Individuals with Schizophrenia: What Role Has the Tobacco Industry Played?" *Schizophrenia Bulletin* 34: 555–67.

Pyles, M. K., and E. J. Hahn. 2009. "Smoke-Free Legislation and Charitable Gaming in Kentucky." *Tobacco Control* 18: 60–62.

Rayens, M. K., E. J. Hahn, R. E. Langley, and M. Zhang. 2008. "Public Support for Smoke-Free Laws in Rural Communities." *American Journal of Preventive Medicine* 34: 519–22.

Reaves, D. W. 1999. "Economic Impacts of Tobacco Industry Changes on Producers and Their Communities: Challenges and Opportunities." Blacksburg: Department of Agricultural and Applied Economics, Virginia Polytechnic Institute and State University.

Repace, J. 2004. "Respirable Particles and Carcinogens in the Air of Delaware Hospitality Venues Before and After a Smoking Ban." *Journal of Occupational and Environmental Medicine* 46: 887–905.

Rezitis, A. N., A. B. Brown, and W. E. Foster. 1998. "Adjustment Costs and Dynamic Factor Demands for US Cigarette Manufacturing." *Agricultural Economics* 18: 217–31.

Ribisl, K. M. 2004. "Retailing." In *Tobacco in History and Culture: An Encyclopedia (Scribner Turning Points Library)*, ed. J. Goodman, M. Norton, and M. Parascandola, pp. 496–504. Farmington Hills, MI: Charles Scribner's Sons.

Ribisl, K. M., A. E. Kim, and R. S. Williams. 2001. "Web Sites Selling Cigarettes: How Many Are There in the USA and What Are Their Sales Practices?" *Tobacco Control* 10: 352–59.

Ribisl, K. M., A. E. Kim, and R. S. Williams. 2007. "Sales and Marketing of Cigarettes on the Internet: Emerging Threats to Tobacco Control and Promising Policy Solutions." In *Ending the Tobacco Problem: A Blueprint for the Nation*, ed. Institute of Medicine, pp. 653–78. Washington, DC: National Academies Press.

Rice, D. P., T. A. Hodgson, P. Sinsheimer, W. Browner, and A. N. Kopstein. 1986. "The Economic Costs of the Health Effects of Smoking, 1984." *Milbank Quarterly* 64: 489–547.

Richter, K. P., C. A. Gibson, J. S. Ahluwalia, and K. H. Schmelzle. 2001. "Tobacco Use and Quit Attempts Among Methadone Maintenance Clients." *American Journal of Public Health* 91: 296–99.

Rigotti, N. A. 2002. "Clinical Practice: Treatment of Tobacco Use and Dependence." *New England Journal of Medicine* 346: 506–12.

Rigotti, N. A., M. A. Stoto, M. F. Bierer, A. Rosen, and T. Schelling. 1993. "Retail Stores' Compliance with a City No-Smoking Law." *American Journal of Public Health* 83: 227–32.

Ring, R. 1999. "Consumers' Share and Producers' Share of the General Sales Tax." *National Tax Journal* 52: 80–90.

Ringen, K., N. Anderson, T. McAfee, S. M. Zbikowski, and D. Fales. 2002. "Smoking Cessation in a Blue-Collar Population: Results from an Evidence-Based Pilot Program." *American Journal of Industrial Medicine* 42: 367–77.

Risch, H. A., G. R. Howe, M. Jain, J. D. Burch, E. J. Holowaty, and A. B. Miller. 1993. "Are Female Smokers at Higher Risk for Lung Cancer Than Male Smokers? A Case-Control Analysis by Histologic Type." *American Journal of Epidemiology* 138: 281–93.

Risch, H. A., G. R. Howe, M. Jain, J. D. Burch, E. J. Holowaty, and A. B. Miller. 1994. "Lung Cancer Risk for Female Smokers." *Science* 263: 1206–8.

Risch, H. A., and A. B. Miller. 2004. "Re: Are Women More Susceptible to Lung Cancer?" *Journal of the National Cancer Institute* 96: 1560–61.

Roberts, E. B., J. Homer, A. Kasabian, and M. Varrell. 1982. "A Systems View of the Smoking Problem: Perspective and Limitations of the Role of Science in Decision-Making." *International Journal of Bio-Medical Computing* 13: 69–86.

Rooney, P., G. Tempel, and J. Small. 2005. "The Impact of Corporate Mergers and Acquisitions on Corporate Giving in an Urban Area." Paper presented at the Association for Research on Nonprofit Organizations and Voluntary Action Annual Conference, Washington, DC, November 17–19.

Rork, J. C. 2003. "Coveting Thy Neighbors' Taxation." *National Tax Journal* 56: 775–87.

Rosenstock, I. M., A. Stergachis, and C. Heaney. 1986. "Evaluation of Smoking Prohibition Policy in a Health Maintenance Organization." *American Journal of Public Health* 76: 1014–15.

Rubin, D. B. 2001. "Estimating the Causal Effects of Smoking." *Statistics in Medicine* 20: 1395–414.

Rucker, R. R., W. N. Thurman, and D. A. Sumner. 1995. "Restricting the Market for Quota: An Analysis of Tobacco Production Rights with Corroboration from Congressional Testimony." *Journal of Political Economy* 103: 142–75.

Ruhm, C. J. 1991. "Are Workers Permanently Scarred by Job Displacements?" *American Economic Review* 81: 319–24.

Ryan, H., P. M. Wortley, A. Easton, L. Pederson, and G. Greenwood. 2001. "Smoking Among Lesbians, Gays, and Bisexuals: A Review of the Literature." *American Journal of Preventive Medicine* 21: 142–49.

Sacco, K. A., K. L. Bannon, and T. P. George. 2004. "Nicotinic Receptor Mechanisms and Cognition in Normal States and Neuropsychiatric Disorders." *Journal of Psychopharmacology* 18: 457–74.

Saffer, H., and D. Dave. 2002. "Mental Illness and the Demand for Alcohol, Cocaine and Cigarettes." NBER Working Paper 8699. Cambridge, MA: National Bureau of Economic Research.

Schauffler, H. H., S. McMenamin, K. Olson, G. Boyce-Smith, J. A. Rideout, and J. Kamil. 2001. "Variations in Treatment Benefits Influence Smoking Cessation: Results of a Randomised Controlled Trial." *Tobacco Control* 10: 175–80.

Schauffler, H. H., J. Mordavsky, and C. T. Orleans. 2001. "State Medicaid Coverage for Tobacco-Dependence in the United States: 1998 and 2000." *MMWR Morbidity & Mortality Weekly Report* 50: 979–82.

Schofield, M., M. Lynagh, and G. Mishra. 2003. "Evaluation of a Health Promoting Schools Program to Reduce Smoking in Australian Secondary Schools." *Health Education Research* 18: 678–92.

Scollo, M., A. Lal, A. Hyland, and S. A. Glantz. 2003. "A Review of the Quality of Studies on the Economic Effects of Smoke-Free Policies on the Hospitality Industry." *Tobacco Control* 12: 13–20.

Secker-Walker, R. H., W. Gnich, S. Platt, and T. Lancaster. 2002. "Community Interventions for Reducing Smoking Among Adults." *Cochrane Database of Systematic Reviews* no. 3: CD001745.

Shavers, V. L., P. Fagan, L. A. Jouridine Alexander, R. Clayton, J. Doucet, and L. Baezconde-Garbanati. 2006. "Workplace and Home Smoking Restrictions and Racial/Ethnic Variation in the Prevalence and Intensity of Current Cigarette Smoking Among Women by Poverty Status, TUS-CPS 1998–1999 and 2001–2002." *Journal of Epidemiology and Community Health* 60: ii34–ii43.

Shimer, R. 2005. "Reassessing the Ins and Outs of Unemployment." Working paper, University of Chicago, Department of Economics.

Shoven, J. B., J. O. Sundberg, and J. P. Bunker. 1990. "The Social Security Cost of Smoking." In *The Economics of Aging*, ed. D. Wise, pp. 231–54. Chicago: University of Chicago Press.

Siegel, M. 2000. "Tobacco Industry Sponsorship in the United States 1995–1999." Boston: Boston University School of Public Health.

Siegel, M., and M. Skeer. 2003. "Exposure to Secondhand Smoke and Excess Lung Cancer Mortality Risk Among Workers in the '5 B's': Bars, Bowling Alleys, Billiard Halls, Betting Establishments, and Bingo Parlours." *Tobacco Control* 12: 333–38.

Skara, S., and S. Sussman. 2003. "A Review of 25 Long-Term Adolescent Tobacco and Other Drug Use Prevention Program Evaluations." *Preventive Medicine* 37: 451–74.

Skeer, M., M. L. Land, D. Cheng, and M. Siegel 2004. "Smoking in Boston Bars Before and After a 100% Smoke-Free Regulation: An Assessment of Early Compliance." *Journal of Public Health Management and Practice* 10: 501–7.

Sloan, F. A., J. Ostermann, G. Picone, C. Conover, and D. H. Taylor. 2004. *The Price of Smoking*. Cambridge, MA: MIT Press.

Sloan, F. A., and J. G. Trogdon. 2004. "The Impact of the Master Settlement Agreement on Cigarette Consumption." *Journal of Policy Analysis and Management* 23: 843–55.

Sly, D. F., R. S. Hopkins, E. Trapido, and S. Ray. 2001. "Influence of a Counteradvertising Media Campaign on Initiation of Smoking: The Florida 'Truth' Campaign." *American Journal of Public Health* 91: 233–38.

Smith, E. A., N. Offen, and R. E. Malone. 2005. "What Makes an Ad a Cigarette Ad? Commercial Tobacco Imagery in the Lesbian, Gay, and Bisexual Press." *Journal of Epidemiology and Community Health* 59: 1086–91.

Smith, R. C., A. Singh, M. Infante, A. Khandat, and A. Kloos. 2002. "Effects of Cigarette Smoking and Nicotine Nasal Spray on Psychiatric Symptoms and Cognition in Schizophrenia." *Neuropsychopharmacology* 27: 479–97.

Snell, W. 2005. "The Buyout: Short-Run Observations and Implications for Kentucky's Tobacco Industry." Working paper, University of Kentucky.

Snyder, L. B., M. A. Hamilton, E. W. Mitchell, J. Kiwanuka-Tondo, F. Fleming-Milici, and D. Proctor. 2004. "A Meta-Analysis of the Effect of Mediated Health Communication Campaigns on Behavior Change in the United States." *Journal of Health Communication* 9, Suppl. 1: 71–96.

Sobel, R. S., and T. A. Garrett. 1987. "Taxation and Product Quality: New Evidence from Generic Cigarettes." *Journal of Political Economy* 105: 880–87.

Social Security Administration. 1996. *Annual Statistical Supplement to the Social Security Bulletin.* Baltimore, MD: Social Security Administration, Office of Research, Evaluation, and Statistics.

Sorensen, G., E. Barbeau, M. K. Hunt, and K. Emmons. 2004. "Reducing Social Disparities in Tobacco Use: A Social-Contextual Model for Reducing Tobacco Use Among Blue-Collar Workers." *American Journal of Public Health* 94: 230–39.

Sorensen, G., K. Emmons, A. Stoddard, L. Linnan, and J. Avrunin. 2002. "Do Social Influences Contribute to Occupational Differences in Quitting Smoking and Attitudes Toward Quitting?" *American Journal of Health Promotion* 16: 135–41.

Sowden, A. J., and L. Arblaster. 1999. "Mass Media Interventions for Preventing Smoking in Young People." *The Cochrane Library* 1: 1–28.

Stark, M. J., and B. K. Campbell. 1993. "Cigarette Smoking and Methadone Dose Levels." *The American Journal of Drug and Alcohol Abuse* 19: 209–17.

St. Clair, P., D. Blake, D. Bugliari, S. Chien, O. Hayden, M. Hurd, S. Ilchuk, F.-Y. Kung, A. Angela Miu, C. Panis, P. Pantoja, A. Rastegar, S. Rohwedder, E. Roth, J. Wedell, and J. Zissimopoulos. 2006. "Health and Retirement Survey Data Documentation, Version F." Santa Monica, CA: RAND Corporation.

Stead, L. F., and T. Lancaster. 2000. "A Systematic Review of Interventions for Preventing Tobacco Sales to Minors." *Tobacco Control* 9: 169–76.

Stead, L. F., and T. Lancaster. 2001. "Telephone Counselling for Smoking Cessation." *Cochrane Database of Systematic Reviews* no. 2: CD002850.

Stead, L. F., R. Perera, and T. Lancaster. 2006. "Telephone Counselling for Smoking Cessation." *Cochrane Database of Systematic Reviews* no. 3: CD002850.

Steger, C. 2006. "Exploring Corporate Philanthropy: A Member Survey." New York: Committee to Encourage Corporate Philanthropy.

Stehr, M. 2005. "Cigarette Tax Avoidance and Evasion." *Journal of Health Economics* 24: 277–97.

Steinberg, M. L., S. M. Hall, and T. Rustin. 2003. "Psychosocial Therapies for Tobacco Dependence in Mental Health and Other Substance Use Populations." *Psychiatric Annals* 33: 469–78.

Steinberg, M. L., J. M. Williams, and D. M. Ziedonis. 2004. "Financial Implications of Cigarette Smoking Among Individuals with Schizophrenia." *Tobacco Control* 13: 206.

Stellman, S. D., and L. Garfinkel. 1986. "Smoking Habits and Tar Levels in a New American Cancer Society Prospective Study of 1.2 Million Men and Women." *Journal of the National Cancer Institute* 76: 1057–63.

Stevens, A. H. 1997. "Persistent Effects of Job Displacement: The Importance of Multiple Job Loss." *Journal of Labor Economics* 15: 165–88.

Stroup, T. S., J. H. Gilmore, and L. F. Jarskog. 2000. "Management of Medical Illness in Persons with Schizophrenia." *Psychology Annals* 30: 35–40.

Stuber, J., and S. Galea. 2009. "Who Conceals Their Smoking Status from Their Health Care Provider?" *Nicotine & Tobacco Research* 11: 303–7.

Stuber, J., S. Galea, and B. G. Link. 2008. "Smoking and the Emergence of a Stigmatized Social Status." *Social Science & Medicine* 67: 420–30.

Stuber, J., S. Galea, and B. G. Link. 2009. "Stigma and Smoking: The Consequences of Our Good Intentions." *Social Service Review* 83: 585–609.

Stull, D. D. 2000. "Tobacco Barns and Chicken Houses: Agricultural Transformation in Western Kentucky." *Human Organization* 59: 151–61.

Substance Abuse and Mental Health Services Administration. 2002. "Report to Congress on the Prevention and Treatment of Co-occurring Substance Abuse Disorders and Mental Disorders." Washington, DC: Substance Abuse and Mental Health Services Administration/U.S. Department of Health and Human Services.

Sullivan, D. 1985. "Testing Hypotheses About Firm Behavior in the Cigarette Industry." *Journal of Political Economy* 93: 586–98.

Sullivan, M. A., and L. S. Covey. 2002. "Current Perspectives on Smoking Cessation Among Substance Abusers." *Current Psychiatry Reports* 4: 388–96.

Sumner, D. A. 1981. "Measurement of Monopoly Behavior: An Application to the Cigarette Industry." *Journal of Political Economy* 89: 1010–19.

Sumner, D. A. 1987. "The Impact of Cigarette Modifications on the Tobacco Production Industry in the United States." Washington, DC: Technical Study Group, Cigarette Safety Act of 1984.

Sumner, D. A., and J. Alston. 1984. "The Impact of Removal of Price Supports and Supply Controls for Tobacco in the United States." In *Research in Domestic and International Agribusiness Management*, ed. R. Goldberg. Greenwich, CT: JAI Press.

Sumner, D. A., and J. Alston. 1987. "Substitutability for Farm Commodities. The Demand for U.S. Tobacco in Cigarette Manufacturing." *American Journal of Agricultural Economics* 69: 258–65.

Sumner, D. A., and M. K. Wohlgenant. 1985. "Effects of an Increase in the Federal Excise Tax on Cigarettes." *American Journal of Agricultural Economics* 67: 235–42.

Sunley, E. M., A. Yurekli, and F. J. Chaloupka. 2000. "The Design, Administration, and Potential Revenue of Tobacco Excises." In *Tobacco Control in Developing Countries*, ed. P. Jha and F. Chaloupka, pp. 409–26. Oxford: Oxford University Press.

Swan, G. E., and D. Carmelli. 1995. "Characteristics Associated with Excessive Weight Gain After Smoking Cessation in Men." *American Journal of Public Health* 92: 990–96.

Swartz, M. S., J. W. Swanson, M. J. Hannon, H. S. Bosworth, F. C. Osher, S. M. Essock, and S. D. Rosenberg. 2003. "Regular Sources of Medical Care Among Persons with Severe Mental Illness at Risk of Hepatitis C Infection." *Psychiatric Services* 54: 854–59.

Swartz, S. H., T. M. Cowan, J. E. Klayman, M. T. Welton, and B. A. Leonard. 2005. "Use and Effectiveness of Tobacco Telephone Counseling and Nicotine Therapy in Maine." *American Journal of Preventive Medicine* 29: 288–94.

Tang, H., D. W. Cowling, J. C. Lloyd, T. Rogers, K. L. Koumjian, C. M. Stevens, and D. G. Bal. 2003. "Changes of Attitudes and Patronage Behaviors in Response to a Smoke-Free Bar Law." *American Journal of Public Health* 93: 611–17.

Tang, H., G. L. Greenwood, D. W. Cowling, J. C. Lloyd, A. G. Roeseler, and D. G. Bal. 2004. "Cigarette Smoking Among Lesbians, Gays, and Bisexuals: How Serious a Problem? (United States)." *Cancer Causes & Control* 15: 797–803.

Task Force on Community Preventive Services. 2005. "Tobacco." In *The Guide to Community Preventive Services: What Works to Promote Health?* ed. S. Zaza, P. A. Briss, and K. W. Harris, pp. 3–79. New York: Oxford University Press.

Tauras, J. A. 2007. "Differential Impact of State Tobacco Control Policies Among Race and Ethnic Groups." *Addiction* 102: 95–103.

Taylor, D. H. J., V. Hasselblad, S. J. Henley, M. J. Thun, and F. A. Sloan. 2002. "Benefits of Smoking Cessation for Longevity." *American Journal of Public Health* 92: 990–96.

Tengs, T. O., S. Ahmad, R. Moore, and E. Gage. 2004. "Federal Policy Mandating Safer Cigarettes: A Hypothetical Simulation of the Anticipated Population Health Gains or Losses." *Journal of Policy Analysis and Management* 23: 857–72.

Tengs, T. O., N. D. Osgood, and T. H. Lin. 2001. "Public Health Impact of Changes in Smoking Behavior: Results from the Tobacco Policy Model." *Medical Care* 39: 1131–41.

Thomas, R., and R. Perera. 2006. "School-Based Programmes for Preventing Smoking." *Cochrane Database of Systematic Reviews* no. 3: CD001293.

Thomas, S., D. Fayter, K. Misso, D. Ogilvie, M. Petticrew, A. Sowden, M. Whitehead, and G. Worthy. 2008. "Population Tobacco Control Interventions and Their Effects on Social Inequalities in Smoking: Systematic Review." *Tobacco Control* 17: 230–37.

Thorndike, A. N., L. Biener, and N. A. Rigotti. 2002. "Effect on Smoking Cessation of Switching Nicotine Replacement Therapy to Over-the-Counter Status." *American Journal of Public Health* 92: 437–42.

Thorndike, A. N., R. S. Stafford, and N. Rigotti. 2001. "US Physicians' Treatment of Smoking in Outpatients with Psychiatric Diagnoses." *Nicotine & Tobacco Research* 3: 85–91.

Thun, M. J., L. F. Apicella, and S. J. Henley. 2000. "Smoking Vs Other Risk Factors as the Cause of Smoking-Attributable Deaths: Confounding in the Courtroom." *Journal of the American Medical Association* 284: 706–12.

Thun, M. J., E. E. Calle, C. Rodriguez, and P. A. Wingo. 2000. "Epidemiological Research at the American Cancer Society." *Cancer Epidemiology, Biomarkers & Prevention* 9: 861–68.

Thun, M. J., C. A. Day-Lally, E. E. Calle, W. D. Flanders, and C. W. J. Heath. 1995. "Excess Mortality Among Cigarette Smokers: Changes in a 20-Year Interval." *American Journal of Public Health* 85: 1223–30.

Thun, M. J., and C. W. J. Heath. 1997. "Changes in Mortality from Smoking in Two American Cancer Society Prospective Studies since 1959." *Preventive Medicine* 26: 422–26.

Thursby, J., and M. Thursby. 2000. "Interstate Cigarette Bootlegging: Extent, Revenue Losses, and Effects of Federal Intervention." *National Tax Journal* 31: 59–77.

Tiller, K. J., W. M. Snell, and A. B. Brown. 2007. "Tobacco Policy." In *2007 Farm Bill: Policy Options and Consequences*, ed. J. Outlaw. Oak Brook, IL: Farm Foundation.

Townsend, J. 1996. "Price and Consumption of Tobacco." *British Medical Bulletin* 52: 132–42.

Travers, M., K. Cummings, A. Hyland, J. Repace, S. Babb, T. Pechacek, and R. Caraballo. 2004. "Indoor Air Quality in Hospitality Venues Before and After Implementation of a Clean Indoor Air Law—Western New York, 2003." *MMWR—Morbidity & Mortality Weekly Report* 53: 1038–41.

Troske, K. R. 1999. "Evidence of the Employer Size-Wage Premium from Worker-Establishment Matched Data." *Review of Economics and Statistics* 81: 15–26.

Unger, J., L. Rohrbach, K. Howard, T. Cruz, C. Johnson, and X. Chen. 1999. "Attitudes Toward Anti-Tobacco Policy Among California Youth: Associations with Smoking Status, Psychosocial Variables and Advocacy Actions." *Health Education Research* 14: 751–63.

Upadhyaya, H. P., K. Rose, W. Wang, K. O'Rourke, B. Sullivan, D. Deas, and K. T. Brady. 2005. "Attention-Deficit/Hyperactivity Disorder, Medication Treatment, and Substance Use Patterns Among Adolescents and Young Adults." *Journal of Child and Adolescent Psychopharmacology* 15: 799–809.

U.S. Census Bureau. 2000. "Components of Change for the Total Resident Population: Middle Series, 1999 to 2100. NP-T6-A." Washington, DC: U.S. Census Bureau.

U.S. Census Bureau. 2006. National Population Projections, Summary Files. http://www.census.gov/population/www/projections/natsum-t3.html.

U.S. Department of Commerce. 2006. "2002 Economic Census-Industry Series Reports: Retail Trade Sector 44-Product Line #20150." http://www.census.gov/econ/census02/guide/INDRPT44.HTM.

U.S. Department of Education. 2006. "Percentage of High School Dropouts (Status Dropouts) Among Persons 16 to 24 Years Old, by Sex and Race/Ethnicity: 1960 Through 2004." http://nces.ed.gov/programs/digest/d05/tables/dt05_105.asp.

U.S. Department of Health and Human Services. 1982. "The Health Consequences of Smoking: Cancer: A Report of the Surgeon General." Washington, DC: U.S. Department of Health and Human Services, Public Health Service, Centers for Disease Control.

U.S. Department of Health and Human Services. 1986. "The Health Consequences of Involuntary Smoking: A Report of the Surgeon General." Washington, DC: U.S. Department of Health and Human Services, Public Health Service, Centers for Disease Control.

U.S. Department of Health and Human Services. 1989. "Reducing the Health Consequences of Smoking: 25 Years of Progress: A Report of the Surgeon General." Atlanta: U.S. Department of Health and Human Services, Public Health Service, Centers for Disease Control, Center for Chronic Disease Prevention and Health Promotion, Office on Smoking and Health.

U.S. Department of Health and Human Services. 1990. "The Health Benefits of Smoking Cessation: A Report of the Surgeon General." Atlanta: U.S. Department of Health and Human Services, Public Health Service, Centers for Disease Control, Office on Smoking and Health.

U.S. Department of Health and Human Services. 1991. "Strategies to Control Tobacco Use in the United States: A Blueprint for Public Health Action in the 1990's." Atlanta: U.S. Department of Health and Human Services, Public Health Service, Centers for Disease Control.

U.S. Department of Health and Human Services. 1994. "Preventing Tobacco Use Among Young People: A Report of the Surgeon General." Atlanta: U.S. Department of Health and Human Services, Centers for Disease Control and Prevention, National Center for Chronic Disease Prevention and Health Promotion, Office on Smoking and Health.

U.S. Department of Health and Human Services. 1996. "Regulations Restricting the Sale and Distribution of Cigarettes and Smokeless Tobacco Products to Protect Children and Adolescents; Final Rule." *Federal Register* 61: 44396–618.

U.S. Department of Health and Human Services. 1997. "Changes in Cigarette-Related Disease Risk and Their Implication for Prevention and Control." Smoking and Tobacco Control Monograph 8. Rockville, MD: U.S. Department of Health and Human Services.

U.S. Department of Health and Human Services. 1999. "U.S. Department of Health and Human Services (USDHHS). Mental Health: A Report of the Surgeon General." Rockville, MD: U.S. Department of Health and Human Services, Substance Abuse and Mental Health Services Administration, Center for Mental Health Services, National Institutes of Health, National Institute of Mental Health.

U.S. Department of Health and Human Services. 2000. "Reducing Tobacco Use: A Report of the Surgeon General." Atlanta: U.S. Department of Health and Human Services, Centers for Disease Control and Prevention, National Center for Chronic Disease Prevention and Health Promotion, Office on Smoking and Health.

U.S. Department of Health and Human Services. 2004a. "The Health Consequences of Smoking: A Report of the Surgeon General." Rockville, MD: Public Health Service, Centers for Disease Control and Prevention, National Center for Chronic Disease Prevention and Health Promotion, Office on Smoking and Health.

U.S. Department of Health and Human Services. 2004b. "News Release Feb 2004." www.hhs.gov/news/press/2004pres.

U.S. Department of Health and Human Services. 2006. "The Health Consequences of Involuntary Exposure to Tobacco Smoke: A Report of the Surgeon General." Atlanta: U.S. Department of Health and Human Services, Centers for Disease Control and Prevention, Coordinating Center for Health Promotion, Office on Smoking and Health.

U.S. Environmental Protection Agency. 1992. "Respiratory Health Effects of Passive Smoking: Lung Cancer and Other Disorders." Washington, DC: U.S. Environmental Protection Agency, Office of Health and Environmental Assessment, Office of Atmospheric and Indoor Air Programs.

U.S. General Accounting Office. 2001. "Synar Amendment Implementation: Quality of State Data on Reducing Youth Access to Tobacco Could Be Improved." Washington, DC: U.S. General Accounting Office.

U.S. General Accounting Office. 2002. "Internet Cigarette Sales: Giving ATF Investigative Authority May Improve Reporting and Enforcement." Washington, DC: U.S. General Accounting Office.

Vanable, P. A., M. P. Carey, K. B. Carey, and S. A. Maisto. 2003. "Smoking Among Psychiatric Outpatients: Relationship to Substance Use, Diagnosis, and Illness Severity." *Psychology of Addictive Behaviors* 17: 259–65.

Van Den Bree, M., M. Whitmer, and W. Pickworth. 2004. "Predictors of Smoking Development in a Population-Based Sample of Adolescents: A Prospective Study." *Journal of Adolescent Health* 35: 172–81.

van Willigen, J., and S. C. Eastwood. 1998. *Tobacco Culture: Farming Kentucky's Burley Belt.* Lexington: University Press of Kentucky.

Viscusi, W. K. 1995. "Cigarette Taxation and the Social Consequences of Smoking." In *Tax Policy and the Economy*, ed. J. M. Poterba, pp. 51–102. Cambridge, MA: MIT Press.

Vollset, S. E., A. Tverdal, and H. K. K. Gjessing. 2006. "Smoking and Deaths Between 40 and 70 Years of Age in Women and Men." *Annals of Internal Medicine* 144: 381–89.

Wakefield, M., and F. J. Chaloupka. 2000. "Effectiveness of Comprehensive Tobacco Control Programmes in Reducing Teenage Smoking in the USA." *Tobacco Control* 9: 177–86.

Wakefield, M., and G. Giovino. 2003. "Teen Penalties for Tobacco Possession, Use, and Purchase: Evidence and Issues." *Tobacco Control* 12: i6–i13.

Warner, K. E., and D. M. Burns. 2003. "Hardening and the Hard-Core Smoker: Concepts, Evidence, and Implications." *Nicotine & Tobacco Research* 5: 37–48.

Warner, K. E., G. A. Fulton, A. Nicolas, and D. R. Grimes. 1996. "Employment Implications of Declining Tobacco Product Sales for the Regional Economies of the United States." *Journal of the American Medical Association* 275: 1241–46.

Warner, K. E., T. A. Hodgson, and C. E. Carroll. 1999. "Medical Costs of Smoking in the United States: Estimates, Their Validity, and Their Implications." *Tobacco Control* 8: 290–300.

Washington State Department of Revenue. 2005. "Major Tribal Internet Cigarette Seller Agrees to Provide Customer Lists" (news release). Tacoma: Washington State Department of Revenue News.

Wasserman, J., W. G. Manning, J. P. Newhouse, and J. D. Winkler. 1991. "The Effects of Excise Taxes and Regulations on Cigarette Smoking." *Journal of Health Economics* 10: 43–64.

Weber, M. D., D. A. S. Bagwell, J. E. Fielding, and S. A. Glantz. 2003. "Long Term Compliance with California's Smoke-Free Workplace Law Among Bars and Restaurants in Los Angeles County." *Tobacco Control* 12: 269–73.

Weiss, W. 1997. "Cigarette Smoking and Lung Cancer Trends: A Light at the End of the Tunnel?" *Chest* 111: 1414–16.

West, R., M. E. DiMarino, J. Gitchell, and A. McNeill. 2005. "Impact of UK Policy Initiatives on Use of Medicines to Aid Smoking Cessation." *Tobacco Control* 14: 166–71.

Wilhelm, I. 2005. "Corporate Giving Rebounds." *The Chronicle of Philanthropy* (Washington, DC), August 4.

Williams, J. M. 2008. "Eliminating Tobacco Use in Mental Health Facilities: Patients' Rights, Public Health, and Policy Issues." *Journal of the American Medical Association* 299: 571–73.

Williams, J. M., K. K. Gandhi, M. L. Steinberg, J. Foulds, D. M. Ziedonis, and N. L. Benowitz. 2007. "Higher Nicotine and Carbon Monoxide Levels in Menthol Cigarette Smokers with and Without Schizophrenia." *Nicotine & Tobacco Research* 9: 873–81.

Williams, J. M., and J. R. Hughes. 2003. "Pharmacotherapy Treatments for Tobacco Dependence Among Smokers with Mental Illness or Addiction." *Psychiatric Annals* 22: 457–66.

Williams, J. M., and D. Ziedonis. 2004. "Addressing Tobacco Among Individuals with a Mental Illness or an Addiction." *Addictive Behaviors* 29: 1067–83.

Williams, J. M., D. M. Ziedonis, F. Abanyie, M. L. Steinberg, J. Foulds, and N. L. Benowitz. 2005. "Increased Nicotine and Cotinine Levels in Smokers with Schizophrenia and Schizoaffective Disorder Is Not a Metabolic Effect." *Schizophrenia Research* 79: 323–35.

Williams, J. M., D. M. Ziedonis, and J. Foulds. 2004. "A Case Series of Nicotine Nasal Spray in the Treatment of Tobacco Dependence Among Patients with Schizophrenia." *Psychiatric Services* 55: 1064–66.

Wilson, N., G. Thomson, M. Tobias, and T. Blakely. 2004. "How Much Downside? Quantifying the Relative Harm from Tobacco Taxation." *Journal of Epidemiology and Community Health* 58: 451–54.

Womach, J. 2005. "Tobacco Quota Buyout." Washington, DC: Congressional Research Service.

Yerger, V. P., and R. E. Malone. 2002. "African American Leadership Groups: Smoking with the Enemy." *Tobacco Control* 11: 336–45.

Yurekli, A., and P. Zhang. 2000. "The Impact of Clean Indoor-Air Laws and Cigarette Smuggling on Demand for Cigarettes: An Empirical Model." *Health Economics* 9: 159–70.

Zagorsky, J. L. 2004. "The Wealth Effects of Smoking." *Tobacco Control* 13: 370–74.

Zang, E. A., and E. L. Wynder. 1996. "Differences in Lung Cancer Risk Between Men and Women: Examination of the Evidence." *Journal of the National Cancer Institute* 88: 183–92.

Zello, J. 2005. "Piecing Together the State-Tribal Tax Puzzle." Denver, CO: National Conference of State Legislatures.

Zhang, X., L. Miller, W. Max, and D. P. Rice. 1999. "Cost of Smoking to the Medicare Program, 1993." *Health Care Financing Review* 20: 179–96.

Zhu, S. H., C. M. Anderson, C. D. Johnson, G. Tedeschi, and A. Roeseler. 2000. "A Centralized Telephone Service for Tobacco Cessation: The California Experience." *Tobacco Control* 9: II48–II55.

Zhu, S. H., C. M. Anderson, G. J. Tedeschi, B. Rosbrook, C. E. Johnson, M. Byrd, and E. Gutierrez-Terrell. 2002. "Evidence of Real-World Effectiveness of a Telephone Quitline for Smokers." *New England Journal of Medicine* 347: 1106–9.

Zickler, P. 2000. "Nicotine Craving and Heavy Smoking May Contribute to Increased Use of Cocaine and Heroine." *NIDA Notes* 15, no. 5: 18–19.

Ziedonis, D. M. 2004. "Integrated Treatment of Co-occurring Mental Illness and Addiction: Clinical Intervention, Program, and System Perspectives." *CNS Spectrum* 9, no. 12: 892–904, 925.

Ziedonis, D. M., and T. P. George. 1997. "Schizophrenia and Nicotine Use: Report of a Pilot Smoking Cessation Program and Review of Neurobiological and Clinical Issues." *Schizophrenia Bulletin* 23: 247–54.

Ziedonis, D., B. Hitsman, J. C. Beckham, M. Zvolensky, L. E. Adler, J. Audrain-McGovern, N. Breslau, R. A. Brown, T. P. George, J. Williams, P. S. Calhoun, and W. T. Riley. 2008. "Tobacco Use and Cessation in Psychiatric Disorders: National Institute of Mental Health Report." *Nicotine & Tobacco Research* 10: 1691–715.

Ziedonis, D. M., T. R. Kosten, W. M. Glazer, and R. J. Frances. 1994. "Nicotine Dependence and Schizophrenia." *Hospital and Community Psychiatry* 45: 204–6.

INDEX

Advertising of tobacco products, restrictions on, 1, 3, 97, 193
Air travel, restriction of smoking during, 342
Alciati index of youth access policy, 216
American Lung Association, 341
Average quantity smoked per smoker (AQSS), 9, 12; projection of, 27, 30–33, 35, 43–44; tobacco control policy and, 13, 16, 21

Bars and clean air laws. *See* Hospitality industry
Beer, wine, and liquor stores: employment in, 132, 135, 140, 141, 143; tobacco control policy and, 149. *See also* Tobacco retailers

Cancer Prevention Study II (CPSII), 238–41, 248, 250–53, 284
Centers for Disease Control and Prevention: funding guidelines for state tobacco control expenditures, 341–42, 346; Smoking-Attributable Morbidity, Mortality, and Economic Costs (SAMMEC) model, 234, 258, 263
Cessation treatment: access to, 386–89; effectiveness of, 17–18; and health disparities, 386–89; insurance coverage of, 18, 387–88; Medicaid coverage of, 18, 377, 387; and the mentally ill population, 376–78; in SimSmoke, 12, 17–18, 27, 42–43; and smoking prevalence, 30
Cigarette manufacturing employees: costs of displacement for, 89–95, 101–3; productivity of, 79–80; projection of employment of, 82, 84, 87–89, 98–101; trends in employment of, 77–80; turnover among, 96; wages of, 80, 82
Cigarettes: domestic consumption of, 33, 55–56, 58–59, 78–79; imported tobacco in, 55, 59, 61, 65, 108; international trade in, 54–55, 78–79, 89; manufacture of, 77–84, 108–9, 111; role of, in mental health treatment settings, 379; smuggling of, 335–37
Clean air laws, 2, 160–61, 181, 342–43, 383; compliance with, 343–45; effectiveness of, 16, 343–44; enforcement cost of, 345–56; and health disparities, 383, 386; and hospitality industry, 161–67, 170, 177, 180–83, 189–90; and the mentally ill population, 374–76; in SimSmoke, 12, 16; and smoking prevalence, 29; and stigma, 353